THE
AIDS
Challenge

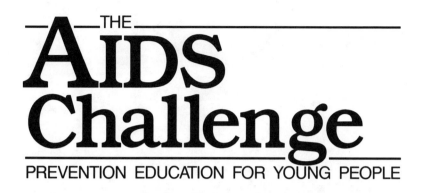

THE
AIDS
Challenge

PREVENTION EDUCATION FOR YOUNG PEOPLE

*Edited by Marcia Quackenbush
and Mary Nelson with Kay Clark*

NETWORK PUBLICATIONS • A DIVISION OF ETR ASSOCIATES
• SANTA CRUZ, CA • 1988 •

10 9 8 7 6 5 4 3 2 1

Cover design: Julia Chiapella
Photo: Comstock Inc./Skip Barron

Title No. 355 (hardbound)
Title No. 356 (softbound)

Library of Congress Cataloging-in-Publication Data

The AIDS challenge: prevention education for young people / [edited
   by Marcia Quackenbush and Mary Nelson, with Kay Clark].

               p. cm.
         ISBN 0-941816-54-0. ISBN 0-941816-53-2 (pbk.)
         1. AIDS (Disease)—Popular works. 2. AIDS (Disease) in
         children—Popular works. 3. AIDS (Disease)—Preven-
         tion. 4. AIDS (Disease)—Study and teaching. I. Quack-
         enbush, Marcia. II. Nelson, Mary. III. Clark, Kay.
         RC607.A26A345725 1988   88-19509
                                                            CIP

Contents

In the Classroom: Students Need to Know

The Religious Setting: A Natural Place for Learning

Facing the Issues: Controversy and AIDS Education

Minority Populations: AIDS Risks and Prevention

Special Populations at Risk

Appendixes

Foreword

In early 1984, I was hired by the University of California at San Francisco AIDS Health Project to help coordinate an AIDS prevention program for teenagers. This was, to my knowledge, the first program in the country specifically founded to promote AIDS prevention for young people. I was excited to be involved in this project, but I was frustrated too—I didn't know what such a program should be doing, and no one else was very clear about it either.

My associate and I tried many approaches. We spoke with youth service providers all over the city and offered to help educate their clients about AIDS. We approached the schools and suggested we be invited to talk about AIDS in classrooms. We went to juvenile hall and requested permission to speak with the young people detained there. We walked through some of the neighborhoods, talking about AIDS to street youth, juvenile prostitutes and drug dealers. We spoke at conferences about our concerns and sometimes pushed our way into agencies to provide inservices about youth and AIDS.

For the most part, people were polite, and some were even interested, but usually they said to us, "We have so many other pressing issues to worry about with our kids. I just can't believe that we need to put a lot of effort into AIDS education—it really isn't that big of a problem."

It was easy to believe them. In early 1984, there were only about 4,000 cases of AIDS nationally. Somewhere along the way I was told that just four diagnoses were among adolescents (adolescent and pediatric AIDS cases were not separated out in the early statistics—"20 and under" was the age category given). Heterosexual transmission was not considered much of a risk at the time, and even gay youth—never a very visible population—were not being diagnosed in any numbers.

We had some naive ideas at that time about *why* adolescents were not being diagnosed with AIDS. My favorite was the suggestion that the immune system of teenagers, because of the hormonal changes during adolescence, was uniquely defended against the organism that caused AIDS (whatever it might be— at that time the AIDS virus had not been identified).* We also thought that cofactors, such as repeated infections with gonorrhea, might be necessary for AIDS to develop, and most teens had not had 10 or 15 bouts with STDs as had many gay men first diagnosed. Never in our wildest imagination did we consider that we were facing a disease with an incubation period that could reach five to ten years or more; that teenagers, even if they *did* become infected, might not become ill until their early adult years. We were to face some real discouragement in the years ahead as some of these facts became known.

It is heartening that today there is much more interest in and responsiveness to the issue of AIDS risks for youth. We have gone from polite detachment to national concern, and there are now many models of what to do to prevent AIDS among young people. Many of the individuals and agencies we approached in 1984 have become leaders in such programs in more recent years. I used to feel isolated in my work and constantly questioned the value of what I was trying to do. Now I feel like I am part of a national community of education and AIDS professionals, of parents, civic and neighborhood leaders, of researchers and scientists, and of teens themselves, raising the awareness of the entire country and promoting effective AIDS prevention education for youth.

Working on this book has been an especially important task for me in light of this history. There is an incredible amount of expertise represented here, and our contributors have all been exceptionally generous in giving their time and efforts to this project. The community represented by the authors of our book speaks with a strong and persuasive voice to these issues, and I am proud to be a part of it.

We have come a long way in a few years, and it is helpful to keep this in mind. We must also remember the reason we have traveled so far in such a short time—the magnitude of this epidemic and the very real dangers it signifies. I hope as readers of this book you will also feel welcomed into this community. There is a lot of work yet to do, and we need your help to get it done well.

–Marcia Quackenbush

* AIDS is certainly, among other things, a disease of ironies. In 1984, I believed the hormonal differences of adolescence were a persuasive consideration in questioning why teenagers were not being diagnosed with AIDS. In spring, 1988, when I wrote these recollections, I included this early idea because it seemed to show how far we were from understanding the true scope and

nature of this epidemic during its early years. Within three days of my first writing this the *New York Times* reported findings that HIV infection in hemophiliac adolescents was progressing significantly more slowly than similar infections in adults, and that hormones were considered a possible cause of this difference.

Preface

In this book, we have followed two editorial guidelines we think are important to note. First, we refer to persons with AIDS, individuals with AIDS, and so forth, rather than AIDS patients (except in a specific medical context), or AIDS victims. Many people diagnosed with AIDS continue to live productive and purposeful lives, and to relegate them to a limited role as a "patient," or disempower them by use of the term "victim," fails to recognize the full range of identities and possibilities available to them.

Second, for the most part we avoid describing AIDS or HIV infection as a "universally fatal disease." We *do* acknowledge the seriousness of AIDS, and it is important, especially with young people, to be clear about how dangerous HIV infection is. At present, the great majority of individuals diagnosed with AIDS will die within two years. However, there are a few individuals who have lived with a diagnosis for as long as six years.

There are people who have been HIV infected for at least nine years, and are still without symptoms. Out of respect for the many people currently living with HIV infection and hoping to prevail over this virus, we would like to support the possibility that a few individuals may succeed in this effort. We prefer such terms as "life threatening" or "usually fatal."

The Human Element:

Real People and
a Real Disease

The Human Element:
Real People
and a Real Disease

The AIDS Challenge brings together a body of specialized knowledge about AIDS education for young people, the scope of which has never been set in one place before. Many chapters are from national and international experts on AIDS with years of experience in the field. Much of the material is so new that no previous writings exist on the subjects. We are impressed by the caliber of expertise represented in this book, by the quality of the information and by the utility of the recommendations and suggestions offered.

We begin, however, with a chapter by an individual who contributes here not in a professional capacity, but from the personal experience of having been diagnosed with AIDS. Jack Balcer tells us what it is like to live with this disease. We feel it is important to begin on this personal, human note. Because what AIDS is about, at the bottom line, is *people*. People with fears, hopes and dreams; with skills and knowledge; with talents and troubles. People who have AIDS or are infected with the AIDS virus; people at risk; people needing to know how to protect themselves. We read about numbers ("60,000 Americans diagnosed," "one and a half million infected," "ten million infections worldwide"), and it is easy to forget that it is not the numbers who are affected by this epidemic, but human beings—all of them, all of you, all of us.

Living with AIDS

Jack Martin Balcer, PhD

L iving with AIDS..." What does it mean? It means many different things to me, and I speak from the personal experience of having lived with the diagnosis for five years. I am lucky—to date, I am doing very well. Others are not so fortunate, and daily the numbers of those dead and ill with AIDS grow and grow.

You may wonder what it is like for the person with AIDS. How does it affect his or her day-to-day life? First, there are the physical concerns: fevers, oral yeast infections, night sweats, aches, pains, fatigue and more—it is different for everyone. The debilitating and relentless fatigue is the hardest. A simple chore—washing some dishes, tidying up the living room—forces you back to bed for the rest of the day to recuperate. It gets harder and harder. The doctor has no cure; no magic pill to give you back your energy. Your time seems limited, and you wonder, "Is this the way I will spend the rest of my life?"

There are emotional concerns that arise for the person with AIDS as well. How frightening this diagnosis is! Images of death, disfigurement and dementia haunt you. Nightmares wrack your sleep, and fears and anguish accompany your waking hours. This is so much to carry, to hold in your consciousness, but for the person with AIDS it is not usually all. Many of us have loving friends and devoted family, fair employers and concerned churches and synagogues. But others are rejected by family and friends, cast out of churches with the pronouncement that they are suffering God's wrath, evicted from apartments, fired from jobs, refused transit by airlines. These are not exceptional stories. Such things happen to people with AIDS all the time.

Abandonment on top of a diagnosis of a life-threatening disease is often more than one can bear. Imagine what it is like, lying in a hospital bed, or homeless, in the streets, removed from familiar surroundings, wasting to a shadow of your former weight, coughing and gasping for air, in terrible pain and discomfort, perhaps with lesions of the cancer Kaposi's sarcoma covering your eyes and face and closing your throat to food and water. People with AIDS have died this way, alone. To reach out and hold a familiar hand, to hear a warm and loving voice, to know someone cares—at such a time, this is important beyond all measure.

Another important concern for the person living with AIDS is the matter of motivation. The desire to live, and the sense that there is meaning and purpose in being alive, contribute immensely to one's physical and mental well-being. For the most part, the person with AIDS who wants to live and has good reason to do so will live longer and better than someone without that will. One group of people with AIDS has found this purpose and will by filling the role of public educator and advocate for better AIDS services and education. There is a small but

4

very active community of persons with AIDS who step out of the crowd and urge wide-scale educational efforts to prevent the spread of HIV. They appear in newspapers, on television and radio. They push back the borders of ignorance and fear.

A second group includes those who cannot care for themselves. They live at home, in a hospital, in their cars, in special residences. These are the very ill and dying. For those who are alone, cast off, abandoned, there will not usually be much motivation to continue. Death is fine and good in its time, but how tragic to see people arrive at this passage early only because they cannot imagine that there are rewards awaiting them if they survive.

The final group of people with AIDS, probably the largest, includes thousands of frightened, angry, sick persons who do not know what to do, where to turn or even how to seek aid. They may be apprehensive about speaking about their illness because of the discrimination they have seen others suffer. They may be uncomfortable asking for help because they have always been the one to help others, or because they think people will reject them. They may avoid talking about their diagnosis because when it comes up they feel nothing but despair and hopelessness. They may deny their anger because they can see no good coming from it.

Fighting back, speaking out, doing something—these three things have kept me going. I am impressed by the power of positive action and positive thinking. Either you can do something about the epidemic and your illness, or you can give up. I have met people with AIDS across this nation, Black, White, Latino, Asian, Native American, women and men, young and old, and they tell me the same thing. With the energy and capabilities they have, they fight. This fight helps keep us alive. I encourage all people with AIDS to be active, to speak up, to take charge.

We have the opportunity, right now, to have a tremendous impact on the future course of the epidemic. We have the knowledge to prevent anyone else from being infected with HIV. What an incredible privilege! This was not the case when I became infected, which was some time before the disease had even been identified by medical science. While people argue about whether to show condom ads on television or talk about safer sex in a high school classroom, people are dying. Let's stop these time consuming arguments and get down to the task of telling teenagers about AIDS.

I know this is a difficult assignment. It will take some effort. And you may have a tendency to think, "Well, yes, AIDS is a problem, but it will mostly be a problem for gay males, for IV drug users, and we don't have those kinds of kids in our schools." You may feel like you need to think it over, plan carefully, send everything through lots of committees for review, stall controversies that might arise. You could do this, but frankly, I don't think you have that much time. If you wait until teenagers in your community have contracted AIDS through sexual activity or IV drug use, you will have waited too long. The epidemic is already brewing. Let me remind you again that I was infected before I even knew this disease existed. Please don't place that same sentence on young people today.

You can implement education programs now. But I want to make another plea here as well. Make AIDS real to the young people in your care; make people with AIDS a focus of their compassion and concern. Encourage them to volunteer to help people with AIDS, to raise donations for AIDS programs. Let them be a vital and active part of a community that supports and encourages people with AIDS to identify themselves, to educate others, to ask for help. Help them create the kind of environment in which people with AIDS will feel useful and needed and motivated to continue their battle with this cunning and dangerous disease. I assure you that this kind of experience will persuade teenagers that they must protect themselves from HIV infection.

The Factual Component:

The Science of AIDS

The Factual Component: The Science of AIDS

P lanning AIDS education programs for youth begins with the task of acquiring solid, basic information about AIDS and HIV infection. It is particularly important to understand how HIV is and is not transmitted, the seriousness of HIV-related diseases, the risks for adolescents, the gravity of the epidemic nationally and worldwide, and our present capabilities and future possibilities in gathering information in the laboratory and research setting. Administrators and educators do not need to become AIDS experts to plan or teach effectively, but they do need to be familiar with this kind of information and be confident of its accuracy.

A good deal of the fear surrounding AIDS stems from the feeling that there is much we do not know about the disease. The fact is, while we do not know how to cure HIV infection, we do have a tremendous amount of information about the virus itself and the diseases it causes. New information is being collected at a remarkable rate, and it usually reinforces the basics we already know, particularly in terms of transmission and prevention.

The authors contributing to this section represent one of the most distinguished assemblies of expertise possible. Each has worked literally thousands of hours in his or her respective AIDS-related field since the earliest months of its existence. We hope the professionalism and expertise of our contributing authors will ensure the level of confidence necessary with this information. A considered review of the chapters in this section should provide a broad and useful foundation of knowledge for educators in many roles and capacities.

2

The AIDS Epidemic: Problems in Limiting Its Impact

Paul A. Volberding, MD

I ncredible strides in our understanding of AIDS at the most basic scientific levels have been made since the disease was first described in 1981. Much has also been learned about the epidemiology of the disease, its routes of transmission, its natural history, and the complex variety of illnesses caused by HIV infection. Newly explored avenues of clinical research are producing more hopeful methods of treating HIV infection and AIDS: antiviral drugs and immune system modulators to halt progression of the infection and correct AIDS-related immune deficiency are being developed and tested as more is learned about the life cycle of the human immunodeficiency virus (HIV). Certainly these are grounds for hope, but there is still no vaccine against AIDS and no cure on the horizon.

Meanwhile, the magnitude of the epidemic increases relentlessly. In the United States more than 50,000 AIDS cases and more than 25,000 AIDS deaths have been recorded (Centers for

Disease Control, 1988). By the end of 1991, these numbers are expected to increase to 270,000 cases and 179,000 deaths (National Academy of Sciences, 1986). One to 2 million people in the United States may currently be infected with the human immunodeficiency virus (HIV), and in Africa and other nations millions more are infected. There are now cases of AIDS in more than 80 countries, clearly showing that the AIDS epidemic is widespread and that HIV infection and its resulting diseases are an international problem.

Estimates of the long-term consequences of HIV infection have increased with the passing of time, and it is now believed that a majority of people with HIV infection will eventually manifest some symptoms of disease (Abrams et al., 1984; Abrams et al., 1986) and that most infected people will eventually develop AIDS (G. Rutherford, personal communication). Thus, the full impact of AIDS in terms of morbidity, mortality, and direct and indirect costs to society has only begun to be felt.

Education continues to be the best defense against AIDS. Educators of all kinds—teachers, parents, board members, administrators, professionals in community agencies, churches, and schools—are in a position to disseminate accurate information about AIDS, and, by presenting facts, to dispel much of the fear this disease has generated. Accurate AIDS information enables people to make informed decisions and to cope rationally with the many-faceted problems this fatal disease presents. To provide this knowledge, educators themselves must be accurately informed. This chapter will present a short history of the disease and a general description of AIDS with its common symptomatology, and focus on the transmission and prevention of AIDS, particularly stressing issues relevant for young people in school and community settings.

History and Definition of AIDS

Several outbreaks of *Pneumocystis carinii* pneumonia and Kaposi's sarcoma in previously healthy young male homosexuals were reported to the Centers for Disease Control (CDC) in 1981 (Centers for Disease Control, 1981a; 1981b). These reports signaled the beginning of a novel syndrome characterized by severely damaged immunologic defenses against a wide range of parasitic, fungal, bacterial, and viral infections, as well as several malignancies.

First seen in homosexual men, the syndrome was soon found in other groups "at risk" for the disease, including intravenous (IV) drug users, recent Haitian immigrants, hemophiliacs, recipients of blood transfusions, sexual partners of persons who had the disease or were at risk, and infants of mothers with or at risk for the disease. At the end of 1982, the CDC established a surveillance definition of AIDS (Centers for Disease Control, 1985) which has changed in only minor ways since then: AIDS is a syndrome characterized by unusual opportunistic infections and rare malignancies in otherwise healthy individuals with no other reason for immune system compromise.

In 1983-84, the retrovirus that causes the underlying immune deficiency in AIDS was independently identified by researchers in France and the United States. Variously named LAV by Luc Montagnier of the Pasteur Institute (Barre Sinoussi et al., 1983), HTLV-III by Robert Gallo of the National Institutes of Health (Gallo et al., 1983), and ARV by Jay Levy of the University of California, San Francisco (Levy et al., 1984), the retrovirus was renamed human immunodeficiency virus (HIV) in 1986 (Coffin et al., 1986). A series of advances, including the ability to grow lymphocytes—the cells in which HIV proliferates—in tissue culture, the finding that an important subset of lymphocytes—the CD4 cells (also known as T4

15

or helper cells) — are the target for HIV infection in the laboratory, the identification of an immortal T-cell line that could be used to grow the virus, and the development of sensitive viral antibody tests made it possible to understand more fully the nature of AIDS and its related syndromes.

HIV infection produces a wide spectrum of disease states ranging from no symptoms and apparent good health in some individuals, to an acute mononucleosis-like illness, to chronic fever, weight loss, malaise, diarrhea, and lymphadenopathy, to rapid disease progression and death from a complicating opportunistic infection or malignancy. Besides AIDS itself, several syndromes have been identified within this clinical spectrum. Persistent generalized lymphadenopathy [swollen lymph glands] (Gottlieb et al., 1985; Metroka et al., 1983), reported even before HIV was isolated and antibody testing became available, was the first element of the broadening clinical spectrum known as AIDS-related complex [ARC] (Abrams, 1986). The definition of ARC is not precise, and it ranges in severity from asymptomatic persistent generalized lymphadenopathy (PGL), to occasional fevers and night sweats, to severe disease courses including dementia and death. ARC can be diagnosed when an individual infected with HIV has persistent clinical problems that do not fit within the CDC's surveillance definition of AIDS. These syndromes are now understood to be stages of progressive retroviral damage to the immune system rather than permanent responses to HIV infection. Most or all patients with ARC will eventually develop AIDS itself.

Because the areas on the clinical spectrum of HIV infection tend to overlap, definitions of AIDS-related syndromes can be arbitrary and misleading, and do not always reflect the HIV-infected person's degree of illness. Some patients infected by HIV who are otherwise without physical symptoms are incapacitated by anxiety. Some individuals diagnosed with ARC have rapidly fatal disease. Others with a diagnosis of an AIDS-related malignancy live in fairly good health for more than five years. Thus, physicians apply definitions to AIDS-related syndromes very cautiously.

Transmission of HIV

HIV is transmitted by direct contact of genital or rectal mucosa with infected semen or vaginal secretions, or by blood. Knowledge of the routes of transmission of HIV is derived primarily from epidemiologic data, which indicate that the virus spreads from infected persons either by anal or vaginal intercourse, or by the introduction of infected blood or blood products through the skin and into the bloodstream. Also, an infected mother can transmit HIV to her infant during pregnancy or at the time of birth. No evidence exists that the virus is transmitted in the air, by sneezing, shaking hands, by sharing a drinking glass, by insect bites, or by being close to or touching an AIDS sufferer or an HIV-infected person. There is no evidence that regular close contact, including sharing accommodations, eating utensils, or even toothbrushes, is a route of transmission of AIDS. Studies of household contacts of AIDS patients demonstrate that what we call casual transmission of the virus does not occur (Friedland et al., 1986; Mann et al., 1986; Fischl et al., 1987).

Although HIV can be grown in many body fluids including saliva, tears, cerebrospinal fluid, breast milk, and urine (Hollander, 1988), these might not carry enough virus to spread the infection. Semen and fluids from the cervix or vagina can, of course, spread HIV to another person in some situations. Through vaginal, anal, or possibly oral intercourse, infected males can transmit the virus to male or female sexual partners, especially if protective barriers such as condoms are not used. Infected females can also transmit the virus sexually to males and can also transmit HIV to their unborn infants. Lesbians who are not bisexual and do not use intravenous drugs are considered to be at low risk for HIV infection. Homosexual men who practice receptive anal intercourse, especially without the protection of condoms, and have many different sexual partners are at very high risk for HIV infection.

The insertion of infected blood or blood products through the skin and into the bloodstream may occur in blood transfusion, IV drug use, or treatment of an inherited blood clotting disorder called hemophilia. In the United States, the risk of infection to recipients of blood transfusion has been dramatically reduced through mandatory HIV antibody testing of all donated blood. There remains only a very small risk of HIV infection in blood transfusion because transmission can occur when the virus is present but HIV antibodies have not yet appeared, and because the sensitivity of the test for detecting antibodies is less than 100 percent (National Academy of Sciences, 1986).

Among IV drug users, blood-borne transmission takes place through sharing hypodermic syringes contaminated with infected blood. HIV can disseminate rapidly if there is sharing of injection equipment outside of small circles of drug users; for example, in "shooting galleries" where equipment is rented and shared among strangers.

Transmission of HIV to hemophiliacs receiving blood-derived clotting factors has also been documented. Hemophiliacs need injections of clotting factors concentrated from human plasma to prevent severe and prolonged bleeding. Until the mid-1980s, the procedures used to manufacture these concentrates allowed HIV to be transmitted from an infected plasma donor to recipients. Since 1984, however, most manufacturers have used a method of treating concentrates with heat to inactivate HIV, and such products no longer cause HIV infection (National Academy of Sciences, 1986).

Health care workers have been concerned about the risk of occupational infection with HIV. This risk appears small but real. In large surveys of doctors, nurses, and other hospital workers, HIV transmission has been seen when a worker is accidentally pricked by a needle used on a patient infected with HIV. The chance of transmission is low (probably less than one percent) but is high enough to have caused fear. Currently, hospitals are working to decrease the likelihood of these injuries by better educational programs.

Apart from needle-stick injuries, the virus may also be spread if fluids like blood that are contaminated with HIV come into contact with skin broken by cuts or rashes. Laboratory workers handling very concentrated HIV fluids have even become infected without breaks in the skin. Again, educational efforts are addressing these issues and these cases should not cause fear in other nonmedical settings where the risk is much reduced.

The risk of infection with HIV relates directly to the frequency of exposure to the virus and varies between different populations. Homosexual men and IV drug users are at very high risk for HIV infection. Heterosexuals who are not IV drug users and who have had long-term monogamous sexual relationships are at very low risk in most parts of the world. When introduced into a susceptible population, as was the case with the homosexual population in San Francisco in the late 1970s, HIV can be spread very rapidly. Epidemiologic studies of AIDS in Central Africa suggest that heterosexual populations may be as susceptible to rapid infection as the homosexual population in San Francisco (Piot et al.,1984; Van de Perre et al., 1984; Clumeck et al., 1985; Kreiss et al., 1986; Mann,

Francis and Quinn, 1986). Retrospective studies of intravenous drug users in New Jersey, in European cities, and in San Francisco also document a rapid spread of HIV infection among these groups (Angarano et al., 1985; Rodrigo et al., 1985; Weiss et al., 1985; Chaisson et al., 1987a).

Clinical Manifestations of AIDS

After being infected with HIV, many people remain healthy and without symptoms for many years (often unaware that they are infected and thereby capable of transmitting the virus to others), whereas others rapidly develop AIDS. Some have chronic symptoms for some time before an opportunistic infection or cancer appears. For others, however, the first manifestation of AIDS may be these cancers or severe (opportunistic) infections. Shortly after infection, some people experience a flu-like illness lasting an average of eight days and characterized by fevers, sweats, malaise, lethargy, swollen glands, and other nonspecific symptoms (Cooper et al., 1985). About half of these patients have a transitory reddish rash. As the immune system becomes more impaired, other clinical symptoms, such as persistent generalized lymphadenopathy, oral candidiasis (a yeast infection), and oral hairy leukoplakia (white patches at the edge of the tongue), may appear.

For reasons that have not yet been explained, the clinical forms of AIDS vary among risk groups. Kaposi's sarcoma (KS) is seen at diagnosis in 30 to 50 percent of cases in gay men (Des Jarlais et al., 1984), whereas only 2 percent of hemophiliacs with AIDS have KS. *Pneumocystis carinii* pneumonia (PCP) is more common in heterosexuals infected through blood transfusions than among gay men. Regional differences also occur in the clinical manifestations of AIDS (Volberding, 1986). The

20

most common manifestations of HIV infection are not the same in all parts of the world; they differ, for example, between the United States and Africa. Whether there are genetic influences on the manifestations of AIDS or regional differences in HIV itself is also not yet known.

Also, the clinical manifestations of AIDS are changing as the epidemic progresses. The incidence of Kaposi's sarcoma accounted for 48 percent of cases in 1981 and decreased to 18 percent of cases in 1986. Ongoing epidemiologic surveillance is necessary to provide an understanding of these changes.

Opportunistic Infections

Opportunistic infections are the most common presenting clinical manifestations that establish a diagnosis of AIDS. Although these infections would seldom cause disease in persons with normal defense mechanisms, they are among the most common causes of death in AIDS patients. They are characterized by an aggressive clinical course, resistance to therapy, a high rate of relapse, and a high incidence of drug toxicity during treatment. Major opportunistic infections are: parasitic (e.g., *Pneumocystis carinii* pneumonia, toxoplasmosis, and cryptosporidiosis), fungal (e.g., oral and esophageal candidiasis), bacterial (e.g., *Mycobacterium* tuberculosis and *Mycobacterium avium intracellulare*), and viral (e.g., infections due to herpes simplex, herpes zoster, and cytomegalovirus). The symptoms experienced by an AIDS patient are most often due to one or more of those infections. In order to present an idea of the incredible range of problems seen in AIDS, some of the more common of these will be reviewed.

PARASITIC (PROTOZOAL) INFECTIONS

Pneumocystis carinii pneumonia is the most common AIDS-related opportunistic infection in the United States (Kaplan, Wofsy and Volberding, 1987). PCP accounts for more than 50 percent of all initial AIDS diagnoses. Patients with PCP typically complain of fever, nonproductive cough, shortness of breath, labored breathing on exertion, and chest tightness. Approximately 80 percent of patients have some or all of these symptoms at the time of diagnosis, and they last from several days to as long as two months (Haverkos, 1984; Kaplan, Wofsy and Volberding, 1987).

Toxoplasmosis is one of the most common causes of central nervous system diseases in AIDS and one of the most treatable AIDS-related opportunistic infections (Haverkos, 1984; Hopewell and Luce, 1987; Kaplan, Wofsy and Volberding, 1987). Clinical features of infection include seizures, focal neurologic deficits, and encephalopathy (Levy, Bredesen and Rosenblum, 1985).

Cryptosporidiosis is a parasitic disease that produces a self-limited diarrhea in animals, travelers, and veterinarians. In persons with AIDS and other immunocompromised individuals, however, it causes sustained, profuse diarrhea, often associated with malnutrition, malabsorption, and substantial weight loss.

FUNGAL INFECTIONS

Oral candidiasis (thrush) is a very common infection in AIDS and in persons at high risk for AIDS. The likelihood that these persons, without AIDS, will subsequently develop a serious opportunistic infection (i.e., AIDS) is very high (Klein et al., 1984; Quintiliani et al., 1984). Thrush is characterized by creamy, curd-like patches on the tongue and buccal mucosa.

Candida esophagitis is a fungal infection of the esophagus. It may be asymptomatic, and most, but not all, patients will have thrush. The most common symptoms include painful swallowing, impairment of speech, retrosternum pain, and nausea.

Cryptococcal disease in patients with AIDS accounts for approximately 5 to 8 percent of all opportunistic infections.

The most common clinical form of cryptococcal infection is a slowly progressive meningitis, although simultaneous or isolated infection of the blood, lungs, or other sites are not infrequent (Zuger et al., 1986). The onset of this infection is usually subtle, and the most common complaint is severe headache and fever. Patients commonly have behavioral changes, memory loss, and confusion.

BACTERIAL INFECTIONS

Mycobacterium tuberculosis is seen with increasing frequency in persons at high risk for AIDS and often precedes the diagnosis of AIDS by several months. In contrast to non-AIDS tuberculosis in the United States, which is pulmonary, tuberculosis in AIDS patients is likely to occur in areas other than the lungs (Pitchenik et al., 1984; Chaisson et al., 1986; Sunderam et al., 1986). In general, it occurs among AIDS patients in those who have had a high rate of TB infection: Haitians, Hispanics, Blacks, and IV drug users (Pitchenik et al., 1984; Sunderam et al., 1986).

Mycobacterium-avium intracellulare (MAI) is usually identified late in the course of disease, in association with fever, wasting, and fatigue, but often without specific organ system failure despite multiple organ involvement. This is an infection with a bacterium that looks like tuberculosis under the microscope, but is much more difficult to treat with antibiotics.

VIRAL INFECTIONS

Cytomegalovirus (CMV) infection is almost universal in homosexual men with AIDS and ARC. Most simply carry the virus without symptoms caused by the infection, but in others it can lead to devastating problems. The most common site of symptomatic CMV infection in AIDS is the eye, where permanent blindness can result. Another common site is the intestine, where CMV can cause diarrhea and bleeding.

Malignancies

Several cancers are associated with HIV infection, including Kaposi's sarcoma and various cancers of the lymphatic tissue (lymphomas). Some of these (Kaposi's sarcoma, central nervous system lymphomas, and high grade peripheral B-cell lymphomas) are believed to be closely related to the immune deficiency caused by HIV infection. Other malignancies, such as Hodgkin's disease, may not be directly attributable to HIV infection, but their clinical course is more complicated and aggressive than when they occur in non-AIDS populations.

KAPOSI'S SARCOMA

One of the first recognized manifestations of AIDS, KS is the second most common clinical manifestation of the disease and is an easily monitored clinical marker of the underlying immune deficiency. KS was a rare cancer in the United States before 1981, and when it did occur, was present in elderly men, especially those of Mediterranean descent, and in black Africans. In these men, there was no sign of underlying immunodeficiency (Ziegler, Templeton and Vogel, 1984). It also occurred in people with severe immunosuppression, such as renal allograft recipients (Taylor et al., 1971; Harwood et al., 1979). Its appearance in young homosexual men in mid-1981 alerted the medical community that a new disease had arrived.

KS is a disease process that produces reddish or purple lesions in various regions of the body simultaneously. The tumors in the early stages are painless, but pain may be present when the disease advances, especially in the feet and lower extremities. Not only are patients with KS disfigured by their visible lesions, they often suffer swelling (lymphedema) of the face and lower extremities caused by blockage of fluid drainage by the tumor. AIDS patients with KS are usually the most stigmatized and isolated and are often rejected by employers, friends, and family members. These patients usually die of opportunistic infections, but this cancer causes many of the most difficult problems associated with AIDS.

Intestinal KS is common, but often produces no symptoms. In contrast, KS in the lungs is less common but more aggressive, and patients with pulmonary KS generally have an extremely poor prognosis and severe symptoms of shortness of breath and coughing.

NON-HODGKIN'S LYMPHOMA

Since the first cases of high grade non-Hodgkin's lymphoma in homosexual men were published (Ziegler et al., 1984), many occurrences of aggressive lymphoma in patients at risk for AIDS have been reported (National Academy of Sciences, 1986). In 1985, the CDC amended its definition of AIDS to include high grade, B-cell non-Hodgkin's lymphoma in the setting of documented AIDS retrovirus infection (Centers for Disease Control, 1985).

In HIV-infected patients as in other patients, lymphomas initially arise in the lymph nodes and often will spread to involve extranodal sites of disease. But clinicians see unusual presentations in AIDS-related lymphoma, such as tumor masses in the arms or legs and other soft tissues, in the common bile duct, the rectum, liver, and lungs. The tumors tend to be aggressive and widespread at the time of diagnosis. People whose first AIDS diagnosis is lymphoma may survive longer than a year, but those who have already had an opportunistic infection or KS have a median survival time of less than two months.

OTHER CANCERS IN AIDS

Squamous cell carcinomas of various sites, malignant melanoma, testicular cancers, Hodgkin's disease, and primary hepatocellular carcinoma are seen in AIDS risk group members (Conant et al., 1982; Purtilo et al., 1984; Ioachim et al., 1985). However, with the exception of Hodgkin's disease in homosexual men, minimal direct evidence exists that these other cancers are caused by HIV-induced immune deficiency or that their mode of presentation or response to therapy has changed.

Prevention of HIV Infection

It is what individuals do and how they do it, not who they are, that is relevant to AIDS prevention. AIDS does not result from the characteristics of persons or groups (e.g., sexual preference, race, ethnicity, or national origin), but rather from specific actions that increase the likelihood of exposure to HIV. Thus, prevention of AIDS involves avoiding or modifying specific risk-related activities, not avoiding or isolating people who are at risk for HIV infection or are already infected with the virus (Heller, 1988). AIDS is a concern of every individual, not only members of high-risk groups. Thus, it is incumbent upon everyone to know specifically the activities that increase the risk of HIV infection.

High-risk sexual practices include activity with numerous sexual partners, especially if unprotected (without a condom), and vaginal or anal receptive sex. Sexual activities that are possibly unsafe include fellatio (sucking the partner's penis and ingesting semen); cunnilingus (oral contact with female genitals without a barrier); and sharing sex toys or implements that have contact with body fluids.

Low-risk sexual practices include anal or vaginal sex with proper use of a high-quality, intact condom (perhaps especially one that is lubricated with a spermicide containing nonoxynol-9). Wet (French) kissing, fellatio interruptus (sucking the partner's penis and stopping before ejaculation), and urine contact, exclusive of contact with mouth, rectum, or cuts or breaks in the skin, are also felt to be unlikely to spread HIV.

Obviously, abstention from sexual contact is an absolutely safe sexual practice. Beyond that, sexual activity that probably involves no risk of transmission includes a mutually monogamous relationship between uninfected partners; self-masturbation; masturbation with a partner if there are no cuts on the hand of either partner; touching, massaging, hugging, and stroking; and social (dry) kissing (Cohen, 1988).

Intravenous drug use with needle sharing carries a high risk for transmission of HIV and should be avoided. The most important potential source of spread of infection to the heterosexual population may be intravenous drug users who sexually transmit HIV to women before or during pregnancy, who in turn pass the infection to their children. Moreover, nondrug using heterosexuals may acquire HIV infection as a sexually transmitted disease. Finally, both habitual and occasional intravenous drug users (IVDUs) may be infected with HIV by sharing contaminated needles and apparatus. The practice of sharing needles is common among all groups of IVDUs. If no intervention occurs, the prevalence of HIV infection in IVDUs will continue to rise (Levy et al., 1986).

Education as a Preventive Strategy

In a statement made in 1986 in Washington, DC, U.S. Public Health Service Surgeon General C. Everett Koop said, "AIDS is not spread by casual, nonsexual contact. It is spread by high risk sexual and drug-related behaviors—behaviors that we can choose to avoid. Every person can reduce the risk of exposure to the AIDS virus through preventive measures that are simple, straightforward, and effective. However, if people are to follow these recommended measures—to act responsibly to protect themselves and others—they must be informed about them. That is an obvious statement, but not a simple one. Educating people about AIDS has never been easy" (Koop and Samuels, 1988).

It has never been an easy matter for several reasons. First, AIDS is a contagious and thus far incurable and fatal disease generating much the same kind of irrational fear as that recorded in previous plagues and pandemics (Simpson, 1988). Second, HIV infection in the United States primarily afflicts groups—homosexuals, IV drug users, minorities—who engage in activities condemned by society at large. Third, sexuality education in this society has always been a controversial issue. The explicit description of certain sexual behaviors is possibly offensive to a majority of people, yet explicit prevention messages are essential to create public understanding of AIDS and halt its spread.

Surveys show that even though most people now know that HIV is transmitted through sexual intercourse, blood transfusions, and sharing contaminated needles during IV drug use, many still hold the erroneous belief that HIV is also spread by donating blood or through casual contact (Heller, 1988). Misunderstanding among high school students about how HIV is transmitted is compounded by ignorance about sexuality in general (Heller, 1988). Misplaced fear and confusion about how HIV is spread can cause people to discriminate against infected people and hamper the development and implementation of effective prevention strategies.

Surveys also show that high-risk behaviors can be modified by education and dissemination of information. Studies show that since 1982, gay men have greatly reduced the number of their sexual contacts and have modified their sexual practices (McKusick et al., 1985; McKusick, Horstman and Coates, 1985). Reports from clinics in San Francisco and around the world show that rates of rectal gonorrhea among men fell dramatically between 1980 and 1984 (Judson, 1983; Centers for Disease Control, 1984; Schechter et al., 1984; Echenberg, 1985). There are indications that the rate of seroprevalence in gay men has fallen in San Francisco and New York, although it is unclear whether this is the result of safer sex practices or a saturation effect. Some evidence exists that education can create changes in the behavior of drug addicts (Froner, 1987). In another survey, investigators found that in 1985, 6 percent of people who said they always or usually shared needles, always sterilized needles with bleach; while in 1987, 47 percent said they always disinfected needles in bleach (Chaisson et al., 1987).

The federal government has been slow to provide leadership or funding for educational programs, partly due to the Reagan administration's fears of appearing to condone homosexuality or drug use and of offending conservative political constituencies through explicit discussions of sexual and drug use practices (Altman, 1986). However, in a report released in 1986, a panel of the National Academy of Science's Institute of Medicine recommended committing 2 billion dollars per year by 1991 to fund a coordinated program of AIDS education, public health and research. The panel stressed the importance of using sexually explicit, easily understood language tailored to various audiences in all communications about AIDS (National Academy of Sciences, 1986). Numerous studies support the fact that prevention messages, in order to be effective, should be framed in the context of the cultural values, language, idioms, and imagery of those one wishes to influence (Richards, 1975; Third World Advisory Task Force, 1987).

Guidelines for Control of Infection

Since no evidence exists that HIV is transmitted by casual contact, the risk of transmission in a classroom, recreational, church, or community setting is extremely low. Young people with HIV infection should be allowed to participate in all classroom and recreational activities; their participation should only be limited by their own clinical and immune status (Grossman, 1988). Spilled blood, body fluids, and secretions may contain many other infectious agents, such as hepatitis; thus, all accidental spills of fluid should be disinfected by washing down with a solution of household bleach (1 part bleach to 10 parts water). As in the hospital setting, school nurses or other personnel who must handle blood should wear gloves to avoid exposure to the variety of infections potentially present in blood. Just as important, however, is the fact that the actual risk of HIV infection is much lower in school age groups than among adults; there is danger of perpetuating unreasonable fear surrounding AIDS if infection control measures are irrationally strict. As with all aspects of this epidemic, the best approach is through education, which is in turn based on facts, not fears.

References

Abrams, D.I., et al. 1986. Antibodies to human T-lymphotropic virus type III and development of the acquired immunodeficiency syndrome in homosexual men presenting with immune thrombocytopenia. *Annals of Internal Medicine* 104:47-50.

Abrams, D.I., et al. 1987. Persistent, diffuse lymphadenopathy in homosexual men: Endpoint or prodrome? *Annals of Internal Medicine* 100:801-8.

Altman, D. 1986. *AIDS in the mind of America. The social, political, and psychological impact of a new epidemic.* Garden City, NY: Anchor Press/Doubleday.

Angarano, G., et al. 1985. Rapid spread of HTLV-III infection among drug addicts in Italy. *Lancet* 2:1302.

Barre-Sinoussi, F., et al. 1983. Isolation of a T-lymphotropic retrovirus from a patient at risk for acquired immune deficiency syndrome (AIDS). *Science* 220:868-71.

Centers for Disease Control. 1981a. Pneumocystis pneumonia—Los Angeles. *Morbidity and Mortality Weekly Report* 30:250-52.

Centers for Disease Control. 1981b. Kaposi's sarcoma and Pneumocystis pneumonia among homosexual men—New York City and California. *Morbidity and Mortality Weekly Report* 30:305-08.

Centers for Disease Control. 1984. Declining rates of rectal and pharyngeal gonorrhea among males—New York City. *Morbidity and Mortality Weekly Report* 33:295-97.

Centers for Disease Control. 1985. *The case definition of AIDS used by CDC for national reporting (CDC reportable AIDS).* Document No. 0312S.

Centers for Disease Control. 1988. Cases of specified notifiable diseases. *Morbidity and Mortality Weekly Report* 37:90-91.

Chaisson, R.E., et al. 1986. *Clinical aspects of tuberculosis in AIDS patients: A population based study.* Paris, France: International Conference on AIDS.

Chaisson, R.E., et al. 1987a. Human immunodeficiency virus infection in heterosexual intravenous drug users in San Francisco. *American Journal of Public Health* 77:169-72.

Chaisson, R.E., et al. 1987b. HIV, bleach and needle sharing. *Lancet* 1:1430.

Clumeck, N., et al. 1985. Heterosexual promiscuity among African patients with AIDS. *Lancet* 2:182.

Coffin, J., et al. 1986. Human immunodeficiency viruses. *Science* 232:697.

Cohen, Philip T. 1988. Safer sex: Risk estimates of sexual practices. In: Cohen, P.T., Sande, M.A., and Volberding, P.A., eds. *San Francisco General Hospital AIDS Knowledgebase* [Computer database]. Waltham, MA: Massachusetts Medical Society.

Conant, M.A., et al. 1982. Squamous cell carcinoma in sexual partner of Kaposi's sarcoma patient [Letter]. *Lancet* 1:286.

Cooper, D.A., et al. 1985. Acute AIDS retrovirus infection: Definition of a clinical illness associated with seroconversion. *Lancet* 1:537-40.

Des Jarlais, D.C., et al. Kaposi's sarcoma among four different AIDS groups. *New England Journal of Medicine* 310:1119.

Echenberg, D.F. 1985. A new strategy to prevent the spread of AIDS among heterosexuals [Editorial]. *Journal of the American Medical Association* 254:2129-30.

Fischl, M.A., et al. 1987. Evaluation of heterosexual partners, children, and household contacts of adults with AIDS. *Journal of the American Medical Association* 256:640-44.

Friedland G.H., et al. 1986. Lack of transmission of HTLV-III/LAV infection to household contacts of patients with AIDS or AIDS-related complex with oral candidiasis. *New England Journal of Medicine* 314:344-49.

Froner, G. 1987. Disinfection of hypodermic syringes by IV drug users [Letter]. *AIDS* 1:133-34.

Gallo, R.C., et al. 1984. Frequent detection and isolation of cytopathic retroviruses (HTLV-III) from patients with AIDS and at risk for AIDS. *Science* 224:500-03.

Gottlieb, M.S., et al. 1985. Persistent generalized lymphadenopathy: The UCLA experience. In: Gupta, S., ed. *AIDS associated syndromes*. New York: Plenum Press, 85-92.

Grossman, Moses. 1988. Infection control for youth facilities/educational institutions. In: Cohen, P.T., Sande, M.A., and Volberding, P.A., eds. *San Francisco General Hospital AIDS Knowledgebase* [Computer database]. Waltham, MA: Massachusetts Medical Society.

Harwood, A.R., et al. 1979. Kaposi's sarcoma in recipients of renal transplants. *American Journal of Medicine* 64:759-765.

Haverkos, H.W. 1984. Assessment of therapy for *Pneumocystis car-*

inii pneumonia. *American Journal of Medicine* 76:501-8.

Heller, Karen. 1988. Public education and prevention strategies. In: Cohen, P.T., Sande, M.A., Volberding, P.A., eds. *San Francisco General Hospital AIDS Knowledgebase* [Computer database]. Waltham, MA: Massachusetts Medical Society.

Hollander, Harry. 1988. Transmission of HIV in body fluids. In: Cohen, P.T., Sande, M.A., and Volberding, P.A., eds. *San Francisco General Hospital AIDS Knowledgebase* [Computer database]. Waltham, MA: Massachusetts Medical Society.

Hopewell, P.C. and Luce, J.M. 1985. Pulmonary involvement in the acquired immunodeficiency syndrome. *Chest* 87:104-12.

Ioachim, H.L., et al. 1985. Lymphomas in men at high risk for acquired immune deficiency syndrome (AIDS): A study of 21 cases. *Cancer* 56:2831-42.

Judson, F.N. 1983. Fear of AIDS and gonorrhea rates in homosexual men [Letter]. *Lancet* 2:159-60.

Kaplan, L.K., Wofsy, C.B. and Volberding, P.A. 1987. Treatment of patients with acquired immunodeficiency syndrome and associated manifestations. *Journal of the American Medical Association* 257:1367-74.

Klein, R.S., et al. 1984. Oral candidiasis in high risk patients as the initial manifestation of the acquired immunodeficiency syndrome. *New England Journal of Medicine* 311:354-58.

Koop, C.E. and Samuels, M.E. 1988. The Surgeon General's report on AIDS. In: Corless, I.B., Pittman-Lindeman, M., eds. *AIDS: Principles, practices, politics.* Washington, DC: Hemisphere Publishing Corporation.

Kreiss, J.K., et al. 1986. AIDS virus infection in Nairobi prostitutes: Spread of the epidemic to east Africa. *New England Journal of Medicine* 314:414-18.

Levy, N. et al. 1986. The prevalence of HTLV-III/LAV antibodies among intravenous drug users attending treatment programs in California: A preliminary report [Letter]. *New England Journal of Medicine* 314:446.

Levy, J.A., et al. 1984. Isolation of lymphocytopathic retroviruses from San Francisco patients with AIDS. *Science* 225:840-42.

Levy, R.M., Bredesen, D.E. and Rosenblum, M.L. 1985.

Levy, R.M., Bredesen, D.E. and Rosenblum, M.L. 1985. Neurological manifestations of the acquired immunodeficiency syndrome (AIDS): Experience at UCSF and review of the literature. *Jour-*

nal of Neurosurgery 62:475.

Mann, J.M., et al. 1986. Prevalence of HTLV-III/LAV in household contacts of patients with confirmed AIDS and controls in Kinshasa, Zaire. *Journal of the American Medical Association* 256:721-24.

Mann, J.M., Francis, H., and Quinn, T.C. 1986. *The natural history of LAV/HTLV-III infection and viraemia in homosexual and bisexual men: A 6-year follow up study* [Abstract P99]. Abstracts of the second international conference on AIDS. Paris.

McKusick, L. et al. 1985. Reported changes in the sexual behavior of men at risk for AIDS. *Public Health Report* 100:622-29.

Simpson, Michael. 1988. The malignant metaphor: A political thanatology of AIDS. In: Corless, I.B., Pittman-Lindeman, M., eds. *AIDS: Principles, practices, politics.* Washington, DC: Hemisphere Publishing Corporation.

McKusick L., Horstman, W. and Coates, T.J. 1985. AIDS and sexual behavior reported by gay men in San Francisco. *American Journal of Public Health* 75:493-96.

Metroka, C.E., et al. 1983. Persistent generalized lymphadenopathy in homosexual men. *Annals of Internal Medicine* 99:585-91.

National Academy of Sciences. 1986. *Confronting AIDS: Directions for public health, health care, and research.* Washington, DC: National Academy Press.

Piot, P.T., et al. 1984. Acquired immunodeficiency syndrome in a heterosexual population in Zaire. *Lancet* 2:65-69.

Pitchenik, A.E., et al. 1984. Tuberculosis, atypical mycobacteriosis, and the acquired immunodeficiency syndrome among Haitian and non-Haitian patients in south Florida. *Annals of Internal Medicine* 101:641-45.

Purtilo, D.T., et al. 1984. Squamous-cell carcinoma, Kaposi's sarcoma, and Burkitt's lymphoma are consequences of impaired immune surveillance of ubiquitous viruses in AIDS, allograft recipients and tropical African patients. *Science* 63:749-70.

Quintiliani, R., et al. 1984. Treatment and prevention of oropharyngeal candidiasis. *American Journal of Medicine* 77:44- 47.

Richards, N.D. 1975. Methods and effectiveness of health education: The past, present and future of social scientific involvement. *Social Science and Medicine* 9:141-56.

Rodrigo, J.M., et al. 1985. HTLV-III antibodies in drug addicts in Spain. *Lancet* 2:156-57.

Schechter, M.T. et al. 1984. Changes in sexual behaviour and fear of AIDS [Letter]. *Lancet* 1:1293.

Sunderam, G., et al. 1986. Tuberculosis as a manifestation of the acquired immunodeficiency syndrome (AIDS). *Journal of the American Medical Association* 256:362-66.

Taylor, J., et al. 1971. Kaposi's sarcoma in Uganda: A clinical pathological study. *International Journal of Cancer* 8:122-125.

Third World Advisory Task Force. 1986. *Proceedings of the western regional conference on AIDS and ethnic minorities.* University of California, San Francisco.

Van de Perre, P., et al. 1984. Acquired immunodeficiency syndrome in Rwanda. *Lancet* 2:62-65.

Volberding, P. 1986. Variations on a theme of cellular immune deficiency. In: Gluckman, J.C. and Vilmer, E., eds. *Acquired immunodeficiency syndrome.* Paris: Elsevier, 191-98.

Weiss, S.H., et al. 1985. *Risk of HTLV-III exposure and AIDS among parenteral drug abusers in New Jersey* [Abstract]. The International Conference on the Acquired Immunodeficiency Syndrome. Philadelphia: American College of Physicians.

Ziegler, J.L., Templeton, A.C. and Vogel, C.L. 1984. Kaposi's sarcoma: A comparison of classical endemic and epidemic forms. *Seminars in Oncology* 11:47-52.

Zuger, A., et al. 1986. Cryptococcal disease in patients with the acquired immunodeficiency syndrome. *Annals of Internal Medicine* 104:234-40.

3

A Dangerous Presence: AIDS in the World Today

Michael J. Helquist

I t was a humble beginning for the new disease, a mere pin-prick in the public consciousness early in June 1981. Media reports mentioned in passing that a physician in Los Angeles had reported to federal health officials the presence of an unexpected disease among young, previously healthy gay men in his practice. Yet from that start the new disease now known as AIDS has assumed a presence so commanding that virtually every government in the world has been forced to cope with its threat. But AIDS touches everyone's lives; not only government leaders. Discussions about AIDS and its prevention can be heard worldwide: among teenagers waiting in line for a movie in Paris, nurses tending patients at a hospital in the African nation of Rwanda, educators trying to reach aborigines in Australia and parents everywhere worrying over the safety of their children.

Students of history, medicine and the social sciences can

already examine how almost every facet of modern day living has been influenced by the presence and the fear of AIDS. Yet the complete story of AIDS is far from being told; it has a future that politicians, physicians, parents and young adults have come to fear. But the unfolding story of AIDS has much more to offer than visions of death and despair. Those people who have worked with AIDS prevention and patient care for many years have learned other lessons from the disease. Their stories are an essential part of any understanding of the worldwide impact of AIDS.

Historical Review

Marion heard the doctor say the words she had expected but had feared for the last two weeks. "The test results came back positive, Marion." She struggled to answer his question, "Do you know what that means?" She looked into his eyes briefly, nodded 'yes' and looked down at her hands. She felt tears come welling up again but forced herself to hold them back. The doctor continued, "This does not mean that you have AIDS, you know. It only means that you have been infected with the virus that can cause AIDS. We will keep a close watch on your health, and if any symptoms occur, there may be treatments available to help you." Marion nodded again, feeling that she should say something but not knowing what to say.

The young doctor knew Marion's situation well, and he was discouraged that so little could be done. She was 22; she lived with her two-year-old daughter in a side building, a shack really, next to the house of distant relatives in the poorer section on the outskirts of the city. The father of her child had abandoned them, and Marion understood from rumors that he had died of AIDS six months earlier. She had not been feeling well for several months; she was scared that she, too, had AIDS. She didn't have a job; there were none to be had. It bothered her that she couldn't buy things for her daughter. Marion saw little promise for herself even before she went to the health clinic. And now this: AIDS. She didn't think it could happen to her.

In the early days of the epidemic, most observers—including scientists, physicians and public health officials—would have agreed with Marion. They did not think the new disease was a threat to women, to heterosexuals, or to anyone outside what was considered the only population at risk for AIDS: gay men, especially those who had been sexually active.

Scientists and most others now know differently. They have found that everyone can be at risk for AIDS if they are exposed to the virus that causes the disease. They also know that there are only a few ways in which the virus can spread from one person to another. But these basic facts about AIDS did not come easily, and the struggle to understand how AIDS is transmitted is an essential element of the history of the disease.

The First Epidemic

Before there was an epidemic of AIDS cases there was first a silent but rapid spread of infection with HIV, the human immunodeficiency virus. At the time, in the 1970s, the virus was not known by scientists. Nevertheless, it spread from person to person, primarily through sexual intercourse. None of these individuals—many of whom would later develop AIDS—knew that a deadly virus was in their midst. None of them knew that their sexual activity was placing them at risk for a devastating disease. Even those who became infected did not develop any symptoms for several years. Scientists discovered only later that it may take many years for symptoms to present themselves to people with the virus. That is why AIDS seemed to appear suddenly and in great numbers.

Research from around the world has revealed that during this early period of the silent epidemic, HIV was spreading not only among young men in urban America but also among young adults in some nations of the Caribbean and in several central African countries. HIV transmission often followed international travel and trade routes; thus AIDS cases were later tracked to major cities in Western Europe, Australia and Asia as well as to villages along the truck and shipping routes in Rwanda, Uganda and Kenya.

Some people who carried the virus were regular blood donors; most did so voluntarily to benefit the community; others did so to earn money for each donation. Whatever the motivation, HIV entered the national blood supplies of the United States and other countries. During the early years of the epidemic, there was no way to screen the donated blood itself for presence of the virus. A portion of this country's blood supply was also regularly sold to other nations; some of that blood we know today was contaminated with HIV. Thus the new virus found another means to gain a foothold around the world. People who needed transfusions and those with hemophilia who need regular infusions of blood products became yet another population at risk for AIDS.

Finally, HIV also entered the population of intravenous substance users who shared needles, a practice that usually includes some blood from one user entering the bloodstream of the next person to share the needle. In the 1970s they shared more than needles and drugs; HIV also spread from one user to another.

Since HIV first spread silently, the exact origin of the virus and where it first began to spread cannot be determined. A few studies found some evidence of HIV contamination in stored blood in Central Africa as early as 1959. However, similar studies of stored blood from elsewhere in the world have not been reported; thus no solid conclusions can be drawn. The available data do indicate that HIV spread within the urban areas of Central Africa, the United States, Western Europe and the Caribbean. Generally, populations in rural areas of the world were not so readily exposed to HIV. Studies in Africa have shown that the rate of HIV transmission may remain stable in the absence of specific conditions that enhance its spread. On the other hand, social changes that might disrupt traditional living patterns and might encourage more urban-rural interaction could have added to the spread of HIV.

It is clear that once introduced into populations where people are likely to have multiple sexual partners, where they may receive contaminated blood, and where needle-sharing IV drug use exists, HIV can spread rapidly. An important lesson from the period of the silent spread of HIV is that the AIDS cases reported today simply reveal what was happening five to ten years ago. And the public should realize that the number of AIDS cases will likely continue to increase for many years after the spread of HIV infection has been controlled or stopped.

The Role of Other Viruses

When the virus that causes AIDS was first identified it was called different names depending on the scientists who claimed to discover it. American scientists generally used the term human T-cell lymphotropic virus (HTLV-3, since it was thought to be the third of its kind in this family) while French researchers preferred the term lymphadenopathy associated virus (LAV). The confusion was finally brought to an end when an international body of scientists chose the term human immunodeficiency virus or HIV, a name that is now accepted worldwide.

In 1985, however, scientists were surprised to discover another human retrovirus, one that appeared to be a genetic cousin of HIV. The new virus was similar to HIV but different enough to consider it a separate and distinct entity. The new discovery was named HIV-2, giving the first retrovirus the distinction of being HIV-1. HIV-2 can also cause disease in humans, yet its actual natural history and the specific diseases to be found with it await further study.

Preliminary research has found HIV-2 primarily in nations of West Africa. It appears that HIV-2 infects those populations generally at risk for HIV-1, with heterosexual activity being the primary route of transmission. HIV-2 appears to spread rapidly, and cases have been identified in Western Europe and, recently, in the United States. HIV-2 poses special problems because the current blood screening tests used to protect against HIV contamination do not effectively screen against HIV-2. Other means of AIDS prevention—use of condoms and other safer sex activities—appear to be adequate to block the spread of this additional viral threat.

The discovery of HIV-2 is just one indication of how much remains unknown about AIDS, its causes, natural history and its variations. Scientists are still at a stage where the more they learn the more they realize they don't know. Nevertheless, most researchers are impressed with the amount of information that has been uncovered about these retroviruses and, perhaps more importantly, the human immune system.

The Statistics: A Part of the Story

There are now more than 100,000 cases of AIDS worldwide, according to estimates of the World Health Organization. The largest number of cases have been found in the United States, Brazil, Western Europe and Central Africa. The actual number of cases may never be known due to difficulties in obtaining accurate diagnoses in addition to some deliberate underreporting by nations reluctant to acknowledge the extent of the disease.

As important as the number of full-blown AIDS cases are the estimates of the incidence and prevalence of HIV infection. WHO believes that there are approximately 100 cases of HIV infection for every one AIDS diagnosis. WHO indicates that there may be from five to ten million people in the world today who are infected with HIV. AIDS cases have been reported from all major areas of the world, and the disease is believed to exist in virtually every country. Currently the United States has reported by far the greatest number of cases, about 70 percent of the worldwide total. Yet on a per capita basis countries like the Bahamas and Bermuda have one of the highest incidences of AIDS.

The Total Impact on Society

Scientists are now trying to determine what proportion of individuals infected with the virus will proceed to full-blown AIDS. Early indications suggest that as many as 75 percent of HIV-infected individuals will develop some AIDS-related symptoms. Even with this threat of a high rate of disease progression, malaria, malnutrition and diarrheal diseases will take a greater toll in Africa and elsewhere in the developing world. Yet AIDS promises to have an especially serious impact because it tends to affect people who are in their most productive years.

The suggested numbers of people ill or dying with AIDS promise to stagger the health care systems of most societies. In the context of available health care services, the countries of Central Africa face the greatest threat from AIDS. Hospitals and clinics in some African cities are already overwhelmed with AIDS patients, who require labor-intensive nursing care, a variety of already-scarce medications and a high proportion of the limited number of hospital beds. In addition, people with HIV infection may experience greater difficulty with other diseases like tuberculosis and syphilis, thus placing an additional burden on health care services.

Other health care programs throughout the world may be affected as well. Childhood and maternal health programs, family planning projects and diarrheal control efforts—all have begun to feel the effect of AIDS on their planning, the availability of funding sources and their effectiveness. Due to the perinatal spread of HIV infection, AIDS may also take a toll on the continuous decline in childhood mortality that had been achieved in the last few decades.

Any devastating disease that sweeps through a population or community will leave in its wake social repercussions that will defy resolution for years to come. AIDS promises to have such an impact as it sets forces in society against each other. Already there have been calls to forbid international travel to HIV infected people, to quarantine them, to withhold basic civil rights and to punish them for acquiring a disease that many did not even know about when they became infected.

AIDS in the world today has managed to expose all the frailties of most of our social institutions: our legal system, the economic structure, religious beliefs and our educational system. AIDS also challenges us to re-examine our belief in the duties of government, the rights of individuals and the meaningfulness of our everyday lives.

Global Cooperation

In the scientific community there has been considerable competition to claim important discoveries about this major threat to the public health. Often this competition has obstructed actual advances in scientific understanding. In the realm of AIDS prevention, however, cooperation has been a predominant theme.

Initially government leaders from various countries were reluctant to acknowledge that there was a problem with AIDS within their borders. They feared being scapegoated or losing valuable foreign income from tourism. As the worldwide dimensions and seriousness of AIDS became more apparent, most countries vowed to cooperate with one another and with the World Health Organization, which assumed leadership of the global effort to stop AIDS.

Today most countries have followed the advice of WHO and have established National AIDS Committees and have developed short-term and medium-term AIDS control plans.

Countries have mounted national information campaigns, improved blood screening programs, involved populations at high risk in special outreach efforts and have exchanged ideas and lessons learned within international forums.

Hanging over all these activities is the fear that prevention efforts represent "too little, too late" for tens of thousands, if not millions, of people infected with HIV-1 or HIV- 2. There remains hope that suitable treatments will be developed that can delay for several years the onset of symptoms for infected individuals. Few scientists indulge in thinking about a cure for AIDS anytime in the near future. And while prevention is the only tool for controlling the spread of AIDS today, researchers worldwide are racing to develop a vaccine that will protect people from infection. Daily news reports seem to follow a roller coaster ride from hopeful predictions for early development of a vaccine to serious doubts that one will ever be available.

Conclusion

AIDS presents a tremendous threat, yet within that threat is also an opportunity to examine the beliefs, attitudes and practices that govern how we relate with each other as individuals and as societies. While AIDS challenges health care systems, it also demands a closer look at how health care is made available in societies. As governments consider whether to impose various restrictions on personal rights, individuals get involved in the debate about their own future.

As a sexually transmitted disease that can only be prevented by sharing information, AIDS has prompted a revolution in open discussion about sexuality and sexual practices. However controversial this discussion, it will likely boost the efforts of family planning programs, STD prevention, health and sexuality education and a greater understanding among men and women, adults and youth. As people with AIDS confront their mortality at an early age, they often take stock of their lives and find previously unknown reservoirs of courage, strength and determination. In so doing, they often become the best educators about AIDS and how to cope with it.

The world was ill-prepared to deal with a new and devastating disease that would shake the very foundations of societies. AIDS will keep its disturbing grip on the world for the foreseeable future. Yet we are not defenseless in its midst; AIDS can be controlled and people can be protected from it if individuals and their governments make a long-term commitment to do so. AIDS is dramatically compelling not because it makes us powerless but rather because it challenges us to use the power that we have.

References

Piot, P., Plumber, F.A., Mhalu, F.S., et al. 1988. AIDS: An international perspective. *Science*: 573-579.

4

The Laboratory Role in the Study of AIDS

Judith C. Wilber, PhD, ABMM

The laboratory has played a very visible role in the evolution of our understanding of human immunodeficiency virus (HIV) infection. The discovery and continuing study of the virus which causes AIDS, the possible role of other factors which cause progression of the disease, and potential treatments and vaccines have all taken place in research laboratories around the world. The public awareness of the laboratory has centered on what has become known as "The Test," the assay for antibody to HIV. This test, which is actually a series of tests, has many uses as well as the potential for misuse.

The identification of HIV as the cause of AIDS led to the development of tests which can determine whether someone has been infected with the virus. The first commercial assays for HIV antibody were licensed by the Food and Drug Administration (FDA) and were available in March, 1985. They were developed specifically to test donated blood to be used for transfusion. Since the virus is known to be transmitted by injection of blood and blood products, an assay identifying donors who are infected with the virus would effectively eliminate infected units from the blood supply.

When it was first announced that there would be an antibody test available to protect the blood supply, there was widespread concern about other uses of the test because:

- We did not know what the results of the test meant prognostically—would an individual who tested positive go on to become ill?
- We were unsure of the accuracy.
- The results could be used for purposes of discrimination.

It was necessary, therefore, to continue to study the immunologic history of HIV infection, to determine the predictive value of the assays and assure quality laboratory work, and to develop the means to assure the confidentiality of the results.

What the Test Is and What It Means

There has always been some confusion about the distinction between HIV infection and the disease called AIDS. Usually, when we talk about an infection, we are also referring to a set of symptoms which we know as a certain disease. Say, for example, an 8-year-old girl is infected with the measles virus. We expect her to have a rash and a fever, and we expect her to be well in a few weeks. There are a few days before there are any symptoms when we know she is infected and we know she might be contagious. We also expect that the virus will be gone when she is well. If she is then tested any time in her life for measles antibody, the test will be positive, and it will mean that she is immune to the disease. Other viruses, such as herpes simplex, produce symptoms again and again, even when the body has antibodies against them. These viruses are said to have latent stages of infection.

HIV infection can have a very long latent stage of infection when there are no apparent symptoms. During this time a person may transmit the virus to others either sexually or through blood. However, a diagnosis of AIDS is not made until there are a very specific set of symptoms and other diseases in the patient.

The most common tests available for evaluating whether a person is infected with HIV are tests for antibody found in the serum, which is the straw-colored fluid that separates from red blood cells when the blood clots. When a person is infected with a virus, his immune system reacts to the infection by producing antibodies. These are proteins that are formed in such a specific way that they can recognize, or fit together with, pieces of the virus called antigens. Sometimes antibodies can "neutralize" or inactivate the virus, and sometimes these proteins stimulate other immune responses, which help the body overcome the infection.

The presence of an antibody can have several meanings, depending on the type of virus being considered. For some types of viruses, the presence of antibody can mean that the person has recovered from an infection and is now immune. In the case of HIV infection, however, these immune mechanisms apparently do not eliminate the virus from the body, and the antibody is found at the same time as the virus. We can, therefore, determine if someone is infected with HIV by looking for either the virus itself, virus antigens, or the antibodies formed in response to the virus infection. HIV virus culture, which will detect the virus itself, is too time-consuming, expensive, and laborious to be used as a routine test. The technology of currently available antigen assays, which will detect small protein components of the virus, cannot detect the virus at all times during infection.

The presence of antibody to HIV has been found to indicate that the person is probably infected with the virus, since it has been shown that HIV can be cultured from at least 90 percent of those who are HIV antibody positive (Gallo et al., 1987). Assays for HIV antibody are technically easier and less expensive than the tests available for the virus itself and are good tests for infection. Assays for antibody will not detect the earliest stages of infection. There is an interval of one to three months and possibly longer after a person becomes infected before antibody can be detected by current assays. However, once this initial period has passed, the antibody test is much more reliable than the antigen assays.

Uses of the Test

Initially, testing was developed for screening blood donations. With improvements in the test procedures and increased knowledge about the infection, diagnostic uses for the HIV antibody test have also been found.

A blood bank wants to find every unit that is infected so that none are used for transfusions. For this purpose, errors on the positive side are acceptable. This means that if there are false positive tests, some blood will be needlessly discarded. But if there were false negative tests, the result might be the transfusion of infected blood. The HIV antibody test was designed so that if there was an error, it would be more likely to be a false *positive* than a false *negative*.

People who donate blood and test positive have to be notified. That makes this a diagnostic test, and a false positive result is not acceptable when it affects someone's life. People with positive HIV antibody tests are told that they are infected with a virus known to cause a devastating disease, that they can no longer donate blood, and that they should take precautions to prevent transmitting the virus to others. Obviously, the laboratory should be as sure as possible that the result is correct before this information is given to the donor. Secondary tests were developed in order to validate the test and give more assurance that positive results are accurate. These secondary tests are less likely to show a false positive, but because they are also considerably more expensive, they are not practical for mass screenings.

The realization that people might want to know their antibody status led to the fear that they would donate blood in order to find out the results of the HIV antibody test. If many high-risk individuals donated blood for this purpose, the likelihood of test errors in screening would be greater. In other words, there would be a greater chance that someone who was infected would donate a unit of blood, the test would mistakenly screen that blood as antibody negative (uninfected), and it would be used in a transfusion, risking transmission of the virus to the transfusion recipient. As a result, health departments established "alternate test sites" as centers where people could be tested voluntarily and anonymously and then counseled about the meaning of the test results in their lives. Knowing that one is infected with HIV can be a powerful motivator in developing behavior that will prevent the transmission of the virus to others. The same behavior may reduce the possibility of becoming infected if the result is negative.

Individuals who are infected should be told that they may transmit the virus to others by sexual intercourse, sharing of needles, or donation of blood, plasma, sperm, or body organs. Women infected with HIV are at risk of transmitting the virus to their babies during pregnancy and should be counseled accordingly.

Many other important applications have been developed for the antibody tests. The ability to identify those who are infected with HIV before there are overt signs of disease is important in epidemiologic surveillance. Anonymous samples which are not linked to identifying information can be tested for research to determine the extent of the infection in different populations. The test is also important in diagnosis and treatment. For example, conventional therapy may not be appropriate if a person has a lymphoma as a result of HIV infection.

There are those who have decided that there should be mandatory HIV tests for various reasons. All of these proposals should be viewed with extreme caution. Most of them purport to prevent the spread of disease, but on closer observation have little to do with what is known about the transmission of HIV. Safeguards to protect confidentiality and to prevent discrimination are very important and should not be breached by the laboratory.

The Tests

The antibody test most commonly used is called the enzyme immunoassay (EIA) or enzyme-linked immunosorbent assay (ELISA). Other tests used to validate the ELISA are the immunofluorescence assay (IFA), and the Western blot (WB). The tests themselves have different technologies, but they all use the same principles.

ELISA

This is a general ELISA procedure:
1. Pieces of the HIV virus, or viral antigens, are coated on a plastic bead, which is placed in a well in a plastic plate.
2. The patient's serum, which contains antibodies to all the

diseases and immunizations the person has had, is allowed to react with the antigens on the bead.

3. Only antibody to HIV will react with the HIV antigens and will, literally, stick to the bead.
4. Everything that is not stuck to the bead is washed away. That means that if this person does not have antibody to HIV, *none* of his/her serum will remain on the bead after this step.
5. Another antibody, called antihuman antibody, is now added. This antibody was made by immunizing goats with human serum. It recognizes and will stick to any human antibody that still remains on the bead after the washing in step 4. Attached to the antihuman antibody is an enzyme that will act as an indicator.
6. Washing as in step 4 is repeated. If there was no antibody remaining on the bead in step 5, there will now be no antihuman antibody with its indicator enzyme attached to the bead. If HIV antibody is present in this serum, none of the reactant will have washed away.
7. A substrate for the enzyme is then added. A chemical reaction takes place, causing a color change. This can happen only if the enzyme is present, and the enzyme will be present only if the serum contained specific antibody to HIV. A positive reaction, therefore, has measurable color, and a negative reaction is colorless.

Summary ELISA Reactions:
- POSITIVE REACTION:
  Bead:HIVantigen:HIVantibody:Antihuman antibody:enzyme: substrate = color change
- NEGATIVE REACTION:
  Bead:HIV antigen:substrate = no color change [no enzyme present to act on substrate]

Immunofluorescence

In the immunofluorescence assay (IFA) the virus is coated on a microscope slide rather than a plastic bead. This is reacted with the patient's serum as described for ELISA. The final step uses an antihuman antibody attached to a fluorescent marker rather than an enzyme. A positive reaction is seen as green fluorescence when the slide is observed through an ultraviolet microscope. The fluorescence is localized in infected cells and has a very typical appearance to a trained observer.

Western Blot

The Western blot (WB) procedure separates all the HIV antigens according to their molecular weights by applying an electrical field to a gel containing disrupted virus. The bands of antigens are transferred to plastic strips. These strips are then reacted with the patient's serum exactly as in the ELISA procedure. Positive results are seen as colored bands on the strips in specific locations known to correspond to the molecular weights of specific HIV antigens. Interpretation of WB results has been the subject of some controversy, but the Public Health Service and other professional groups are working on guidelines which will help to standardize the procedure.

Assuring the Quality of Testing

A test for antibody to HIV carries a great deal of impact whether it is positive or negative. Every effort should be made to ensure accurate results. Every positive ELISA test should be performed twice on the same specimen by the same method. A single reactive (positive) ELISA should never be reported, even as a "preliminary result." Laboratory procedural errors such as inadequate washing and incorrect dilution may cause falsely reactive tests. Repeating the procedure in duplicate reduces this source of error. If one or both repeat tests are reactive, or positive, the ELISA is called "repeatably reactive." The specimens should then be tested by another type of test, usually IFA or WB, before the patient or donor is informed of the results (Centers for Disease Control, 1987).

IFA and WB are not necessarily better tests than ELISA. They have gained confidence as tests that validate ELISA because they enable us to *see* the reaction between the patient's specimen and the virus in more detail than a colored well in ELISA. The designation "confirmatory" test has been avoided by the FDA because in blood bank parlance a blood unit which has a negative confirmatory test can be used for transfusion. No one is willing to place a unit of blood into the blood supply that has the slightest chance of being infected. The term used by the FDA is "additional, more specific" tests. In public health they are generally called "supplemental" tests. Whatever the term, the process of repeating HIV antibody tests by methods which measure the result in a different way greatly decreases the likelihood of error.

Laboratories doing HIV testing should be licensed and should have rigorous quality control procedures in place. These should be reviewed by the licensing agency. Unfortunately, at the time of this writing such licensing requirements are not in place in most states. For-profit businesses promoting home testing and mail-in procedures are growing in number. They are being scrutinized by the FDA, but given the need for accuracy and counseling, home testing and mail-in procedures are not appropriate.

Accuracy

The goal of the testing process is to be as sensitive and specific as possible. Sensitivity measures the ability to detect all of the true positives tested and, therefore, will not result in false negatives. Specificity measures the ability to call all truly negative specimens negative and, therefore, eliminate false positives.

False Positives

The fact that HIV antibody assays are used most widely in screening populations with the least risk of being infected (blood donors, military recruits) has led to some misleading conceptions about the rate of false positivity. There are seven manufacturers of licensed ELISAs for antibody to HIV, and all of them have clinical trial data and independent published studies showing sensitivity and specificity of over 98 percent, many approaching 100 percent. This is better than almost any other existing diagnostic test. However, statistically, the majority of false positive results will be found in the groups which have little likelihood of being infected, leading to predictions that most results will be wrong in low-risk populations. Even the general public now has an awareness, though not necessarily an understanding, of the concept of predictive value of tests in different populations (*The New York Times,* 1987). Meyer and Pauker (1987) gave this explanation:

> Imagine testing 100,000 people, among whom the prevalence of disease is 0.01 percent. Of the 100,000, 10 are infected; 99,990 are not. A combination of tests that is 100 percent sensitive will correctly identify all 10 who are infected. If the joint false positive rate is 0.005 percent, the tests

will yield false positive results in 5 of the 99,990 people who are not infected. Thus, of the 15 positive results, 10 will come from people who are infected and 5 from people who are not infected, and the probability that infection is present in a patient with positive tests will be 67 percent.

Even though the positive predictive value is only 67 percent in the defined population, this does *not* mean, as the public and many officials assume, that 33 percent of all of the results were wrong. Looking at the uninfected people tested, there were 5 errors out of 99,990 tests run, less than 0.005 percent.

Many investigators have attempted to identify factors which cause false reactivity in the ELISA procedures. Since the HIV antigen is produced in cultured human cells, occasional problems have been reported with sera from individuals with autoimmune diseases, history of multiple pregnancies, antibody to class II histocompatability antigens (especially HLA-DR4), or hypergammaglobulinemia. Aware of these problems, manufacturers have developed methods to avoid reaction with most sera of these types and have incorporated these improvements into newly licensed versions of the ELISA test kits (generally referred to as "second generation ELISAs"). As a result, even in extremely low prevalence populations, the specificity has been greatly improved.

Specimens which cause problems in one test generally are not falsely positive in another type of assay. This is the basis for doing assays such as immunofluorescence (IFA) or WB in addition to ELISA on reactive specimens (Wilber, 1987). Testing a new blood specimen is a good idea in order to be even more sure of the results. A second specimen may also clear up questions if a test is neither clearly positive nor clearly negative (indeterminate).

False Negatives

The sensitivity of the current generation ELISAs is close to 100 percent when the antibody is present in peripheral blood. However, assays for antibody will not detect the earliest stages of infection. There is an unknown interval during which antibody is formed. There is also a period of time when the antibody may be undetectable because it is complexed with excess antigen. From a compilation of HIV studies and observation of other viral diseases, the time interval between actual infection and the first positive antibody tests, called seroconversion, is estimated to be from 1 to 3 months, possibly up to 6 months. The difficulty in being more definitive is in pinpointing exactly when a person became infected. This has been possible only in well-documented cases of transmission by a single event, such as an accidental needle-stick, blood transfusion, or transplanted organ from an infected person. Even in these cases, if specimens are not collected frequently, the time to seroconversion may appear longer than it actually is. For example, if the first specimen is not taken until three months after the infecting event, a positive test shows only that the seroconversion took place some time during those three months.

Any time interval between infection and seroconversion, however, presents a problem in interpreting negative HIV antibody tests. Even with an antibody assay with 100 percent sensitivity, there will be a "window" period before any tests become positive. Therefore, it should be understood by the physician and by the patient that follow-up testing may be necessary if the exposure to HIV was recent.

Caution

The consequences of testing errors are great. The blood bank can use a blood unit for transfusion if it incorrectly tests negative. A person receiving an incorrect positive test result is being told he or she is infected with a virus known to cause devastating disease. Every effort should be made to assure the accuracy of the tests. With extremely careful monitoring of quality control, proper use and interpretation of supplemental tests, and the realization that a single blood specimen may not give the final answer, HIV antibody testing is one of the most accurate laboratory procedures.

Research on Development of Vaccines and Treatment of HIV Infection

When she announced the U.S. discovery of the AIDS virus in 1984, Margaret Heckler, who was then Secretary of Health and Human Services, predicted that a vaccine would be developed within two years. Now scientists are being more and more pessimistic, doubting that there will be an effective vaccine before the mid-1990s, if then. The development of a successful vaccine would be very helpful in preventing further spread of HIV because it would prevent infection with the virus, rather than trying to kill the virus once it has infected someone. There are many successful virus vaccines including those for measles, polio and rubella. However, HIV is a very different kind of virus because it attacks the immune system itself and can evade the usual mechanisms set up to fight off infection. There are several problems hindering the development of an effective HIV vaccine:

- The only animal that can be used to study HIV vaccines is the chimpanzee, which is an endangered species. There are several vaccine developments that have not yet been tested because of the shortage and expense of using these animals.
- HIV has a changing genetic makeup. Therefore, a vaccine may work against one strain and not another. Research is focusing on development of vaccines to the parts of the virus that seem to change the least.
- Antibodies developed against HIV may not neutralize or inactivate the virus. A recent study showed that a chimpanzee infected with one strain of HIV actually became infected with another strain at the same time.

Clinical trials are now in progress with vaccines that have shown promise in the laboratory. These are expected to test whether the vaccines are safe, not whether they will prevent HIV infection. For obvious reasons, we cannot challenge the efficacy of the vaccine by trying to infect a person.

Treatment of HIV infection—that is, aiding the individual already infected with the virus—is also a challenging concern for researchers. It is very difficult to kill viruses with drugs because viruses incorporate directly into the machinery of a person's own cells. Once the virus is in the cell, a drug that successfully deactivates the virus may well damage or destroy the cell as well. These and other problems make the cost of developing safe, effective medications for viral diseases (including HIV infection and AIDS) immense. Unfortunately, even when research has tremendous commercial potential—such as a cure for the common cold would have—we have seen little success and few adequate offerings on the market.

There are many drugs that will prevent HIV from growing in human cells in a laboratory test tube, but these may be ineffective or very toxic in a person infected with the virus.

Several avenues of attack are being explored:
- Blocking the virus from entering cells in the first place;
- Preventing the activity of reverse transcriptase, which gives the virus the ability to translate its information into human genes or DNA;
- Boosting the immune system so that it will be able to fight the virus. There is a study giving vaccine to people who are already infected in the hope that it will stimulate an immune response to rid the cells of HIV infection;
- Preventing new viruses from forming from the information in the virus DNA, which has become part of the human DNA in the white blood cells.

The last method is the one exploited by the drug that has shown the most promise so far, AZT (also known as azidothymidine, Retrovir or Zidovudine). AZT helps block the spread of HIV to uninfected cells by attaching itself to the DNA chain of the virus and terminating its copy before it can be inserted into the DNA of another cell. AZT is not a cure for AIDS because it does not kill the virus. AZT has shown promise in prolonging the lives of people with AIDS and ARC. There is also hope that treating people before they start showing symptoms of the disease may be even more effective. AZT can cause considerable toxicity, but physicians are learning ways of alleviating some of the problems.

This sounds like a rather bleak picture of the prospects of research into ways of preventing and curing HIV infection. Great breakthroughs have been made, but the process takes time no matter how urgent the problem. For this reason, prevention education is supremely important. Preventing transmission of the virus can be achieved if people are aware of the precautions that need to be taken.

References

Centers for Disease Control. 1987. Public Health Service guidelines for counseling and antibody testing to prevent HIV infection and AIDS. *Morbidity and Mortality Weekly Report* 36:509-515.

Gallo D., Diggs J.L., Shell G.R., et al. 1987. Comparative studies on use of fresh and frozen peripheral blood lymphocyte specimens for isolation of Human Immunodeficiency Virus and effects of cell lysis on isolation efficiency. *J Clin Microbiol* 25:1291-1294.

Meyer K.B., Pauker S.G. 1987. Screening for HIV: Can we afford the false positive rate? *NEJM* 317(4):238-241.

The New York Times. Editorial: A treacherous paradox: AIDS tests.

Wilber J.C. 1987. Serologic testing of Human Immunodeficiency Virus infection. *In* W.L. Drew (ed.) *Diagnosis and treatment of viral infections*. Clinics in Laboratory Medicine 7(4):777-791.

5

Acquired Immunodeficiency Syndrome in Infants, Children and Adolescents

**Sandra K. Schwarcz, MD, MPH,
and George W. Rutherford, MD**

A cquired immunodeficiency syndrome (AIDS) was first
described as a disease of homosexual men in the United
States in 1981 (Centers for Disease Control, 1981). Since that
time, the causative agent of the disease, human immunodeficiency virus (HIV), has been well characterized (Barre-Sinoussi et al., 1983; Gallo et al., 1983; Levy et al., 1984; Coffin
et al., 1986), and AIDS has been described in intravenous drug

Editors' note:
Epidemiology is the study of the incidence and prevalence of disease. It
allows us to consider who gets what, where, when and how. Drs. Schwarcz
and Rutherford offer an excellent example of the sort of knowledge and
conclusions we can derive from sound epidemiologic studies. Their report
on AIDS among infants, children and adolescents is based on statistics gathered as of January, 1987. Therefore, one might conclude that this material is

users (Gottlieb et al., 1981; Centers for Disease Control, 1982a), Haitians (Centers for Disease Control, 1982b), hemophiliacs (Centers for Disease Control, 1982c; 1982d), blood transfusion recipients (Centers for Disease Control, 1982e), infants of mothers at increased risk for AIDS (Centers for Disease Control, 1982f), and sexual partners of HIV-infected persons (Masur et al., 1982; Centers for Disease Control, 1983). These patient groups are now known to reflect three different patterns of HIV transmission—sexual, parenteral, and perinatal (Curran et al., 1985; Peterman and Curran, 1986; Peterman, Drotman and Curran, 1985; Rogers, 1985).

The first cases of AIDS in children were reported in 1982 and involved a transfusion recipient and four infants of mothers

---

dated. In fact, while the number of actual cases has increased significantly, the trends reported here continue to the present time. Percentages given are still accurate. The facts about transmission modes remain unchanged.

These authors refer in several places to preliminary findings that await further study for verification. Once again, as new data has been reported, it has been consistent with the material in this chapter. For example, Drs. Schwarcz and Rutherford cite three studies that show the risk of perinatal HIV infection for newborns of HIV-infected mothers to be in the range of 20-65 percent. Present estimates based on further studies continue to suggest a range in this area. Most physicians would counsel the actual risk to be approximately 50-60 percent.

Another question raised in this chapter and by many other researchers concerns the number of children HIV infected at birth who will go on to develop clinical AIDS. This figure is still not known, though it appears that a majority of such children will become ill.

Finally, our authors also make reference to the fact that there have been no cases of HIV transmission in school, day-care or foster care settings or through other casual person-to-person contact. At the time of this writing, there are 62,740 reported cases of AIDS in this country and we continue to see no cases of household or casual transmission.

at increased risk for AIDS (Centers for Disease Control, 1982e; 1982f). Subsequent series and case reports have established that HIV infection can be transmitted to infants perinatally (Cowan et al., 1984; Joncas et al., 1983; Lapointe et al., 1985; Oleske et al., 1983; Rubinstein et al., 1983; Scott et al., 1984; Scott, Fischl, Klimas et al., 1985; Sprecher et al., 1986; Thomas et al., 1984), and possibly through breast milk in the immediate postpartum period (Thiry et al., 1985; Ziegler et al., 1985), and parenterally to infants, children, and adolescents through blood, blood products, and factor concentrates (Curran et al., 1984; Peterman et al., 1985; Evatt et al., 1984; Centers for Disease Control, 1984). Additionally, HIV can be transmitted sexually and through shared needles among adolescents.

This article reviews the current epidemiology of AIDS in infants, children, and adolescents in the United States and examines prospects for prevention of HIV transmission.

Epidemiology of AIDS and HIV

Definition and Classification

For surveillance purposes, the Centers for Disease Control (CDC) defines a case of pediatric AIDS as the presence of a disease moderately predictive of an underlying cellular immunodeficiency with the exception of congenital immunodeficiency syndromes and secondary immunodeficiency from medication, lymphoreticular malignancy, or starvation in a child less than 13 years old (Centers for Disease Control, 1985a). The diseases included in the definition of pediatric AIDS are the same as those used for the definition of adolescent and adult AIDS with the addition of chronic interstitial pneumonitis in the absence of negative HIV serology (Centers for Disease Control, 1985a, Table 1).

Table 1
Surveillance Case Definition of Pediatric AIDS

A case of AIDS is defined as a reliably diagnosed opportunistic disease in an adult or child at least moderately indicative of underlying cellular immunodeficiency and with no other known cause of underlying cellular immunodeficiency or any other reduced resistance reported to be associated with an opportunistic disease, including secondary immunodeficiencies associated with immunosuppressive therapy, lymphoreticular malignancy, or starvation, and, in children, primary immunodeficiencies, including severe combined immunodeficiency syndrome, DiGeorge syndrome, Wiskott-Aldrich syndrome, ataxia-telangectasia, graft-versus-host disease, neutropenia, neutrophil function abnormalities, agammaglobulinemia, and hypogammaglobulinemia with elevated IgM.

Opportunistic Diseases
Cryptosporidiosis
Pneumocystis carinii pneumonia
Strongyloidosis - pulmonary, central nervous system,
or disseminated
Toxoplasmosis - encephalitis or disseminated (≥ 1 month old)
Candidiasis - esophagitis
Cryptococcosis - meningitis or disseminated
Atypical mycobacteriosis - disseminated
Herpes simplex virus infection - chronic mucocutaneous
or disseminated (≥ 1 month old)
Cytomegalovirus infection - pulmonary, gastrointestinal,
or central nervous system (≥ 6 months old)
Papovavirus infection - progressive multifocal
leukoencephalopathy
Kaposi's sarcoma (<60 years old)
Primary lymphoma - limited to brain

Opportunistic Diseases Requiring Virologic or Serologic Evidence of HIV Infection
Histoplasmosis - disseminated
Isosporiasis - chronic diarrhea
Candidiasis - bronchial or pulmonary
Non-Hodgkin's lymphoma - diffuse, undifferentiated
Kaposi's sarcoma (≥ 60 years old)
Lymphoid interstitial pneumonitis (<13 years old)

To account for the full range of HIV-related disease, CDC has recently developed a classification system for HIV infection in children (Centers for Disease Control, 1987). Unlike the AIDS case definition, this classification system includes asymptomatic infection and less severe manifestations of HIV infection as well as the secondary opportunistic infections and malignancies currently required for the diagnosis of AIDS (Table 2).

Descriptive Epidemiology

Of the 29,137 cases of AIDS reported to CDC through January 6, 1987, 410 (1.4 percent) were in children less than 13 years old, and 127 (0.4 percent) were in adolescents 13 to 19 years old. Sixty percent of pediatric and 52 percent of adolescent AIDS patients have died. Cases in both children and adolescents have increased steadily since 1981, but the proportion of total AIDS cases in children and adolescents has remained constant over time (Figure 1).

Children Less Than 13 Years Old. Of the 410 children with AIDS less than 13 years old, 325 (79 percent) acquired HIV infection perinatally, 74 (18 percent) acquired it parenterally through infected blood or blood products, and for 11 (3 percent) the route of acquisition was undetermined (Table 3). Overall, 57 percent were Black, 23 percent were Hispanic, and 20 percent were White; the male-to-female ratio was 1.2:1. Cases were reported from 30 states, Puerto Rico, and the District of Columbia, and were concentrated in New York (150, 37 percent), New Jersey (60, 15 percent), Florida (54, 13 percent), California (23, 6 percent), and Puerto Rico (18, 4 percent).

Of the 325 infants who were perinatally infected, 190 (58 percent) had mothers who were intravenous drug users, 101 (31 percent) had mothers who were sexual partners of men in risk groups, 18 (6 percent) had mothers who were from Haiti or

69

Table 2
Classification of HIV Infection in Children less than 13 Years Old.

Class P-0. Indeterminate Infection

Class P-1. Asymptomatic Infection
    Subclass A. Normal Immune Function
    Subclass B. Abnormal Immune Function
    Subclass C. Immune Function Not Tested

Class P-2. Symptomatic Infection
    Subclass A. Nonspecific Findings
    Subclass B. Progressive Neurologic Disease
    Subclass C. Lymphoid Interstitial Pneumonitis
    Subclass D. Secondary Infectious Diseases
        Category D-1. Specific secondary infectious diseases listed in the CDC surveillance definition for AIDS
        Category D-2. Recurrent serious bacterial infections
        Category D-3. Other specified secondary infectious diseases
    Subclass E. Secondary Cancers
        Category E-1. Specified secondary cancers listed in the CDC surveillance definition for AIDS
        Category E-2. Other cancers possibly secondary to HIV infection
    Subclass F. Other Diseases Possibly Due to HIV Infection

Central Africa, 13 (4 percent) had mothers who themselves had AIDS, and 3 (1 percent) had mothers who had been infected through blood or blood products. Two hundred eight (64 percent) of these perinatally infected infants were Black, 79 (24 percent) were Hispanic, and 35 (11 percent) were White. Moreover, among the 190 cases acquired from an intravenous-drug-using mother, 119 (63 percent) were Black and 53 (27 percent) were Hispanic (Table 4).

Adolescents. Unlike children with AIDS, adolescents tend to follow adult patterns of transmission. Of the 127 adolescents with AIDS, 65 (51 percent) acquired HIV infection sexually, 36 (28 percent) acquired it through transfusion of blood or blood products, 9 (7 percent) acquired it through intravenous drug use, 8 (6 percent) acquired it either sexually or through intravenous drug use, and for 9 (7 percent) the route of acquisition was undetermined (Table 3). Seventeen (13 percent) patients had histories of intravenous drug use. Overall, 39 percent were Black, 39 percent were White, and 20 percent were Hispanic; the male-to-female ratio was 4.5:1. Of the 54 homosexual and bisexual adolescent males with AIDS, 26 (48 percent) were Black, 15 (28 percent) were White, and 12 (22 percent) were Hispanic. Cases were reported from 27 states, the District of Columbia, and Puerto Rico, and were concentrated in New York (31, 24 percent), California (18, 14 percent), New Jersey (9, 7 percent), and Puerto Rico (8, 6 percent).

Additionally, 1,295 (4.4 percent of total) AIDS cases have been reported in 20-24 year olds, a high proportion of whom were likely infected with HIV during adolescence. Of these 1,295, 902 (70 percent) acquired HIV infection sexually, 195 (15 percent) acquired it parenterally, 136 (11 percent) acquired it either sexually or parenterally, and for 62 (5 percent) the route of acquisition was undetermined (Table 3). Importantly, in 283 (22 percent) cases the patients had histories of intrave-

Table 3
AIDS Cases by Transmission Category and Age Group, United States*

Route of Transmission	CASES							
	Age Group (years)						Total	
	0 - 12		13 - 19		20 - 24			
Transmission Category	N	(%)	N	(%)	N	(%)	N	(%)
Sexual								
Homosexual/bisexual male	0	(0)	54	(43)	793	(61)	847	(46)
Heterosexual	0	(0)	11	(9)	109	(8)	120	(7)
Parenteral								
Intravenous (IV) drug user	0	(0)	9	(7)	147	(11)	156	(9)
Transfusion, blood/ components	51	(12)	6	(5)	19	(1)	76	(4)
Hemophilia/coagulation disorder	23	(6)	30	(24)	29	(2)	82	(4)
Perinatal								
Parent with/at risk for AIDS	325	(79)	0	(0)	0	(0)	325	(18)
Sexual or parenteral								
Homosexual/bisexual male and IV drug user	0	(0)	8	(6)	136	(11)	144	(8)
Undetermined	11	(3)	9	(7)	62	(5)	82	(4)
Total	410		127		1,295		1,832	

* Provisional data through January 6, 1987

nous drug use, and of the 147 heterosexual intravenous drug users, 67 (46 percent) were Hispanic and 45 (31 percent) were Black (Table 5).

Clinical Course and Prognosis

The true risk of perinatal transmission from an infected mother to her child remains unknown (Centers for Disease Control, 1985b). Three studies have evaluated this risk and conclude that 20-65 percent of the children born to infected mothers will become infected before or during delivery (Scott, Fischl, Klimas et al., 1985; Scott, Fischl, Klimas, Fletcher et al., 1985; Stewart et al., 1985). Prospective studies are currently in progress and should provide more accurate estimates of the transmission rate.

The proportion of infants infected at birth who will develop clinical AIDS is currently not known. Since passively acquired maternal antibody may persist in an infant for up to 15 months (Centers for Disease Control, 1987), these children must be retested after this time to assess their true risk of disease. For those who do progress to disease, prodromal symptoms will usually develop by 4 months of age, with most infants progressing rapidly to clinical AIDS (Rogers, 1985). The majority (62-70 percent) of children with AIDS develop *Pneumocystis carinii* pneumonia (Rogers, 1985).

In contrast to perinatally acquired infection, transfusion-associated disease in infants manifests itself at approximately 8 months of age. Hemophiliacs, infected through transfusions of blood products, present in the second decade of life at a median age of 14 years (Rogers, 1985). Unlike AIDS in adults, 41 percent of children with AIDS present with lymphoid interstitial pneumonia, a diffuse interstitial and peribronchiolar pneumonia without identifiable pathogens (Scott and Parks, 1986). The prognosis for children with AIDS is poor, and, although

Table 4
Perinatally Transmitted Pediatric AIDS Cases
by Maternal Transmission Category and Race, United States*

Maternal Transmission Category	Race of Child				
	White N (%)	Black N (%)	Hispanic N (%)	Other N (%)	Total N (%)
Intravenous drug user	17 (49)	119 (57)	52 (66)	2 (67)	190 (58)
Heterosexual partner of male in risk group	13 (37)	63 (30)	24 (30)	1 (33)	101 (31)
Haitian/Central African	1 (3)	16 (8)	1 (1)	0	18 (6)
Mother with AIDS	2 (6)	9 (4)	2 (2)	0	13 (4)
Transfusion, blood/ components	2 (6)	0	0	0	2 (1)
Hemophilia/coagulation disorder	0	1 (0)	0	0	1 (0)
Total	35	208	79	3	325

*Provisional data through January 6, 1987

prophylactic therapy with intravenous immune globulin, treatment of secondary opportunistic diseases, and aggressive nutritional support may prolong survival, they do not provide a definitive cure for the underlying immunodeficiency.

Public Health Issues

Prevention of Perinatal Transmission

Reduction of perinatal transmission requires the reduction of HIV infection in sexually active and drug-using women of child-bearing age. Specifically, linguistically and culturally appropriate risk-reduction educational campaigns targeted at sexually active and drug-using women at highest-risk must be provided. This education should include clear information on safe sexual practices and how a woman's risk of acquiring HIV infection can be reduced (Rutherford et al., 1987). In addition, intravenous drug use is currently the major risk factor for HIV infection in women and their children and must be addressed through substance abuse prevention and treatment programs.

Special efforts should be aimed at identifying women at risk who may be contemplating pregnancy. These may include the development and implementation of educational and antibody testing programs at family planning, drug treatment, and sexually transmitted disease clinics. Infected women should be encouraged to delay pregnancy until therapies are available to reduce the risk of perinatal transmission (Centers for Disease Control, 1985b; Rutherford et al., 1987). Pregnant women should receive special counseling and evaluation regarding the high risk of infection in their children and the possibility that pregnancy may affect their own health. Options regarding continuation of the pregnancy should be discussed (Rutherford et al., 1987).

Table 5
Adolescent* AIDS cases by Transmission Category and Race, United States**

	White N (%)	Black N (%)	Hispanic N (%)	Other N (%)	Total N (%)
Homosexual/bisexual male	15 (31)	26 (52)	12 (48)	1 (33)	54 (43)
Intravenous (IV) drug user	1 (2)	2 (4)	3 (12)	1 (33)	9 (7)
Homosexual/bisexual male and IV drug user	3 (6)	1 (2)	4 (16)	0	8 (6)
Hemophilia/coagulation disorder	22 (45)	4 (8)	3 (12)	1 (33)	30 (24)
Heterosexual	3 (6)	8 (16)	0	0	11 (9)
Transfusion, blood/ components	3 (6)	3 (6)	0	0	6 (5)
Undetermined	2 (4)	6 (12)	1 (4)	0	9 (7)
Total	49	50	25	3	127

*13-19 years of age
**Provisional data through January 6, 1987

Prevention of Sexual and Drug-Abuse-Associated Transmission among Adolescents

Reduction of HIV transmission in the adolescent population involves risk reduction programs aimed at sexual and drug-use-associated transmission. Specifically, all adolescents should receive accurate and comprehensive sex education in the schools or at agencies serving the homeless and truant youth (San Francisco Department of Public Health, 1987a; 1987b; U.S. Department of Health and Human Services, 1986). The curriculum should include standard family life education as well as information regarding mechanisms of transmitting and preventing HIV infection and other sexually transmitted diseases (San Francisco Department of Public Health, 1987b).

Curricula aimed at preventing and reducing drug abuse should also be developed and implemented. In addition, youth as well as parents and teachers should be informed regarding the education and treatment of individuals with substance abuse problems. Strong efforts should be made to refer youth in need of services for drug abuse counseling and treatment (San Francisco Department of Public Health, 1987b).

Education and Foster Care of Children with HIV Infection

None of the identified cases of HIV infection in the United States are known to have been transmitted in school, day-care, or foster-care settings or through other casual person-to-person contact (Centers for Disease Control, 1985c). Other than sexual partners of HIV-infected patients and infants born to infected mothers, none of the family or household members of the over 29,000 AIDS patients reported to CDC have developed AIDS or been infected with HIV (Centers for Disease Control, 1985c). Two cases involving nonparenteral transmission of HIV from a patient to persons providing extended nursing care have been cited in the literature (Centers for Disease Control,

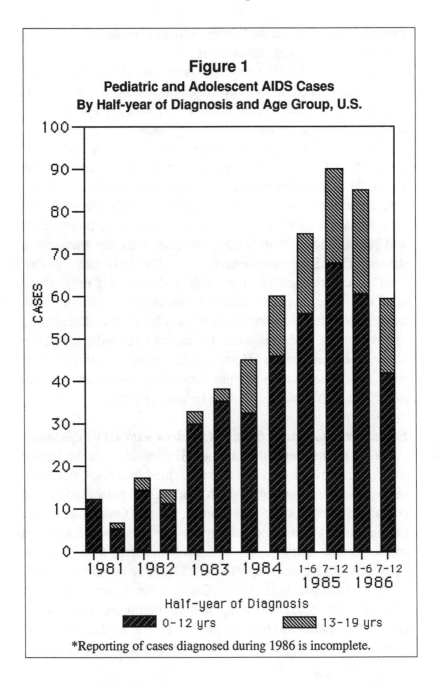

Figure 1
Pediatric and Adolescent AIDS Cases
By Half-year of Diagnosis and Age Group, U.S.

*Reporting of cases diagnosed during 1986 is incomplete.

78

1986; Grint and McEvoy, 1985). Studies of family members of patients with AIDS in the United States and Africa have failed to demonstrate HIV transmission to adults who are not sexual contacts of the infected patients or to children who have not already been infected perinatally (Fischl et al., 1986; Friedland et al., 1986; Jason et al., 1986; Kaplan et al., 1985; Lawrence et al., 1985; Lewin, Zack and Ayodele, 1985; Mann et al., 1986; Peterman, Stoneburner and Allen, 1986; Redfield et al., 1985; Rogers et al., 1986; Saltzman et al., 1986; Thomas et al., 1985).

Theoretically, if casual person-to-person transmission were to exist, the risk of transmission would probably be greatest in young children. This theoretical transmission would most likely involve exposure of open skin lesions or mucous membranes to blood and possibly other body fluids of an infected person. There is, however, no evidence of this type of transmission occurring in any setting. On the other hand, HIV-infected children are at greater risk for serious infection from a variety of common childhood pathogens than non-HIV-infected children (Rutherford et al., 1987; San Francisco Department of Public Health, 1987a). The risk of acquiring infectious agents probably increases in schools, day-care, and foster-care settings with increasing numbers of children, especially young children who are not toilet trained.

Guidelines for the education and foster care of HIV-infected children have been developed by CDC (Centers for Disease Control, 1985c), the American Academy of Pediatrics (American Academy of Pediatrics, 1986; 1987), and local health departments (Rutherford et al., 1987; San Francisco Department of Public Health, 1987a). In general, decisions regarding educational and foster-care of HIV-infected children should be made by an interdisciplinary team that considers the age, behavior, and neurologic development of the child. For school-age children who do not exhibit behaviors such as drooling, mouthing, and incontinence, the benefits of unrestricted placement outweigh the risk of acquiring serious infections. Preschool children under three years of age with age-appropriate development should be educated and cared for in settings which minimize their exposure to serious infectious agents. Although live virus vaccines are contraindicated for symptomatic HIV-infected children, inactivated vaccines are clearly indicated as is postexposure prophylaxis for measles, chickenpox, meningococcus, and *Haemophilus influenzae* infection (Rutherford et al., 1987; San Francisco Department of Public Health, 1987a; American Academy of Pediatrics, 1986; ACIP, 1986). Mandatory screening for HIV infection is not appropriate as a condition for school entry (San Francisco Department of Public Health, 1987a; Centers for Disease Control, 1985c).

When there is high risk of a mother having been infected with HIV, to ensure proper medical care, screening of children awaiting foster-care placement or adoption should be considered. Mandatory screening of children without known risk factors is not indicated.

Conclusion

HIV infection in children occurs primarily through perinatal transmission with drug abuse as the major maternal risk factor for infection. In adolescents, the majority of infections have occurred in homosexual or bisexual youth through sexual transmission and in hemophiliacs through transfusion of infected blood products. As the prevalence of HIV infection rises, increases in drug-use-associated transmission in women with secondary perinatal transmission and sexual transmission in adolescents seem likely to occur. To prevent further spread of infection to children and adolescents, health agencies must target extensive linguistically and culturally appropriate educational campaigns at all adolescents, young adults, and sexually active women.

Reprinted with permission from the *Journal of Drug Issues*.

References

American Academy of Pediatrics. 1986. School attendance of children and adolescents infected with T-lymphotropic virus type III/lymphadenopathy-associated virus. *Pediatrics* 77:430-2.

American Academy of Pediatrics. 1987. Health guidelines for the attendance in day-care and foster care settings of children infected with human immunodeficiency virus. *Pediatrics* 79:466-9.

ACIP. 1986. Immunizations of children infected with human T-lymphotropic virus type III/lymphadenopathy-associated virus. *Morbidity and Mortality Weekly Report* 35:595-8, 603-6.

Barre-Sinoussi, F., Chermann, J.C., Rey, F. et al. 1983. Isolation of a T-lymphotropic retrovirus from a patient at risk for acquired immune deficiency syndrome (AIDS). *Science* 220:865-7.

Centers for Disease Control. 1981. Pneumocystis pneumonia - Los Angeles. *Morbidity and Mortality Weekly Report* 30:250-2.

Centers for Disease Control. 1982a. Update on Kaposi's sarcoma and opportunistic infections in previously healthy persons-United States. *Morbidity and Mortality Weekly Report* 31:294, 300-1.

Centers for Disease Control. 1982b. Opportunistic infections and Kaposi's sarcoma among Haitians in the United States. *Morbidity and Mortality Weekly Report* 31:353-4, 360-1.

Centers for Disease Control. 1982c. *Pneumocystis carinii* pneumonia among persons with hemophilia A. *Morbidity and Mortality Weekly Report* 31:365-7.

Centers for Disease Control. 1982d. Update on acquired immunodeficiency syndrome (AIDS) among patients with hemophilia A. *Morbidity and Mortality Weekly Report* 31:664-6, 652.

Centers for Disease Control. 1982e. Possible transfusion- associated acquired immunodeficiency syndrome (AIDS) — California. *Morbidity and Mortality Weekly Report* 31:652-4.

Centers for Disease Control. 1982f. Unexplained immunodeficiency and opportunistic infections in infants—New York, New Jersey, California. Morbidity and Mortality Weekly Report 31:665-7.

Centers for Disease Control. 1983. Immunodeficiency among female sexual partners of males with acquired immunodeficiency syndrome. *Morbidity and Mortality Weekly Report* 31:697-8.

Centers for Disease Control. 1984. Update: Acquired immunodeficiency syndrome (AIDS) in patients with hemophilia. *Morbidity and Mortality Weekly Report* 33:589-91.

Centers for Disease Control. 1985a. Revision of the case definition of acquired immunodeficiency syndrome for national reporting—United States. *Morbidity and Mortality Weekly Report* 34:373-5.

Centers for Disease Control. 1985b. Recommendations for assisting in the prevention of perinatal transmission of human T-lymphotropic virus type III/lymphadenopathy-associated virus and acquired immunodeficiency syndrome. *Morbidity and Mortality Weekly Report* 34:721-32.

Centers for Disease Control. 1985c. Education and foster care of children infected with human T-lymphotropic virus type III/lymphadenopathy-associated virus. *Morbidity and Mortality Weekly Report* 34:517-21.

Centers for Disease Control. 1986. Apparent transmission of human T-lymphotropic virus type III/lymphadenopathy-associated virus from a child to a mother providing health care. *Morbidity and Mortality Weekly Report* 35:76-79.

Centers for Disease Control. 1987. Classification system for human immunodeficiency virus (HIV) infection in children under 13 years of age. *Morbidity and Mortality Weekly Report* 36:225-30, 235-6.

Coffin, J., Haase, A., Levy, J.A. et al. 1986. Human immunodeficiency viruses [Letter]. *Science* 232:697.

Cowan, M.J., Hellman, D., Chudwin, D., Wara, D.W., Chang, R.S. and Amman, A.J. 1984. Maternal transmission of acquired immune deficiency syndrome. *Pediatrics* 73:382-6.

Curran, J.W., Morgan, W.M., Hardy, A.M., Jaffe, H.W., Darrow, W.W. and Dowdle, W.R. 1985. The epidemiology of AIDS: Current status and future prospects. *Science* 229:1352-7.

Curran, J.W., Lawrence, D.N., Jaffe, H.W. et al. 1984. Acquired immunodeficiency syndrome (AIDS) associated with transfusions. *New England Journal of Medicine* 310:69-75.

Evatt, B.L., Ramsey, R.B., Lawrence, D.N., Zyla, L.D. and Curran, J.W. 1984. The acquired immunodeficiency syndrome in patients with hemophilia. *Annals of Internal Medicine* 100:499-504.

Fischl, M.A., Dickinson, G.M., Scott, G.B., Klimas, N., Fletcher,

M.A. and Parks, W. 1986. Heterosexual and household transmission of the human T-lymphotropic virus type III. International Conference on AIDS. Paris, France.

Friedland, G.H., Saltzman, B.R., Rogers, M.F. et al. 1986. Lack of transmission of HTLV-III/LAV infection to household contacts of patients with AIDS or AIDS-related complex with oral candidiasis. *New England Journal Medicine* 314:344-9.

Gallo, R.C., Sarin, P.S., Gelmann, E.P., Robert-Guroff, M. and Richardson, E. 1983. Isolation of human T-cell leukemia virus in acquired immune deficiency syndrome (AIDS). *Science* 220:863-5.

Gottlieb, M.S., Scroff, R., Schanker, H.M. et al. 1981. *Pneumocystic carinii* pneumonia and mucosal candidiasis in previously healthy homosexual men. *New England Journal of Medicine* 305:1425-31.

Grint, P. and McEvoy, M. 1985. Two associated cases of the acquired immune deficiency syndrome (AIDS). *Communicable Disease Reports* 42:4.

Jason, J.M., McDougal, J.S., Dixon, G. et al. 1986. HTLV-III/LAV antibody and immune status of household contacts and sexual partners of persons with hemophilia. *Journal of the American Medical Association* 255:212-15.

Joncas, J.H., Pelage, G., Chael, Z. and Lapointe, N. 1983. Acquired (or congenital) immunodeficiency syndrome in infants born of Haitian mothers [Letter]. *New England Journal of Medicine* 308:842.

Kaplan, J.E., Oleske, J.M., Getchell, J.P. et al. 1985. Evidence against transmission of HTLV-III/LAV in families of children with AIDS. *Pediatr. Infect. Dis.* 4:468-71.

Lapointe, N., Michaud, J., Pekovic, D., Chausseau, J.P. and Dupuy, J.M. 1985. Transplacental transmission of HTLV-III virus [Letter]. *New England Journal Medicine* 312:1325-6.

Lawrence, D.N., Jason, J.M., Bouhasin, J.D. et al. 1985. HTLV-III/LAV antibody status of spouses and household contacts assisting in home infusion of hemophilia patients. *Blood* 66: 703-5.

Levy, J.A., Hoffman, A.D., Kramer, A.D., Landis, J.A. and Shimbukuro, J.M. 1984. Isolation of lymphocytopathic retrovirus from San Francisco patients with AIDS. *Science* 225:840-2.

Lewin, E.B., Zack, R. and Ayodele, A. 1985. Communicability of AIDS in a foster care setting. International Conference on Acquired Immunodeficiency Syndrome (AIDS). Atlanta, GA.

Mann, J.M., Quinn, T.C., Francis, H. et al. 1986. Prevalence of HTLV-III/LAV in household contacts of patients with confirmed AIDS and controls in Kinshasa, Zaire. *Journal of the American Medical Association* 256:721-4.

Masur, H., Michelis, M.A., Wormser, G.P. et al. 1982. Opportunistic infection in previously healthy women: Initial manifestations of a community-acquired cellular immunodeficiency. *Annals of Internal Medicine* 97:533-9.

Oleske, J., Minnefor, A., Cooper, R.J. et al. 1983. Immune deficiency syndrome in children. *Journal of the American Medical Association* 249:2345-9.

Peterman, T.A., Drotman, D.P. and Curran, J.W. 1985. Epidemiology of the acquired immunodeficiency syndrome (AIDS). *Epidem. Rev.* 7:1-21.

Peterman, T.A., Jaffe, H.W., Feorino, P.M. et al. 1985. Transfusion-associated AIDS in the United States. International Conference on Acquired Immunodeficiency Syndrome (AIDS). Atlanta, GA.

Peterman, T.A. and Curran, J.W. 1986. Sexual transmission of human immunodeficiency virus. *Journal of the American Medical Association* 256:2222-6.

Peterman, T.A., Stoneburner, R.L. and Allen, J.R. 1986. Risk of HTLV-III/LAV transmission to household contacts of persons with transfusion-associated HTLV-III/LAV infection. International Conference on AIDS. Paris, France.

Redfield, R.R., Markham, P.D., Salahuddin, S.Z. et al. 1985. Frequent transmission of HTLV-III among spouses of patients with AIDS-related complex. *Journal of the American Medical Association* 253:1571-3.

Rogers, M.F. 1985. AIDS in children: a review of the clinical, epidemiologic and public health aspects. *Pediatr. Infect. Dis.* 4:230-6.

Rogers, M.F., White, C.R., Sanders, R. et al. 1986. Can children transmit human T-lymphotropic virus type III/lymphadenopathy-associated virus (HTLV-III/LAV) infection? International Conference on AIDS. Paris, France.

Rubinstein, A., Sicklic, M., Gupta, A. et al. 1983. Acquired immunodeficiency with reversed T4/T8 ratios in infants born to promiscuous and drug-addicted mothers. *Journal of the American*

Medical Association 249:2350-6.

Rutherford, G.W., Oliva, G.E., Grossman, M. et al. 1987. Guidelines for control of perinatally transmitted human immunodeficiency virus infection and care of infected mothers, infants and children. *West. J. Med.* 146.

Saltzman, B.R., Friedland, G.H., Rogers, M.F. et al. 1986. Lack of household transmission of HTLV-III/LAV infection. International Conference on AIDS. Paris, France.

San Francisco Department of Public Health. 1987a. Education of children infected with human immunodeficiency virus. *San Francisco Epidemiologic Bulletin* 3 (suppl 1):1s-6s.

San Francisco Department of Public Health. 1987b. Guidelines for the control of human immunodeficiency virus infection in adolescents. *San Francisco Epidemiologic Bulletin* 3 (suppl 2).

Scott, G.B., Buck, B.E., Letterman, J.G., Bloom, F.L. and Parks, W.P. 1984. Acquired immunodeficiency syndrome in infants. *New England Journal of Medicine* 310:76-81.

Scott, G.B., Fischl, M.A., Klimas, N. et al. 1985. Mothers of infants with the acquired immunodeficiency syndrome: evidence for both symptomatic and asymptomatic carriers. *Journal of the American Medical Association* 235:363-6.

Scott, G.B., Fischl, M.A., Klimas, N., Fletcher, M., Dickinson, G. and Parks, W. 1985. Mothers of infants with the acquired immunodeficiency syndrome: Outcome of subsequent pregnancies. International Conference on Acquired Immunodeficiency Syndrome (AIDS). Atlanta, GA.

Scott, G.B. and Parks, W.P. 1986. An overview of pediatric AIDS: Approaches to diagnosis and outcome assessment. In: Broder, S. (ed.). *AIDS: Modern Concepts and Therapeutic Challenges.* New York: Marcel Dekker. 245-62.

Sprecher, S., Soumenkoff, G., Puissant, F. and Delgueldre, M. 1986. Vertical transmission of HIV in 15-week fetus [Letter]. *Lancet* 2:288-9.

Stewart, G.J., Tyler, J.P.P., Cunningham, A.L. et al. 1985. Transmission of human T-lymphotropic virus type III (HTLV-III) by artificial insemination by donor. *Lancet* 2:581-5.

Thiry, L., Sprecher-Goldberger, S., Jonckheer, T. et al. 1985. Isolation of AIDS virus from cell-free breast milk of three healthy virus carriers [Letter]. *Lancet* 2:891-2.

Thomas, P.A., Jaffe, H.W., Spiva, T.J., Reiss, R., Guerrero, I.C. and

Aurbach, D. 1984. Unexplained immunodeficiency in children: A surveillance report. *Journal of the American Medical Association* 252:639-44.

Thomas, P.A., Lubin, K., Enlow, R.W. and Getchell, J. 1985. Comparison of HTLV-III serology, T-cell levels, and general health status of children whose mothers have AIDS with children of healthy inner-city mothers in New York. International Conference on Acquired Immunodeficiency Syndrome (AIDS). Atlanta, GA.

United States Department of Health and Human Services. 1986. *The Surgeon General's report on acquired immune deficiency syndrome*. Washington, DC: Author.

Ziegler, J.B., Cooper, D.A., Johnson, R.O. and Gold, J. 1985. Postnatal transmission of AIDS-associated retrovirus from mother to infant. *Lancet* 1:896-8.

A Framework:

Essential Elements
for Prevention Education

A Framework: Essential Elements for Prevention Education

B ecause AIDS raises a broad spectrum of issues—sexuality, drug use, mortality, values—no organization or entity can single-handedly provide the comprehensive education needed. We believe AIDS education for young people must result because of a unified message and concern expressed throughout a community, and be a responsibility shared among many.

To have the greatest possible impact and assure that a program will succeed, several factors must be considered. We must strengthen community support for AIDS education; deepen the commitment and involvement of parents; train educators thoroughly; evaluate programs thoughtfully; provide AIDS education in a variety of settings; and collaborate with medical providers to reinforce prevention.

When these elements are in place, a framework is set that we can build upon, thereby responding better to future areas of need. We must allow ourselves the opportunity to share our concern and regard for young people in many ways and at many moments in their lives. A strong framework for AIDS prevention helps us accomplish this.

6

Developing Community Support for School-Based AIDS Education

Debra W. Haffner, MPH

Information about AIDS *could* be taught without controversy, but it would probably not be very effective. Basic information about the disease's epidemiology, virology, and disease symptoms could easily be integrated into a biology class without much discomfort. However, AIDS education that appropriately emphasizes safer behaviors over biomedical topics is more likely to raise concerns among some sectors of the population.

Communities need to anticipate opposition to AIDS education and develop proactive plans for introducing programs. It is important to remember that 91 percent of the American public supports AIDS education in the school (National Broadcasting Corp., 1987). Yet, the small minority of organizations that oppose AIDS education may preempt it.

A few groups have announced opposition to AIDS education. The United Families Foundation states that "sexuality education should simply teach that sex can lead to AIDS. AIDS leads to death (Bartleson, 1987)." Phyllis Schlafly's group, the Coalition for Teen Health, says that AIDS education is "a violation of the First Amendment rights of children whose religion teaches that nonmarital sex acts are morally wrong" (Schlafly, 1987). Indeed the Secretary of Education, William Bennett, when asked about teen sex on a NBC television documentary said, "AIDS may give us an opportunity to discourage it, and that would be a good thing" (NBC News Special, 1987).

AIDS education is raising many old controversies and fueling old fights. Anyone who has been involved in sexuality education will find many of the current controversies familiar. Educators have a great deal of experience in overcoming barriers to sexuality education. In developing AIDS prevention programs for teens, these ten principles may help foster community-based support.

Educate! Educate! Educate!

The general public is both scared and confused about AIDS. They are largely misinformed about AIDS and its transmission, especially about ways it is *not* transmitted. Almost half of Americans believe that they are likely or somewhat likely to get AIDS by sharing utensils with a sick person, 38 percent believe in mosquito transmission, 21 percent that they can get AIDS from a coworker, and 31 percent from public toilets (APHA, 1987). The community at large needs to know the facts about the virus and to understand why some teens are potentially at risk.

Prepare written information to help support your efforts and distribute it widely. Survey the community's feelings about AIDS education and document the results. Develop fact sheets on the AIDS epidemic and why young people are at risk. The Center for Population Options' fact sheet "AIDS and Adolescents" can easily be adapted for local use (CPO, 1988).

School administrators need special support and education efforts. At the time of this writing, 18 states and the District of Columbia have mandated AIDS education. The personal support of local school board members, curriculum superintendents, and school principals is crucial to your program's success. Be sure administrators are involved in the program's design and plans for implementation. Provide them with information on how to handle difficult questions.

Enlist the help of the local media (newspapers, radio and television) in disseminating correct information. Hold seminars for media leaders on the AIDS epidemic and its impact in your community. Ask them to air the many excellent public service announcements on AIDS, and to consider running ads for contraceptive products.

Hold a series of community forums for the public, press and parents. Introduce the program's philosophy, discuss the core content and introduce the teachers. Have key community supporters publicly endorse the program. Provide an opportunity for questions to be raised. It is important to anticipate potentially controversial questions and be prepared to calmly answer them (see p. 96). Some suggestions for handling questions include clarifying and validating the question; steering clear of arguments; showing respect for the questioner; and following-up on concerns (CPO, 1986).

Develop a Community Task Force or Advisory Committee

Involve school administrators, teachers, medical profes-

Possible Answers to Common Questions About AIDS Education

Will talking to teenagers about sex encourage them to have it?
No. Studies have clearly indicated that sex education does not lead to higher or earlier rates of teen sexual activity.

Will telling teens about condoms promote promiscuity?
No. Half of all teenagers are having sexual intercourse, and they need to know that condoms are the best protection available for sexually active teens. All teenagers will be told that abstinence and long-term mutual monogamy with an uninfected partner are the only 100 percent effective methods of AIDS prevention.

Will AIDS education scare teens about sex?
Good programs will underscore that sexuality is an integral, positive part of life. Students will learn that it is important to make responsible decisions about sexuality. Further, students will learn the facts about transmission which should reduce panic and misinformation.

Will AIDS education promote homosexuality?
No. Programs will teach young people about the behaviors that could put them at risk of contracting HIV. Programs will not promote sexual practices, but will encourage respect for a diversity of values and ideas.

Why can't we just tell teens not to have sex?
Abstinence *is* the best method of AIDS prevention for teenagers, but half of teens are already sexually active. These

teens need information to protect their lives.

Are condoms really safe?
For sexually active people who are not involved in long-term monogamous relationships, condoms are the best protection against AIDS and other sexually transmitted diseases. In the laboratory, condoms are found to be 100% effective in preventing transmission.

sionals, clergy, parents, and teenagers as you design your program. Strive for diversity to assure broad support. Ask the group for input into the program, assistance in recruiting participants, and support during program implementation.

The Advisory Board can serve multiple functions. It can help assess community needs and desires for AIDS education, survey current levels of knowledge and attitudes, help identify community resources, and review materials and curricula. Most important, members are advocates for your program and can address any concerns which arise.

Identify Community Support

Many groups are already concerned about AIDS education and prevention, and many other organizations have the potential to become involved. Develop lists of potential supporters and meet with them. Consider developing a community coalition or network. Community coalitions for AIDS prevention could include religious organizations, youth organizations like the Girls Club, YWCA and YMCA, the local chapter of the Red Cross, the PTA, civic organizations, businesses and local government organizations.

Resolve Key Questions

Certain questions are sure to be raised as AIDS education programs are being developed and need to be discussed and resolved before the program begins. Educators, health professionals, and school administrators should meet to develop a consensus on these issues. Key questions in some communities have included:

- What subjects should be included in AIDS education and at what level? What should happen when students ask questions on subjects that are not included?
- Who will teach the AIDS unit? Will outside speakers be used? How will they be selected? Monitored? Can persons with AIDS be invited to speak to classes?
- How will the school link to existing community AIDS resources for students who request counseling, testing or additional information?
- How will parents be involved in the program? Will parental permission be required for participation?
- What training will teachers receive before they teach the program? What quality control will there be?
- How will sensitive issues, like homosexuality, condom use, anal intercourse, and mutual masturbation, be handled in the classroom?

Involve Parents

Parents must be included not just in the planning stages, but in all aspects of the program. Encourage parents to preview the curriculum and meet the teachers. Hold parent seminars. Encourage parents to call with any questions.

Remember that parents will support your efforts. Eighty

percent of parents agree that it is their responsibility to provide sexuality education to their children (General Mills, 1979), yet few actually offer adequate information (Roberts, Kline and Gagnon, 1981). Only one-quarter of adults say that they learned about sex from their mother or father (Roberts, Kline and Gagnon). More than 8 in 10 parents say they would like help in providing sexuality education to their children (Alan Guttmacher Institute, 1981), and most support AIDS education in public schools (National Broadcasting Corp., 1987).

Involve Teenagers

Teens can be important advocates for themselves and also can provide input into what they *really* need to know. Survey teens and ask them what to teach in prevention programs. Use their anecdotes to substantiate the need for your program. Ask for their testimony at community meetings.

Teenagers themselves can be very effective AIDS educators. Teens can:
- Serve as role models for other teens.
- Educate each other.
- Act as peer counselors.
- Design materials.
- Serve on advisory boards.
- Conduct needs assessments.
- Organize student AIDS prevention groups.
- Conduct other innovative projects that they design.

Develop Reasonable Expectations for the Program

It is important that we not build false hopes for the efficacy of school-based AIDS education programs in changing young people's behaviors. Evaluations of sexuality education programs have found that they are quite effective in increasing knowledge, but significantly less effective in changing behaviors or attitudes. Existing attitudes can be reinforced, and communication between parents and children can be improved. However, a national study of sexuality education found that unless the education is combined with services, there is little likelihood that sexual behaviors will be affected (Kirby, 1984).

Numerous studies have shown that teenagers take risks even when they are well-informed about the consequences. Providing facts is not enough. The majority of teenage pregnancies are unintended, even though most teenagers are well-acquainted with the facts about how pregnancies occur (Zabin et al, 1984).

It is important then to not promise that school-based AIDS education will *by itself* stop the spread of HIV infection. Rather, this type of education can realistically increase teenagers knowledge and assist in attitudinal changes. School-based programs, however, will need to be supplemented by such community efforts as increasing teens' access to condoms.

State the Values of the Program

AIDS education cannot be value free because of its connection with the most intimate part of people's lives. Develop and then share the program's philosophy. For many AIDS education programs, these values will include that abstinence is the best method of AIDS prevention for teenagers, that sexually active teenagers need access to information and services, and that compassion and respect for a diversity of individual and family values underlie the program.

Programs can clearly state that abstinence from IV drug use and sexual intercourse of any kind is the only completely effective method of AIDS prevention, and that long term mutual monogamy with an uninfected partner is also effective. However, given the large number of young people involved in risky behaviors, most programs will also want to adopt the value that it is immoral to tell students "just say no or die." Many educators believe they have a moral obligation to provide young people with complete information on AIDS prevention, including information on safer sex practices.

Recognize that AIDS Education Has Political Dimensions

Dr. Nicholas Freudenberg of Hunter College stated, "The AIDS epidemic first hit the US just as a social and political backlash to the changing sexual values of the sixties and seventies was winning new political power." He goes on to state that it is imperative to acknowledge the political dimensions of AIDS, i.e. its relationship to such issues as racism, inadequate health care, sexual politics, public distrust and homophobia (Freudenberg, 1987).

The political dimensions of AIDS require educators to develop skills that may be new to them. Educators will need to learn to lobby, advocate, testify, organize, and use the media. Program planners and educators need to anticipate the potential opposition. It is most likely to come from those small ad hoc groups that have fought in the past against sexuality education, women's rights and gay rights.

Opposition groups are often very small, but their threat remains large because proponents for programs are often not organized or local. Do your homework. Involve parents, students, educators, press, and clergy in designing the program and reviewing all materials. Document community support for the program. Be prepared.

Make a Long Term Commitment

AIDS prevention cannot be this year's fad. Prevention of an epidemic among the nation's young people will require a sustained effort.

A Challenge

The AIDS epidemic demands the best from all of us. Educators have a major role to play in fighting the spread of HIV infection. We must develop programs that will be effective not only in providing information but in changing behaviors. We must develop community support and be prepared to fight the small but vocal opposition. Our children's lives depend on it.

This chapter is adapted from Haffner, Debra. 1987. *AIDS and adolescents: The time for prevention is now.* Washington, DC: Center for Population Options.

References

The Alan Guttmacher Institute. 1981. *Teenage pregnancy: The problem that hasn't gone away.* New York: Alan Guttmacher Institute.

American Public Health Association. 1987. *The Nation's Health.* Washington, DC, December, 1987.

Bartleson, B. 1987. United Families Foundation, Coalition for Teen Health. Press Conference. Washington, DC, March 13.

Center for Population Options. 1988. *AIDS and adolescents: The facts.* Washington, DC: CPO.

Freudenberg, N. 1987. *AIDS educator's perception of political barriers.* Presented at the American Public Health Association Annual Meeting, New Orleans, October.

General Mills, Inc. 1979. *Family health in an era of stress.* Minneapolis, MN: General Mills, Inc.

Hadley, E. et al. 1986. *School-based health clinics: A guide to implementing programs.* Washington, DC: Center for Population Options.

Kirby, D. 1984. *Sexuality education: An evaluation of programs and their effects, an executive summary.* Santa Cruz, CA: Network Publications.

National Broadcasting Corporation, Inc. 1987. *NBC News poll results.* New York, January 16.

NBC News Special, December 30, 1987.

Roberts, E.S., Kline, D. and Gagnon, J. 1981. *Family life and sexual learning of children,* Vol. 1. Cambridge, MA: Population Education, Inc.

Schlafly, P. 1987. *Eagle Forum, open letter to Surgeon General C. Everett Koop.* Washington, DC.

Zabin, L.S., Hirsch, M.B., Smith, E.A. and Hardy, J.B. 1984. Adolescent sexual attitudes and behaviors: Are they consistent? *Family Planning Perspectives* 16:4:181-185.

7

Involving Parents in AIDS Education Programs

Manya Ungar

P arents play a pivotal role in AIDS education for teenagers and younger children. In any program planning for AIDS education, we hope that parents' needs and concerns will be carefully considered and well addressed. With parents as allies, schools and other youth-serving groups will be assured much greater success in communicating necessary messages to young people.

The National PTA has developed a program which supports parent involvement in AIDS education, with the theme *AIDS Education at Home and School—PTAs Respond to the Need*. (To receive a packet of information about this program, write The National PTA, 700 N. Rush Street, Chicago, IL 60611-2571.) We believe this program addresses three concerns of particular note. First, parents should be encouraged to provide AIDS education for their children at home. Second, parents should be involved in promoting appropriate AIDS education in the nation's schools. And third, children with AIDS or HIV infection are deserving of an education and should not be hindered in any way from attending school if that is considered by the child's physician, the public health officers, selected school officials and parent or guardian to be the appropriate setting.

AIDS Education at Home

Home education about AIDS is extremely important. AIDS brings up many questions related to personal values, and children learn values most powerfully and effectively from their parents. While children may seem disinterested or uncomfortable when parents bring up sensitive topics (i.e., sex, love, drugs, death), they do respond positively to the expression of concern and caring that such an effort represents. When parents have established an open line of communication with their children on such topics, their children will feel free to come to them when other equally sensitive questions arise.

Parents cannot control their children's behavior, but they can help protect them through education. Although most parents have a hard time talking with their children about sex, death and drugs, such matters will come up in discussing AIDS. The National PTA offers the following recommendations to parents embarking on this task:

- The most important step is the first one. Start talking. Don't wait for your teens and children to begin.
- Provide and discuss information at a level that's understandable and suitable to your child's age.
- Learn accurate information about AIDS. Teach your children how they can and can't get AIDS.
- Be aware of some children's worries, such as that they may catch AIDS and die. Reassure them that while AIDS

is dangerous, they can avoid it and stay safe.

- Find out what your teens and children think they know about AIDS. Correct misinformation or wrong ideas.
- Tell your children that casual contact with a person who has AIDS has been shown to be risk-free. It is also not possible to get AIDS from a family member of someone with AIDS.

Teenagers face special AIDS-related risks because of high levels of sexual activity and drug use. Teens need to know detailed facts about AIDS. Most importantly, teens should understand that they can avoid getting AIDS by making good decisions, using sound judgment, and refraining from high-risk behavior. Parents should discuss frankly with teens the specific modes of AIDS transmission and what activities, including sexual, do and do not put a person at risk for infection. In talking with teenagers, parents should avoid acting shocked by what they hear or responding with lectures or frightening stories. An atmosphere of concern and acceptance will allow teens to continue to discuss their questions with parents.

Schools or other organizations providing AIDS education can offer help to parents learning to talk about AIDS with their children. The National PTA has developed a meeting agenda titled, "Talk to my child about AIDS? How do I begin?" Such meetings, which distribute educational literature, provide information about AIDS and have a speaker or speakers discuss the issue, accomplish several goals. First, parents are educated about potential risks. Second, parents' efforts to educate their children at home are endorsed and supported. Third, parents learn that they are not alone in having questions or uncertainties about how to proceed with home education about AIDS. And, finally, parents are encouraged to become involved with school-based education.

The PTA has developed a series of copy-ready ads encouraging parents to talk about AIDS with their children (with such headlines as, "AIDS Education: Homework for Parents," and "Five things to tell your preteens and teens about AIDS"). These can be printed in newsletters or submitted to local newspapers or magazines for public service publication. Such efforts expand the reach of this message to parents who do not ordinarily attend community meetings.

Parent Support for School-Based AIDS Education

Parent involvement in school-based education programs is extremely important. The National PTA supports having a wide range of health topics—including alcohol, drug abuse and AIDS— in comprehensive, continuing, age-appropriate school health education programs. We promote AIDS education in all schools in the United States. We know the endorsement of supportive parents can both motivate administrators to act in this area, and assuage their concerns about discord and controversy. The participation of parents in curriculum development and review can help ensure the appropriateness and effectiveness of the educational programs.

Parent groups or organizations like the PTA should sponsor parent meetings to review the status of AIDS education in the schools. If AIDS education is being offered, school personnel should be asked to inform parents about the curriculum and educational materials being used. If there is no AIDS education program in place, parents should advocate for the establishment of an AIDS curriculum committee consisting of a PTA representative, health professionals, teachers and other appropriate individuals.

The committee should first adopt guidelines acceptable to the committee and the community at large. A curriculum and other materials should be evaluated carefully and adapted as necessary to meet these guidelines. Questions to be considered include:

- Are teachers being given special training to teach this new material?
- Are the materials age appropriate?
- Does the teaching emphasize the behaviors that put one at risk for infection and how to avoid infection, rather than focusing exclusively on biomedical facts?
- What reviews and updates of the curriculum are planned? How often will reviews take place?
- Do skills-based learning activities teach problem-solving and decision-making skills to help students avoid risk?
- Does the classroom environment support students who choose to abstain from or delay sexual activity while also informing all students about effective ways to prevent infection if and when they become sexually active?

When any school is offering lessons on issues that address human sexuality or drug use, as AIDS education certainly does, parents should be able to review lesson plans and any materials used in the classroom. They should also be allowed to observe classes in session if they request to do so.

General community support for school-based AIDS education can be organized. Many different organizations and individuals can work together to see such programs established.

The HIV-Infected Student in School Settings

The National PTA is on record supporting suitable school placement for HIV-infected students. In our Resolution, on Acquired Immune Deficiency Syndrome, (See Appendix D.) adopted by the 1986 National PTA convention delegates, we acknowledge that though there are a significant number of children under the age of 18 diagnosed with AIDS, none of these cases in the United States is known to have been transmitted in school, day care or foster care settings. We believe that a child's suitable placement is best determined by the child's physician, public health officials, the parents or guardians of that child and the appropriate school personnel. We discourage any social displays that would seek to segregate, persecute or ban children with AIDS or HIV infection from school. Following these guidelines helps achieve our goal of promoting the welfare of children, youth and the community.

Conclusion

The National PTA program on AIDS Education at Home and School is a wide-scale effort to reach parents and involve them in this crucial task. The breadth of our organization (30,000 local units in 50 states, Washington, DC and Europe totaling 6.2 million members) makes this specific program accessible to communities throughout the country. It is our goal that many parents and schools will be served directly by the PTA program. We also hope that the principles of this program will be considered in nonschool settings and in locales without strong local PTA organizations. The effective partnership of parents and schools offers the HIV epidemic a formidable opponent, and with these combined resources and commitment we can have the only reasonable hope of slowing the spread of this frightening disease.

8

Teacher Training
for AIDS Education

Ellen Wagman, MPH, and Sandra Orwitz Ludlow

Teacher training is a critical component of effective school-based AIDS education programs (Davidson, 1988; Centers for Disease Control, 1988. See also Appendix A.). The fact that HIV infection is a critical health issue with social, moral, legal and ethical ramifications confirms and compounds the need for careful preparation of teachers prior to classroom implementation of AIDS prevention units.

Preparing teachers to conduct effective AIDS education is similar to preparing them to teach about other sensitive, family life or sexuality education content. The lessons learned from years of experience training family life instructors and more recent experience with AIDS training serves as the basis for the recommendations presented in this chapter.

Context of Teacher Training

The ultimate goal of training is to provide teachers with the knowledge, attitudes and skills to effectively teach about AIDS. Having well-trained teachers alone, however, does not ensure that programs will be implemented and sustained. Experience in family life education program development has demonstrated the necessity for three additional factors: (1) involvement of the community, (2) support of administration and school board, (3) approved curriculum (Krebill and Wagman, 1986). Ideally, each of these components will be addressed prior to teacher training.

Development of a Broad Range of Parent and Community Involvement and Support

In many communities, parent and community involvement is accomplished by using an existing health or family life education advisory committee. If none exists, a committee representing a broad range of views and comprised of parents, students, school staff, health professionals, physicians and other community leaders should be convened. This standing committee is generally charged with the responsibility for defining AIDS education goals and approach; reviewing, adapting or developing curriculum materials; and providing information about the program to the community at large.

Informing parents and other interested community members and incorporating their feedback into implementation plans is critical. Mechanisms used to communicate with these groups include presentations at regularly scheduled meetings of the PTA, Home and School Association, school site councils, civic organizations, etc.; individual meetings with parent and community leaders; articles in school or district newsletters; mailings outlining details of the classes; and invitations to parents and community leaders to attend a teacher training or parent preview night.

Development of Administrative and School Board Support and Commitment

In order to ensure their support and commitment, school board members should be involved from the earliest stages. School board support can be demonstrated on several levels including: (1) the adoption of a policy concerning students and employees infected with HIV; (2) the mandate or directive for implementation of appropriate AIDS prevention education, and (3) support for teacher training (Hooper and Gregory, 1986).

Administrative support can be built through their participation in fundamental decisions about curriculum and class scheduling. Another crucial administrative decision is the selection of appropriate teachers. Because of the sensitive nature of this subject, educators charged with the responsibility of teaching about AIDS should be committed, should have good rapport with their students, and should be respected by parents and community members. Ideally, the regular classroom teacher at the elementary level, and the health or family life education teacher at the secondary level, will integrate AIDS instruction into their regular courses of study. (See Appendix A.)

Additionally, administrators can enhance faculty support and understanding of the AIDS education program by providing a staff orientation focusing on basic information about the transmission and prevention of HIV, and school and community resources for dealing with this problem. (See Appendix A.) The goals and content of the curriculum should also be explained.

Development and Adaptation of Curriculum Materials

Goals for AIDS instruction developed by the advisory committee and approved by the school board should serve as the basis for district instructional materials. Curricula and resource guides are available for secondary level students (Quackenbush and Sargent, 1988; Sroka, 1987; Yarber, 1987; Oatman, 1988); middle school (Post and McPherson, 1988; Meeks and Heit, 1988) and primary grades (Quackenbush and Villarreal, 1988). District curriculum writers may choose to expedite the development process by adapting one of these resources to the needs of their students and community. It is especially important in AIDS education that materials, whether they be a comprehensive curriculum guide or of a more general scope and sequence, provide adequate guidelines for teachers to use in making decisions about content and methodology appropriate to developmental levels of their students. (See Appendix A.)

Program Development Training

Implementation of the key factors and processes described above can be facilitated by conducting a Program Development Training for school-community teams. At minimum, each team should consist of: (1) an administrator who will be responsible for program development, (2) a parent leader or school board member who will coordinate parent and community communication and involvement, (3) a teacher who will be responsible for teaching about AIDS, and (4) a local public health or AIDS professional who will contribute information and resources expertise.

The purpose of this training is to provide specific guidelines for developing and implementing AIDS prevention education programs. Content for the training can include:
  • basic information about the transmission and prevention

114

of AIDS
- local, state and national resources for assisting with AIDS prevention education program development
- rationale for providing elementary and secondary students with AIDS prevention education
- policies and guidelines for establishing school-based prevention programs and for dealing with students and staff with AIDS and HIV infection
- the role of the administration, parents, teachers, public health and AIDS organizations in the development and implementation of AIDS prevention programs
- the relationship between behavior and health and the importance of AIDS prevention as part of a comprehensive health or family life education program
- the need to incorporate a method for involving parents and community members in the development and implementation of prevention programs and in dealing effectively with AIDS-related controversies
- formulation of an action plan for developing and implementing AIDS prevention education in each participating school or district
- curriculum guidelines for each grade level.

Content of Teacher Training

Ideally teacher training will be part of this comprehensive AIDS curriculum implementation process. In addition to the district's progress in accomplishing all of the implementation steps, the actual content of a teacher training will depend on a number of factors. These factors include participants' previous experience teaching health or family life education; their current knowledge about AIDS content, instructional methods and resources; grade level of students whom participants instruct; curriculum guidelines from participants' districts; and amount of time available for the training.

Training that provides basic preparation for teachers should include content to address the following objectives:

- to increase teachers' basic knowledge about AIDS, including its transmission and prevention
- to increase teachers' ability to integrate AIDS instruction into health and family life education curricula
- to reduce teachers' fears and prejudices that may hinder their effectiveness as AIDS prevention educators
- to increase teachers' comfort and skills to teach sensitive subject matter and support family values
- to increase teachers' knowledge about HIV risk-taking behaviors and increase teachers' competencies to teach risk-reduction skills
- to increase teachers' knowledge of age-appropriate and sensitive teaching activities and resource materials.

Although content should be tailored to match the specific needs of each teacher-participant audience, it should, on some level, address these objectives by providing content in the cognitive, affective and behavioral domains.

Cognitive Objectives

Participants will know: (1) the methods of transmission and guidelines for the prevention of AIDS, (2) district, state and federal policies and guidelines related to teaching about AIDS, and (3) sources for resource materials, professional services and personal support.

Content that addresses cognitive objectives should include several categories of information. First, training should provide accurate, up-to-date information about AIDS and HIV infection including:

- its cause
- its frequency and expected progression
- the ways it is transmitted (including sexual contact with an infected person, sharing needles or other injection equipment with an infected person, from an infected mother to her infant before or during birth)
- the ways it is not transmitted (emphasizing the fact that HIV is not transmitted through casual contact)
- the behaviors that put people more at risk (including having multiple sexual partners and sharing IV drug needles and other injection equipment)
- the ways in which people can protect themselves (including abstention from sexual activity, consistent use of condoms and spermicides with sexual activity, and abstention from IV drug use or use of sterile needles)
- information about HIV antibody testing.

In order to reduce their own anxieties teachers want and need more detailed information about AIDS than their students require. Therefore, the training must clarify and separate background information for teachers from content that can be presented in classrooms. This, of course, will vary with the age, developmental and environmental needs of their students, and the curriculum guidelines adopted by their school districts.

A second category of information is guidelines and policies related to teaching AIDS prevention. Training should thoroughly acquaint teachers with any existing, approved district curriculum or policy regarding students and staff infected with HIV. Teacher training should also provide information about other support for teaching AIDS prevention education, including the Surgeon General's Report (U.S. Department of Health and Human Services, 1986), the Centers for Disease Control guidelines (1988), and U.S. Conference of Mayor's Report (1987), state education guidelines, policies from national education and health organizations (Hooper and Gregory, 1986), and national and local parent groups. (See Chapter 7 and Appendix D.)

A third category is information about resources. Teachers should learn about local, state and national AIDS organizations, audiovisual materials, background and curricula materials, as well as guidelines for selecting and using these resources.

Finally for teachers who are new to health or family life education, the training should address the placement of AIDS within the broader context of health education and human sexuality. Important topics include reproductive anatomy and physiology, the range of human sexual behavior and orientation, risk-taking behaviors including unprotected intercourse and intravenous drug use, communicable diseases including STDs, and decision-making and assertive communication skills.

Affective Objectives

Participants will: (1) feel comfortable teaching about AIDS, and (2) understand the potential impact of their personal feelings, fears, attitudes and values about AIDS on their role as effective prevention educators.

For teachers to be leaders in providing school-based programs, they must feel comfortable teaching about this sensitive subject. Teachers must, therefore, overcome any fears or prejudices they may have about AIDS and HIV infection to prepare them to effectively dispel the fears or prejudices of students and parents. In addition, teachers should be prepared to reduce unfounded fears and deflect emotional responses away from detrimental associations sometimes made between AIDS and various lifestyles or ethnic populations. All information should be presented in a manner that increases compassion for persons with AIDS.

Teachers' comfort will also grow as they become aware of and acknowledge their personal feelings, fears, resistances, attitudes and values related to AIDS. This awareness is a starting point for assuming two important roles of the AIDS educator: (1) facilitator of objective classroom discussions, and (2) supporter of family/community values. Thus, training, especially for secondary level teachers, should include discussions of value-laden issues such as sexual behavior, homosexuality, premarital sex, substance abuse, availability of contraceptives for teens, condom use, personal privacy versus public health, and death and dying.

Once teachers have a clear knowledge of their own personal belief system and areas of discomfort, they should be able to accept and validate the diversity of beliefs of their students and thus be able to establish a learning environment in which young people feel free to explore these issues. This is not to say that teaching about AIDS should be value free. In fact, there appears to be strong agreement that teachers must present clear values messages related to sexual behavior and substance abuse in order to help prevent the spread of AIDS. What is not universally agreed upon is exactly what these messages should be. Should we advocate: abstention from sexual intercourse until the establishment of mutually monogamous marital relationships? delay of the initiation of sexual relationships? use of safer sex techniques? abstention from all illicit drug use? use of clean needles?

If no district curriculum or guidelines currently exist, training should prepare teachers to work with their advisory committees to establish guidelines upon which to build AIDS instruction. It is important that these guidelines both reflect the values within that community and meet the needs of the student population. When curricula or guidelines do exist, training should prepare teachers to implement these guidelines, even if the values-base differs from their own. In either case, training should prepare teachers to refer students to their parents in order to stimulate intrafamily communication.

Educators new to the teaching of health or family life education may need additional training to enhance their ability to support parents as the primary value educators of their own children. Training should identify common parental concerns (i.e., who is the teacher? what content and values will be taught? how can I help my child understand about AIDS if I've never been educated about it myself?), ways to inform parents about AIDS instruction; and methods for facilitating parent-child communication about values issues.

Skills Objectives

Training participants should become skilled in selecting and using developmentally appropriate and culturally sensitive classroom activities and materials about AIDS and risk-reduction behaviors.

Training to teach AIDS prevention education requires more than the provision of information; it requires that teachers understand and teach in a manner that facilitates the adoption of positive health behaviors by students.

Teacher training content should address relevant learning theory, including social learning theory, skills-based instruction, and cognitive-behavioral theory. Content of training should be provided to teachers in support of concepts that include (1) the personalization and integration of information as part of classroom instruction, (2) the provision of relevant, culturally and ethnically sensitive information, and (3) the enhancement and practice of social skills that are critical to the adoption of positive health behaviors.

Risk reduction behavior includes abstaining from sexual

activities or commitment to use condoms and spermicides with sexual activity, and abstaining from IV drug use or commitment to use sterile needles with drug use. Critical skills for enacting risk reduction behaviors include effective problem-solving, decision-making, communication, assertiveness and refusal skills.

Training content should provide practical guidelines and examples that assist teachers in teaching critical skills and in determining the age appropriateness and cultural sensitivity of various classroom activities and materials.

Teacher Training Methodologies

The methodologies for training teachers correspond to the concept of what constitutes effective AIDS education for young people. The methodologies employed to train teachers parallel—and therefore model—those methodologies thought to be useful as classroom teaching techniques: (1) present information, (2) process feelings and (3) address skills for positive health behavior.

Presentation of information can employ a variety of methodologies. Traditional lecture followed by a question/answer session is effective for presenting basic AIDS information. This is especially effective when the presenter is an AIDS expert (i.e., a guest speaker from the public health agency or local AIDS organization), who can respond authoritatively to teachers' fears and misinformation, including those generated by the "latest study" reported in that morning's newspaper. Guest speakers offer additional advantages. They familiarize teachers with community resources, provide a change of pace during the training (and thus reduce potential boredom with one trainer's style), and are an excellent means of filling gaps in a trainer's expertise. Thus, using guest speakers reinforces the message that teachers don't need to be medical experts to teach about AIDS since such expertise is close at hand. Films and videos can also be used to present AIDS information and to familiarize teachers with potential classroom resources.

Training (and classroom teaching) methodologies that more actively involve participants and hence increase the likelihood of information personalization and retention include: (1) true-false quizzes, (2) practice answering typical student questions, (3) use of flash cards (teachers define the AIDS-related terms written on each card), (4) use of information games, (5) information-processing (participants in small groups first identify their questions about AIDS; a speaker covers the topic by responding to these questions; participants, again in small groups, identify their remaining questions; and the speaker concludes the session by answering the final questions), and (6) information-sharing (information is requested from teachers to develop, for example, a chart listing the modes of transmission and methods of preventing the spread of AIDS. The trainer fills in detail and adds pertinent information where necessary).

In order to process the feelings of teachers, to increase teachers' awareness of their personal values, and to increase comfort teaching about AIDS, training should present many opportunities for teachers to share their own beliefs, to hear the diversity of beliefs that exist amongst their colleagues, and to practice communicating about AIDS and related sensitive issues. Methods for stimulating such discussions include the use of films and videos and traditional values clarification techniques such as incomplete sentences, values continuums and ambiguous questionnaires (Simon, Howe and Kirshenbaum, 1973). Presentations by persons with AIDS are especially effective. In addition, panels consisting of representatives of the major religious denominations within a particular community can be used to present the views of these denominations regarding any AIDS-related values issues.

Techniques for preparing teachers to be effective supporters of parents include the fishbowl technique in which a small number of teachers, who themselves are parents, form an interactive group (fishbowl) that is encircled by a large group of observers. Fishbowl participants candidly discuss the concerns they would have if they learned their children were about to receive AIDS instruction at their schools. Parents can also be invited to participate in the training to bridge the communication gap that may exist between parents and educators. A third training methodology is to have teachers participate in and then discuss their feelings about using parent-child homework activities designed to facilitate family discussion.

As a methodology for addressing skills enhancement, modeling effective classroom activities remains one of the most useful training strategies. This is especially important for teachers lacking previous health or family life education training or teaching experience. Watching a skilled trainer address controversial topics or conduct and process a participatory activity greatly enhances participant learning and reduces the apprehensions that surround the adoption of a new skill or teaching strategy.

Modeling of classroom activities will address not only skill objectives but also two affective objectives (increasing teacher comfort and awareness) mentioned earlier. Participation in sample student activities designed, for example, to enhance awareness of personal risk behaviors and vulnerability to AIDS or to teach communication skills for refusing undesired or unprotected sexual behavior, will generate strong feelings in teachers as well as stimulate their participation in discussions of difficult-to-talk-about topics. Therefore, it is important to process these activities on two levels. The personal level: What did you learn about yourself from this activity? And the class-room application level: How do you think your students would react to this activity? Are you aware of other activities or re-sources that accomplish the same objective?

Equally important to skills modeling is skills practice. Skills practice is an often overlooked, yet essential element in the adoption of a new skill or learned behavior. Providing teachers with an opportunity to practice new teaching skills or answer difficult questions and receive constructive feedback will facilitate their adoption of new techniques. Similarly, an opportunity in the classroom to practice new decision-making, communication or assertive skills will facilitate the adoption or use of these skills by students.

Summary

Safeguarding our youth from the threat of AIDS requires a multidimensional approach involving parents, health and youth-serving organizations and schools. In order to participate in this critical effort, classroom teachers must be supported by their school boards, administration and communities, and trained to teach about this sensitive topic. Support will be en-gendered through a program development process that involves decision-makers, parents and community leaders. Training will have impact when it provides teachers with up-to-date informa-tion about AIDS and HIV infection, relevant guidelines, poli-cies and resources; when it addresses attitudes and fears that may interfere with effective communication with students and parents; and when it demonstrates and provides opportunities to practice recommended teaching activities that increase stu-dent knowledge and decrease risk-taking behaviors.

References

Centers for Disease Control. 1988. Guidelines for effective school health education to stop the spread of AIDS. *Morbidity and Mortality Weekly Report* 37(S-2):1-4.

Davidson, D. 1988. *Guidelines for selecting teaching materials.* Boston, MA: National Coalition of Advocates of Students.

Hooper, S. and Gregory, G. 1986. *AIDS and the public schools.* Alexandria, VA: National School Boards Association.

Krebill, J. and Wagman, E. 1986. *An evaluation of the family life education and training program.* Report submitted to the Office of Family Planning, California Department of Health Services. Santa Cruz, CA: ETR Associates.

Meeks, L. and Heit, P. 1988. *AIDS: What you should know.* Websterville, OH: Merrill Publishing Company.

Oatman, E. 1988. *AIDS and your world.* New York: Scholastic, Inc.

Post, J. and McPherson, C. 1988. *Critical issues in human sexuality: AIDS module.* Santa Cruz, CA: Network Publications.

Quackenbush, M. and Sargent, P. 1988. *Teaching AIDS: A resource guide on acquired immune deficiency syndrome* (Revised Edition). Santa Cruz, CA: Network Publications.

Quackenbush, M. and Villarreal, S. 1988. *"Does AIDS Hurt?" Educating Young Children About AIDS.* Santa Cruz, CA: Network Publications.

Simon, S., Howe, L. and Kirshenbaum, H. 1973. *Values clarification.* New York: Hart Publishing Company.

Sroka, S. 1987. *Educator's guide to AIDS and other STDs.* Lakewood, OH: Author.

United States Department of Health and Human Services. 1986. *The Surgeon General's report on acquired immune deficiency syndrome.* Washington, DC: Author.

United States Conference of Mayors. 1987. Local school districts active in AIDS education. *AIDS Information Exchange* 4(1):1-10.

Wagman, E., Cooper, L. and Rodenberg-Todd, K. 1982. *Family life education teacher training manual.* Santa Cruz, CA: Network Publications.

Yarber, W. 1987. *AIDS: What young adults should know.* Reston, VA: American Alliance for Health, Physical Recreation and Dance.

9

Evaluation of
AIDS Education Programs

Joyce V. Fetro, PhD

In the Surgeon General's report on Acquired Immune Deficiency Syndrome, Dr. Koop emphasized the role of education in controlling the spread of AIDS and dispelling fear-provoking myths concerning the disease (U. S. Department of Health And Human Services, 1986). Since Koop's recommendation, a wide variety of educational materials for school children has been developed by local, state and federal agencies, voluntary health organizations, and commercial publishers (e.g. Meeks and Helt, 1988; Quackenbush, 1988; Yarber, 1987).

A survey of local school districts, conducted by the United States Conference of Mayors (1986), indicated that 54 percent of the districts surveyed were providing some form of AIDS education. The Combined Health Information Database identified 21 AIDS curricula/teaching guides developed for school AIDS education (Centers for Disease Control, 1987). However, subsequent review of AIDS-related literature revealed few evaluation studies related to these newly developed programs.

In these early stages of school AIDS education program development and implementation, there are many unanswered questions related to program effectiveness. Do these programs increase student knowledge about AIDS, its transmission, and high-risk behaviors? Do they alleviate fears and discount myths about AIDS? Do they change student perceptions about suscep-tibility to the AIDS virus? Do they affect student attitudes about people with AIDS? Will they reduce the spread of AIDS in high-risk youth?

Program evaluation is a valuable means for finding answers to these questions and determining if newly-developed and existing AIDS education programs are actually doing what they were designed to do. Simple, carefully designed evaluations can yield important information that can be used in making decisions about future program directions. This chapter will discuss the importance of program evaluation, summarize re-cent evaluative efforts of school AIDS programs, describe cri-teria for evaluating AIDS curricula, and outline comprehensive evaluation procedures for school AIDS education programs.

Implicit in program development is the belief that certain educational methods will produce certain outcomes (Windsor et al., 1984). However, few educational programs are actually evaluated and when evaluations are conducted, they are often included as an afterthought to program development and im-plementation.

Program evaluation can be the primary channel through which educators learn whether or not programs are working. What educators learn through evaluations of their school AIDS education programs will enable them to increase what students learn about AIDS and its transmission and, hopefully, to help stu-dents modify behaviors to prevent the spread of the AIDS virus.

Several studies have been conducted to determine the need for educating young adults about AIDS. Recent surveys of high school students' perceptions about AIDS showed marked variability in knowledge about AIDS and its transmission and minimal worries about contracting AIDS (DiClemente, Zorn and Temoshek, 1986; Price, Desmond and Kukulka, 1985; Strunin and Hingson, 1987). Similar surveys of university students indicated that many students lack accurate information about AIDS and most fail to see any relevance between the growing incidence of AIDS and their personal behaviors (Caron, Bertran and McMullen, 1987; Goodwin and Roscoe, 1988; McDermott et al., 1987).

Thus far, efforts to determine effectiveness of school AIDS education programs have been limited to measuring the number of students receiving AIDS education. Very few AIDS education programs have been implemented and evaluated. Recent evaluation research by DiClementi and others (cited in Kirby, 1987) measured changes in knowledge and attitudes of middle and high school students after a three-hour AIDS education program. Statistically significant increases in AIDS-related knowledge and decreases in misconceptions about transmission of the AIDS virus were found. Similarly, Miller and Downer (cited in Kirby, 1987) measured knowledge and attitudes of high school students before and after a 50-minute AIDS education program. Statistically significant changes were shown in both knowledge about AIDS and attitude about people with AIDS.

Although AIDS-related literature identified few evaluative studies of the efficacy of existing AIDS education programs, the National Coalition of Advocates for Students (1987) has established criteria for evaluating an AIDS curriculum. (See Appendix A.) These criteria provide parents, child advocates, school board members and educators with a checklist for evaluating existing curricula relative to content, development and implementation. The National Coalition of Advocates for Students (NCAS) recommends that AIDS curricula provide simple, clear and direct information, focus on teaching healthy behavior, and emphasize high-risk behavior rather than high-risk groups. The NCAS also recommends that curricula be developed with participation/support of parents, students and other community members and that adequate training be provided for teachers.

Similarly, the Centers for Disease Control (1988) listed nine assessment criteria to monitor the extent to which local school AIDS programs are providing effective health education about AIDS. (See Appendix A.) These assessment criteria include, but are not limited to: presenting essential knowledge to students at appropriate grades; designing programs to describe the benefits of abstinence and mutually monogamous relationships within the context of marriage; providing adequate training to school personnel; and involving parents, teachers, students and community representatives in program development, implementation and assessment.

The NCAS and CDC recommendations provide school districts with important guidelines about program content, development, implementation and assessment. These documents do not, however, provide educators with information about how to conduct program evaluations.

Although evaluation studies require careful thought and effort, they can be completed by school personnel and do not necessarily require a thorough knowledge of measurement theory and statistics. Evaluation research includes activities related to collecting, analyzing and interpreting information about the need for, implementation of and impact of intervention efforts (Rossi and Freeman, 1982). The evaluation process should be built into the developmental stages of a program as well as during implementation and after program completion. Evaluations of educational programs answer questions such as: what should be included in the program, have the students learned anything from the program, how much did they learn, and did they learn what was intended?

Three major classes of evaluation are used in educational settings: evaluation of educational needs, formative evaluation and summative evaluation. Individual scope and focus of evaluations within school districts depend on the purposes for which the evaluations are being conducted. Although it is not always possible in educational settings, comprehensive evaluations should include all three classes of evaluations (see Figure 1).

Evaluation of educational needs is a prerequisite to effective program planning. In designing AIDS education programs

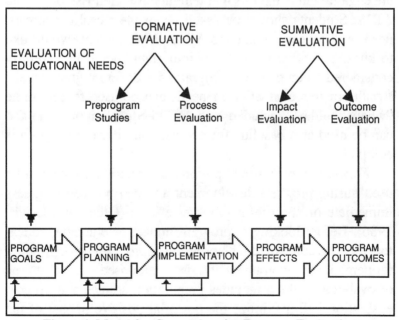

Figure 1. Model for Comprehensive Program Evaluation

school districts should plan carefully including the establishment of detailed program goals and objectives as well as explanations of how they will be achieved. Tailoring these goals and objectives to individual school districts requires an evaluation of student needs.

An evaluation of needs can determine gaps between "what is" and "what should be" (Kaufman and English, 1979; Stufflebeam et al., 1985). Surveys have been developed to assess student knowledge and attitudes concerning AIDS (e.g. DiClementi, Zorn and Temoshek, 1986; Goodwin and Roscoe, 1988; Strunin and Hingson, 1987). These and other available questionnaires can be adapted by school districts to identify "what is." However, a needs assessment should not be limited to finding out what students know about AIDS and its transmission, how they feel about people with AIDS, and whether or not they are engaging in behaviors that will increase their risk of getting AIDS. Students should be asked about their health interests, needs and concerns related to AIDS. What students would like to know and what they feel is important should be carefully considered when planning programs for different grade levels. Results of this evaluation of needs can be used to determine "what should be" included in the AIDS education program and can be used as a baseline for comparison after the program is completed.

Formative evaluations provide information which can be used during program development and can be used to assess immediate or short-term program effects (Green and Lewis, 1986). Before looking at program impact or outcome, educators must be concerned with program appropriateness, program refinement and program receptivity at proposed sites. This type of evaluation which includes preparation studies and process evaluation will maximize the potential positive impact of the educational process.

132

Formative evaluations are crucial for school AIDS education programs because "educating young people about becoming infected through sexual contact can be controversial" (Centers for Disease Control, 1988, p.2). Lack of receptivity of administrators, teachers, students and community members could be detrimental to the effectiveness of school health education programs to prevent the spread of AIDS.

Initial stages of formative evaluation include pretesting activities, conducting focus groups and pilot testing the implementation process. Each of these preparation studies can help program developers determine if content, language and process of proposed student activities are appropriate.

Individual lessons can be taught by experienced teachers to see if they work. Problem areas can be identified and reviewed. Teacher suggestions can be utilized to make lessons more appropriate and effective.

Focus group interviews with students of various ages can provide important information about student needs and student response to proposed activities. Students often are an underutilized resource in curriculum development. Student questions and concerns can be identified in focus groups and incorporated during program planning.

Pilot testing the entire curriculum in one or two classes can provide information about how well lessons and student activities fit together. In addition, instruments to measure student knowledge, attitudes and behavior can be tested for reliability and validity during the pilot program.

Results of all preprogram studies can be used to make program revisions and refinements before program implementation in school districts. This preliminary data collection should precede implementation of any new AIDS education program.

Process evaluations are conducted during initial implementation phases of newly-developed programs and on a regular basis in existing programs. They monitor the implementation process, site response, student response, teacher response and teacher competency (Green and Lewis, 1986).

Once new programs are developed, it is important that they are delivered as planned. In addition, the implementation process should be evaluated to determine whether the AIDS-related information and classroom activities are being integrated into existing health education programs. Other important assessments include whether enough time was allotted for each activity; whether adequate directions were given; whether directions were clearly written; and whether enough background information was provided for teachers.

Site response evaluates how well the program is being accepted at the implementation site. Factors which can affect site response include: administrative concerns related to scheduling, facilities and cost; compatibility of AIDS education program with existing programs; school climate in response to education about AIDS; perceived staff response; perceived parent/guardian response; perceived community response. Evaluation of the site response will identify obstacles to effective program implementation.

Three levels of student response can be assessed during the program. First, actual participation in the program is measured by the number of students reached and the number of hours of AIDS education received per student on each grade level. Second, quality of participation can be assessed with written/oral measures of student comprehension, attitudes and skills. In other words, are the students learning what was intended during program planning stages? Third, but equally important to program success, is student satisfaction. Students should be given an opportunity to evaluate their own experience in the program. For example, did they like the program? Did they feel the activities were worthwhile? Did discussions about AIDS make them uncomfortable? Were activities compatible with multiple ethnic groups? Would they recommend the AIDS education program to other students?

Teachers implementing the AIDS education program can also contribute to its refinement. During the process evaluation, teachers can identify weak areas and make suggestions for improvement. They can respond to the appropriateness of both AIDS-related content and process to student developmental levels and unmet student needs. This feedback can be used to make program revisions that will ultimately increase program impact.

Oftentimes, new programs are implemented with little or no teacher training. The Centers for Disease Control (1988) recommend training for educational personnel about the nature of the AIDS epidemic as well as educational methods to provide effective AIDS education programs. Self-assessment of teacher knowledge, skills and performance can provide feedback about teacher competency. These measures are important indicators of staff needs for continuing education and in-service training.

Formative evaluations are considered the "quality control" of programs in practice. Information gained from preprogram studies feeds back to program planning; information gained from process evaluations feeds back to program implementation. This feedback can be used to improve the program.

Although formative evaluations do not demand the same degree of precision as summative evaluations, they have equal importance. Decisions about the amount of time and effort devoted to formative evaluations should be based on program goals/objectives and available funding. However, program planners should realize that conducting a formative evaluation will increase validity of measured impact in the summative evaluation.

Summative evaluations provide a summary about program effectiveness over a period of time (Green and Lewis, 1986; Windsor et al., 1984). Summative evaluations allow program planners to draw conclusions about program impact and program outcomes. In other words, is the AIDS education program reaching the intended target population? And is it providing the services and benefits envisioned by the program planners? Decisions about future program directions and resource allocations are usually based on these results.

Program impact evaluations assess the overall effectiveness of school AIDS education programs in producing some change in cognitive, affective or behavioral measures in school children. Again, individual program goals and objectives usually determine which effects should be measured. To determine program impact, questionnaires should be administered before and after the AIDS education program. If possible, the same questionnaires should be administered to students not receiving the AIDS education program. Students' scores are then compared to determine changes as a result of the program. (School districts wishing to conduct more scientific educational research should consult: Babbie, 1986; Borg and Gall, 1986; Campbell and Stanley, 1963; Isaac and Michael, 1984; Posavac and Carley, 1980; Windsor, et al., 1984).

There are five major categories of effects on program participants: knowledge, perceptions/beliefs, attitudes, skills and behaviors. Although categories are interrelated, school districts may choose to measure some effects and not others. Examples of questions that could be included in each category follow.

- *Student knowledge about AIDS*: What is AIDS? What causes AIDS? How can a person become infected with AIDS? What are the symptoms of AIDS? What is ARC? What is an AIDS antibody test? How can AIDS be prevented?

136

- *Student perceptions/beliefs about AIDS:* Do students perceive themselves at risk for contracting AIDS? Do students perceive homosexuality as wrong? Do students believe that they can get AIDS from casual contact with another infected student?
- *Student attitudes about AIDS:* Do students feel that people who get AIDS deserve it? Are students afraid of getting AIDS? Do they think that AIDS is a smaller problem than media suggests? Are students afraid to have casual contact with people they suspect are homosexuals?
- *Student skills:* Do students have the skills to make informed decisions? Do students have the communication skills to avoid behaviors which may lead to exposure to the AIDS virus?
- *Student behaviors related to transmission of AIDS virus:* Are students engaging in sexual behaviors which place them at-risk for getting AIDS? Are students engaging in drug behaviors which place them at-risk for getting AIDS?

Several questionnaires have been developed to measure knowledge about AIDS and attitudes/beliefs about AIDS and people with AIDS (Caron, Bertran and McMullen, 1987; DiClementi, Zorn and Temoshek, 1986; Goodwin and Roscoe, 1988; McDermott, Hawkins, Moore and Cittadino, 1987; Price, Desmond and Kukulka, 1985; Strunin and Hingson, 1987). Additionally, a three-part questionnaire developed to measure AIDS knowledge, attitudes and behaviors of adolescent populations is included in Appendix F. Content of evaluation instruments could be locally determined. School districts can develop their own questionnaires to match their program objectives. In all cases, care should be taken to assure that questions are developmentally appropriate for students.

Program outcome evaluations assess changes or improvements in health status indicators for specific target populations, i.e., rates of HIV infection in heterosexual adolescents. Since changes in health status occur after long periods of time, outcome measures are seldom examined in educational settings. Hopefully, long-term effects of school AIDS education programs will include a decrease in the number of heterosexual adolescents infected with the AIDS virus.

Results of summative evaluations can be used to determine whether a program has succeeded or failed (based on previously established criteria). Although many school districts are not able to devote staff time or district funds to conduct carefully designed quasi-experimental evaluation studies, the value of summative evaluations should not be minimized. They are a valuable means of improving the program planning process and impacting school district policy.

In summary, evaluation is an integral part of program planning and development. A comprehensive program evaluation model contains an evaluation of educational needs, a formative evaluation, and a summary evaluation (see Figure 1). The evaluation of educational needs identifies what AIDS-related knowledge and process ought to be addressed by program goals and objectives. These goals and objectives are used in the program planning process to develop classroom strategies. Preprogram studies, such as discussion groups and pilot studies, assess immediate effects of the program; results of preprogram studies are used to make improvements before full implementation. A process evaluation during program implementation identifies defects or "bugs" by monitoring what is actually happening in the classroom and by assessing school/community response to the AIDS education program. The program design and procedures are then refined based on the process evaluation. After completion of the program, the impact evaluation determines whether changes in knowledge, attitudes and behaviors related to AIDS have occurred as a result of the program. The outcome evaluation determines whether changes in health status indicators have occurred. Finally, results of the impact and outcome evaluations are used to make decisions about future program directions.

School districts nationwide have "a strategic role to play in assuring that young people understand the nature of the epidemic they face and the specific action they can take to protect themselves" (Centers for Disease Control, 1988). In fulfilling that role, schools must assume the responsibility of providing students with AIDS education programs that are carefully designed and comprehensively evaluated.

References

Babbie, E. 1986. *The practice of social research.* Belmont, CA: Wadsworth.

Borg, W.R. and Gall, M.D. 1986. *Educational research: An introduction.* New York: Longman.

Campbell, D.T. and Stanley, J.C. 1963. *Experimental and quasi-experimental designs for research.* Boston, MA: Houghton Mifflin.

Caron, S.L., Bertran, R.M. and McMullen, T. 1987, July-August. AIDS and the college student: The need for sex education. *SEICUS Report,* 6-7.

Centers for Disease Control. 1987, October. *AIDS school health education subfile on the combined health information database.* Atlanta, GA: Author.

Centers for Disease Control. 1988. Guidelines for effective school health education to stop the spread of AIDS. *Morbidity and Mortality Weekly Report.* 37(S-2):1-14.

DiClementi, R.J., Zorn, J. and Temoshek, L. 1986. Adolescents and AIDS: A survey of knowledge, attitudes and beliefs about AIDS in San Francisco. *American Journal of Public Health.* 76:1443-1445.

Goodwin, M.P. and Roscoe, B. 1988. AIDS: Students' knowledge and attitudes at a midwestern university. *Journal of American College Health.* 36:214-222.

Green, L.W. and Lewis, F.M. 1986. *Measurement and evaluation in health education and health promotion.* Palo Alto, CA: Mayfield.

Isaac, S. and Michael, W.B. 1984. *Handbook in research and evaluation for education and the behavioral sciences.* San Diego, CA: Edits.

Kaufman, R. and English, F. 1979. *Needs assessment: Concept and application.* Englewood Cliffs, NJ: Educational Technology.

Kirby, D. 1987. *The effectiveness of educational programs to help prevent school-age youth from contracting AIDS: A review of relevant research.* Paper presented at the Office of Technology Assessment, U.S. Congress, Washington, DC.

McDermott, R.J., Hawkins, M., Moore, J.R. and Cittadino, S.K. 1987. AIDS awareness and information sources among selected university students. *Journal of American College Health* 35:222-226.

Meeks, L. and Heit, P. 1988. *The Merrill wellness series: AIDS: Understanding and prevention.* Columbus, OH: Merrill.

National Coalition of Advocates for Students. 1987. *Criteria for evaluating an AIDS curriculum.* Boston, MA: Author.

Patton, M.Q. 1980. *Qualitative evaluation methods.* Beverly Hills, CA: Sage.

Posavac, E.J. and Carley, R.G. 1980. *Program evaluation: Methods and case studies.* Englewood Cliffs, NJ: Prentice-Hall.

Price, J.H., Desmond, S. and Kukulka, G. 1985. High school students' perceptions and misperceptions of AIDS. *Journal of School Health* 55(3):107-109.

Quackenbush, M. and Sargent, P. 1988. *Teaching AIDS* Revised 1988 Edition. Santa Cruz, CA: Network Publications.

Rossi, P.H. and Freeman, H.E. 1982. *Evaluation: A systematic approach.* Beverly Hills, CA: Sage.

Strunin, L. and Hingson, R. 1987. Acquired immune deficiency syndrome and adolescents: Knowledge, beliefs, attitudes, and behaviors. *Pediatrics* 79(5):825-828.

Stufflebeam, D.L., McCormick, C.H., Brinkerhoff, R.O. and Nelson, C.O. 1985. *Conducting educational needs assessments.* Boston, MA: Kluwer-Nijhoff.

United States Conference of Mayors. 1987. Local school districts active in AIDS education. *AIDS Information Exchange* 4(1):1-10.

United States Department of Health and Human Services. 1986. *The Surgeon General's report on acquired immune deficiency syndrome.* Washington, DC: Author.

Windsor, R.A., Baronowski, T., Clark, N. and Cutter, G. 1984. *Evaluation of health promotion and education programs.* Palo Alto, CA: Mayfield.

Yarber, W.L. 1987. *AIDS: What young adults should know: Instructor's guide.* Reston, VA: American Alliance for Health, Physical Education, Recreation, and Dance.

---------- 10 ----------

Natural Allies: Youth Organizations as Partners in AIDS Education

Jane Quinn, MA

At a meeting on adolescent pregnancy prevention, the national executive director of one of the country's major youth agencies quipped that "although our groups are usually described as 'traditional' organizations, we prefer to think of ourselves as 'contemporary.'" The AIDS crisis in the United States has confronted the country's youth agencies with both a challenge and a test of their ability to respond effectively to a truly contemporary issue. The news to date is heartening, although much work remains to be done.

This chapter will offer an overview of the youth-agency community and an analysis of this sector's potential role in providing AIDS education. The chapter will then move from theory to practice with a description of how several specific organizations have begun to address the AIDS issue through programmatic efforts.

A Brief Overview of American Youth Agencies

Youth-serving agencies in the United States rank second only to the public school system in the number of young participants they serve. Collectively such organizations as Girls Clubs, Boys Clubs, Girl Scouts, Boy Scouts, Camp Fire, 4-H, the YWCA, and the YMCA reach an estimated 25 million young people each year. On the national level, fifteen of those agencies work together through an interagency council known as the National Collaboration for Youth, which serves as a forum for the exchange of information and, occasionally, as a vehicle for conducting joint programs. While some competition definitely exists among these groups locally and nationally for resources and even for members, their relationships are also marked by a spirit of cooperation. And despite the programmatic and policy differences that exist between these groups, there is also a shared sense of overall mission.

Most American youth organizations consider health education to be an important part of that mission, and an increasing number are including—and even emphasizing—sexuality education in their programming. This trend did not occur accidentally. Twenty of the nation's major youth organizations have, since 1977, voluntarily participated in a Program to Expand Sexuality Education in Cooperation with Youth Serving Agencies, initiated and sponsored by the Center for Population Options (Washington DC). This project has offered consultation, technical assistance, training and educational resources to members of the staffs and boards of these national organizations in an effort to harness their potential as providers of effective sex education. Other more general factors also contribute to this positive trend. Most youth organizations work hard to stay abreast of current research on youth issues. The burgeoning professional literature on adolescent sexuality, beginning with the 1976 landmark study, *11 Million Teenagers* (Alan Guttmacher Institute, 1976), has helped to spur several organizations into action. The findings of this body of research have been corroborated by studies initiated by individual agencies themselves. For example, membership surveys conducted by the YWCA and 4-H during the 1970s revealed that sex education was a major unmet need among respondents.

The organizations that have already accepted a role in providing sexuality education to young people have found themselves well-positioned to respond to the AIDS issue, at least from a programmatic point of view. For example, Girls Clubs of America's existing policy statement on sexuality education, passed by its Board and Council in 1981, was comprehensive enough to permit the agency to begin offering AIDS education without establishing new or separate policy. In theory, organizations with less clear-cut policies on sexuality education might choose to incorporate AIDS education into existing health, safety or life-skills courses (Haffner, 1987). However, the necessary sexual education might get short-changed by nervous program administrators in such a situation. In many ways, the planning of successful AIDS education programs should follow the basic rules of sound programming in general. A key tenet is that good programming is rooted in good policy.

Characteristics of the Youth Agency Setting

The same factors that make youth agencies appropriate providers of sexuality education serve to make those settings effective in delivering AIDS education. Youth membership organizations provide an already-existing network for reaching large numbers of young people on a regular basis. Because their members choose to belong to these groups, they are willing participants in program activities. The adults who work with youth in such settings usually have established a high level of trust and possess good communication skills, which enables members to feel comfortable exploring sexual issues with these leaders. And, because secular and religious groups are respected by parents and the larger community, they tend to be viewed as credible, safe sources of sexual information for young people.

Other characteristics enhance the usefulness of youth agencies as sex education providers. For example, parents are often involved in the program as group leaders or program advisors. This factor can assist in discouraging opposition to proposed programs and in encouraging dialogue within families. Youth organizations also serve significant numbers of youth that tend to be underserved by traditional sex education sources including preadolescents, males and out-of-school youth. In addition to these several characteristics that apply to the provision of sexuality education in general, there are a few characteristics of the youth agency that are particularly relevant to the provision of AIDS education specifically. One of the special challenges in teaching young people about AIDS is their tendency to disbelieve the information. The hidden and long-term nature of the disease, coupled with young people's developmentally-appropriate feeling of invulnerability, combine forces to lead adolescents to conclude that "it won't happen to me." The hardwon credibility of the youth worker can serve to help convince young people of the very real threat of AIDS. Also, the information can be reinforced over a long period of time and through both structured and informal interaction. Most youth organizations regularly employ a wide repertoire of active, experiential teaching techniques to convey program content (Pagano, 1987). Such techniques have been demonstrated as a necessary component of effective programs in which behavioral change is an intended outcome (Kirby, 1984). Although the goals of AIDS education may vary from agency to agency, most programs seek to decrease high-risk behavior as well as to increase accurate information. Experiential learning using a small group format is particularly suited to such behavioral goals.

Youth agencies also tend to be good collaborators. Many organizations have already established solid working relationships with other community agencies, including health departments and similar medical resources. This factor has enabled many agencies to respond quickly to the AIDS crisis, and to offer multifaceted services that include accurate information, skills practice directed toward behavioral outcomes, counseling, and (in some cases) health services.

While many youth agencies find themselves well-positioned and well-equipped to offer effective AIDS education, others face formidable barriers, including political, financial and technical obstacles. Those agencies for whom sex education remains controversial have tended to be inactive on the AIDS issue. The dependence on outside funding sources that characterizes most youth organizations is an additional barrier—while an agency may recognize its role and responsibility in providing AIDS education, it may encounter difficulty in raising the necessary funds to do so. Technical barriers faced by youth agencies in developing AIDS education programs include deciding on appropriate program content, evaluating and selecting educational resources, and ensuring that program instructors are adequately trained. An analysis of this set of barriers has led several of the national youth agencies to develop targeted services designed to assist their local affiliates in overcoming such obstacles.

From Theory to Practice—What Specific Youth Agencies Are Doing

The responses to date of agencies on the national level seem to fall into four categories: (1) offering targeted program services to affiliates; (2) implementing special projects; (3) developing resource materials; and (4) developing policies and administrative procedures. On the local level, many excellent AIDS education programs have been developed and are being offered to young people and, in some cases, their parents. This section will provide highlights of national and then local initiatives organized by youth agencies to date. It is not intended as an exhaustive list, but rather as a set of examples of work very much in progress.

Targeted Program Services Offered by National Agencies
Girls Clubs of America is considered a leader among national youth organizations in its commitment to providing health promotion, sexuality education, and pregnancy prevention services to its members. GCA's most recent survey data indicate that 91 percent of its affiliates offer health education and 83 percent provide sexuality education. On the national level, health and sexuality programs have been a stated priority for the past decade, and the organization currently conducts major national-level programs in health promotion and pregnancy prevention.

Against this backdrop, GCA began early in 1986 to develop a set of services designed to encourage and enable local Girls Clubs to expand their current health and sexuality programs to include AIDS education. These services include incorporating AIDS education into National Girls Clubs health curricula. GCA has developed *Girl Power: Health Power*, a health promotion course for preadolescent girls; *Growing Together*, a

148

parent-child communication course for early adolescents; and *Health Bridge*, a program geared toward helping adolescent girls understand and utilize community health services. The organization has also developed and can deliver training on AIDS transmission and prevention to local executive and program staff; collected, reviewed, and disseminated the best available AIDS information and resource materials to local Clubs; and created incentives for Clubs to develop and implement high-quality AIDS education programs. GCA has established a technical advisory committee to guide this work and has generated start-up funds from private foundation sources to underwrite these activities.

Similar approaches have been taken by the Young Women's Christian Association and Boys Clubs of America. The YWCA is expanding its national-level peer education course to include AIDS education. Its national program department is coordinating the evaluation and dissemination of appropriate AIDS education resource materials. Boys Clubs of America is adding AIDS education units to its *Body Works* health promotion program and its *Smart Moves* substance abuse/pregnancy prevention course. The BCA national office is also working to apprise its affiliates of the best available educational resources on the topic.

Staff training is a major focus of Camp Fire, Inc.'s targeted program services to its Councils nationwide. Camp Fire's national office has incorporated AIDS information into all professional staff training courses, focusing on both programmatic and administrative issues.

The Center for Population Options based in Washington, DC is providing technical assistance and educational resources to these and other youth agencies through a project funded by the Centers for Disease Control.

Nationally-Initiated Special Projects

In September 1987, the National Network of Runaway and Youth Services, Inc. launched the "Safe Choices" Program, a five-year effort directed toward increasing the number of AIDS education/prevention programs within runaway centers and other National Network member agencies. With funding from the Centers for Disease Control, the organization is developing six program modules for use by member agencies. These modules concentrate on six sets of issues: corporate/board policies; staff training; group sessions; street outreach; counseling outlines; and individual/family counseling. Network member agencies in New York, Los Angeles, Seattle, Miami, Des Moines, and Boston are participating as field-test sites in "Safe Choices."

Nationally-Developed AIDS Education Resource Materials

The American Red Cross is widely considered to have developed the most comprehensive organizational response to the AIDS crisis. Only a part of its efforts have been directed toward youth, but these efforts have been significant in scope and have provided assistance to other organizations, as well as to the youth programs of local Red Cross chapters. The goal of the American Red Cross' AIDS Prevention Program for Youth is "to develop a family and school-based program that will provide junior and senior high school students with the information they need to choose behaviors that reduce their risk of contracting the AIDS (HIV) virus." Its objectives are to increase the acceptance by educators of the need for AIDS education in schools; to increase teachers' abilities to provide AIDS education; to increase parental ability to discuss AIDS with their children; to increase youth knowledge about the risk of AIDS; and to increase young people's skills in and positive attitudes toward risk avoidance. The AIDS prevention program

150

consists of a 25-minute video/film, entitled *A Letter from Brian*, a student workbook, a leader's/teacher's guide, and a parent support brochure. The program components work well together to demonstrate to youth that they can avoid AIDS by saying no to sex and drugs. The resource materials are made available to schools, families, and community agencies through the American Red Cross' local chapters.

Development of Policy Statements and Administrative Procedures

The AIDS crisis has caused national and local youth agencies to clarify their policies and procedures, focusing on personnel and administrative issues as well as on program topics. Camp Fire, Inc. and the National Network of Runaway and Youth Services were the first of the national youth agencies to develop specific policy statements regarding AIDS. Other agencies, such as Boys Clubs of America, refer to AIDS in broader administrative policies. The national office of the Young Men's Christian Association issued a set of operating guidelines for use by its member associations, as well as resource information and a listing of suggested education and communications strategies.

The National Collaboration for Youth sponsored a special leadership seminar on AIDS and agency operations in January 1988. Designed especially for the top professional and volunteer leadership of national human service organizations, this session focused on a set of practical issues concerning AIDS faced by executives, managers and policymakers of these agencies. The issues included the following: (1) the applicability of current laws governing safety, health, labor relations, civil rights and privacy; (2) liability of board members, executives, staff and volunteers; (3) nationally-generated standards and guidelines for affiliates; (4) AIDS testing; (5) dealing with employees or members who have AIDS; (6) the board's role in policy-setting and other decision making; (7) special issues in relation to facility-centered programs; (8) confidentiality; and (9) public/community relations.

The Local Focus

There is no doubt that, in addition to all the national activity, many excellent locally-developed programs are also taking place, although there does not appear to be any systematic documentation of such efforts. Two such nationally-recognized programs are: a multifaceted initiative organized in 1986 by the Girls Club of New York, with separate components for early adolescents, older adolescents and parents; and a targeted outreach program organized by the Sequoia YMCA in Redwood City, California, which provides AIDS education to out-of-school, homeless, delinquent, and incarcerated youth. (This latter program was the subject of testimony before the House Select Committee on Children, Youth and Families in July 1987.)

Conclusion—A View Toward the Future

Although the youth agency community has been quick to respond to the AIDS epidemic, much work remains to be done. The process of translating national guidelines and services into local program activity takes time and financial resources. However, strong networks are in place to channel information and assistance. These networks, coupled with their strong sense of responsibility to assist young people, make youth agencies a powerful and viable partner in the work of educating America's adolescents about the threat of AIDS.

References

The Alan Guttmacher Institute. 1976. *11 million teenagers: What can be done about the epidemic of adolescent pregnancies in the United States?* New York: Alan Guttmacher Institute.

Haffner, D. W. 1987. *AIDS and adolescents: The time for prevention is now.* Washington, DC: Center for Population Options.

Kirby, D. 1984. *Sexuality Education: An Evaluation of Programs and Their Effects.* Santa Cruz, CA: Network Publications.

Pagano, A. 1987. Community service groups enhance learning. *Learning Opportunities Beyond the School.* Wheaton, MD: Association for Childhood Education International.

U.S. House of Representatives, Select Committee on Children, Youth, and Families. July 18, 1987. Hearing Summary. *AIDS and Teenagers: Emerging Issues.*

AIDS Education in a Medical Setting

Sylvia F. Villarreal, MD

E ducation is the primary tool available to pediatric providers in preventing life threatening diseases and injuries. Through routine health care maintenance and specialty clinics, health providers can discuss issues that impact on a child's life with both parent and child. At San Francisco General Hospital's Children's Health Center, education and prevention of HIV infection is implemented in multiple settings.

Pediatric Staff Education

Education to inform residents in pediatrics, family practice and primary care medicine; medical students; fellows; attending staff; nurse practitioners and nurses about the signs and symptoms of AIDS is vital and ongoing. In addition to this important technical training, two issues of an emotional nature must be addressed. The first is the small but real risk of occupational exposure to HIV. If clinicians' fears about becoming infected with HIV in the course of their work are not acknowledged and considered, their apprehensions may ultimately compromise the health and well-being of one of their patients. Careful training on infection control practices and rigorous observance of guidelines for body substance isolation (Lynch et al., 1987) significantly lower clinician risk and reassure most staff. Further discussions validating a reasonable level of anxiety usually help the staff to come to terms with their concerns and carry forth their duties appropriately.

A second issue arises from the need to follow infection control guidelines. It is now assumed that all patients undergoing examinations have infection potential. Thus, staff have had to change the routine ways of drawing blood, starting IVs and changing diapers. Thorough hand washing is emphasized more than ever. These practices are time-consuming and may be cumbersome. Pediatric providers have entered their profession in large part because of their love for and enjoyment of children. They often find the idea of suiting up with gown, mask, goggles and gloves to examine a child or perform simple procedures a little far-fetched. Many clinicians who chose this specialty because they would have direct and personal contact with their patients experience legitimate feelings of loss. This reaction must also be acknowledged, even while infection control guidelines are enforced.

Education is crucial and critical to the smooth running of an extremely busy pediatric emergency clinic. (Ours sees, on the average, 200 children a day.) Once the staff is educated, the work of caring for children can go on.

Pediatric Patient Education

Our pediatric population is similar to that of any county hospital. We serve poor and lower middle class families of diverse ethnic and racial background. Often English is the second language or patients are monolingual in a language other than English. Therefore, relevant AIDS education must be bilingual and bicultural. Some patients have come from Third World countries where hypodermics are routinely re-used. Many of the families coming to the clinic are worried about the sterility of needles used in giving routine immunizations. Through a parent survey, we found some think the needles are contaminated with AIDS or that they can catch AIDS from the toilets in the clinic. Personnel from the Ross Center for Patient Education, a San Francisco General Hospital program, have spent time with families in the waiting room explaining the fundamentals of HIV infection. This is a captive population waiting to be seen and often worried about the safety of the hospital itself. Through listening to the concerns of families we are able to address misinformation about HIV infection.

Informative posters and pamphlets are available in the waiting and examination rooms. But what seems to work best is verbal reassurance by the providers that Carlos' cold is not a sign of AIDS.

Routine Health Maintenance

Beginning at the two-week well baby visit, extensive histories of the child's mother and father concerning potential drug abuse, hemophilia, transfusions, and sexual high risk behavior are taken. Many of the mothers have been previously identified in the obstetrical clinic or nursery as being at risk for HIV infection, and some of these mothers and babies have been tested for HIV antibodies.

Kempe High Risk Clinic

High risk infants and families are then placed in specialty clinics such as the Kempe Clinic. (C. Henry Kempe was a leader in the identification and prevention of child abuse. The name is a euphemism for a clinic which examines potential abuse or neglect.) This is a multidisciplinary clinic that closely follows teenage mothers, infants of addicted mothers, infants who fail to thrive, and potential HIV infected infants. Using social workers, nutritionists, AIDS and substance abuse counselors, nurse practitioners and pediatricians, this clinic offers a comprehensive health setting for high risk families. AIDS prevention education is given to all families, including instruction on the use of safer sex, testing alternatives, enrollment in substance rehabilitation programs, participation in schools for the teens, and job training for others. We believe that the issue of AIDS in our clinic population is one of poverty. By offering health, educational and economic alternatives, we hope to prevent child abuse, failure to thrive and HIV infection.

Young Adult Health Care

Teen and family planning clinics become a natural place to provide AIDS education. There has been an alarmingly high rate of increase in syphilis and gonorrhea in urban minority teens (DiClemente, Zorn and Temoshok, 1986). Many teens are sexually active at an early age and need education to make appropriate decisions about whether or not to engage in sexual

behavior. The double edged sword of sexual and drug explorations put many young people at risk for HIV and other dangers.
Worrisome or dangerous behaviors may manifest in other aspects of the teen's life. Such circumstances make this an especially crucial time for providing education and health services.
We can respond by establishing a clinic environment in which a
teen can speak freely about sexually transmitted infections, at
risk behavior, gender identity issues, substance use and AIDS
issues. Every visit can be used as a time when behavioral
choices, including abstinence, can be discussed with the teen.

At teen family planning clinics, indepth sex histories can be
taken, especially covering safer sex guidelines and condom
use. Minority youth, including gay identified youth and those
involved in prostitution, need a place where they can discuss
their concerns and be fairly treated. Liaison work with other
agencies dealing with teens is an important facet of the SFGH
Children's Health Center. For example, Larkin Street Youth
Center, a San Francisco outreach program for street youth, re-
fers clients to us for medical specialty backup. Specially trained
staff at San Francisco's Youth Guidance Center (juvenile hall)
provides health care and AIDS education to incarcerated youth,
and these teens are also referred to the Center as needed for
backup medical care. Such collaborations allow us to work
with and monitor hard-to-reach youth at very high risk for HIV
infection.

Children in Foster Care

The Children's Health Center also provides special HIV-
related interventions for children in foster care. The inter-rela-
tionships of minority populations (especially Black and Hispanic), IV drug use and HIV infection become manifest when

looking at the problem of HIV infection in newborns (Villar-real, 1987). Minority children are overrepresented among foster care children, and a remarkable number are placed because their mothers are IV drug users considered to be unable to care adequately and appropriately for the child. The Center provides medical clearance for foster children and performs HIV antibody tests either with permission of a parent or by court order on selected children believed to be at high risk.

A number of health policy issues arise with testing of these children. Primary among these is the possibility a child will actually be HIV-infected. This raises concerns regarding approaches to routine health care, such as the use of immunizations and the treatment of infections. Another issue is the reticence of some foster parents to care for a known HIV- infected child. There is concern about the risk of an HIV- infected child being with other children, especially toddlers and infants in diapers. This relates both to fears that other children will acquire HIV infection through this contact (even though to date no such cases are reported) and concerns for the health of the infected child who will inevitably be exposed to a number of typical childhood diseases that could be life-threatening.

The foster parent with a known HIV-infected child clearly needs instruction on care and infection control. In addition, however, we find some foster parents of children without known risk to be unreasonably anxious and fearful, insisting sometimes that the child be tested, or taking unnecessary precautions in the home.

Once again the importance of liaison with agencies such as departments of social services, Children's Home Society, foster parents organizations, and health care providers is critical.

Conclusion

The pediatric medical setting is an especially ideal arena for AIDS education and the provision of preventive health measures for children, youth and their families. Health care providers can offer non-judgmental AIDS information to parents, teens and agencies while providing the necessary health care. Unfortunately, this takes time, energy, money and patience (Smith and MacDonald, 1987). One agency cannot attempt to do all. Only by practicing true community oriented health care can this epidemic be appropriately addressed.

Pediatrics supports the concept of education and prevention in the earliest stages of a person's development. Community public health clinics, private pediatrics offices, health maintenance organizations and military health facilities can incorporate AIDS education and prevention into their health maintenance protocols. By preparing children and their parents to master the complexities of healthy living, health care providers will diminish the ultimate impact of the AIDS epidemic.

References

DiClemente, R.J., Zorn, J. and Temoshok, L. 1986. Adolescents and AIDS: A survey of knowledge, beliefs and attitudes about AIDS in San Francisco. *Am J Pub Health* 76:1443-1445.

Lynch, P., Jackson, M.M., Cummings, M.J. and Stamm, W.E. 1987. Rethinking the role of isolation practices in the prevention of nosocomial infections. *Annals of Internal Medicine* 107:243-246.

Smith, W.A. and MacDonald, G.B. 1987. The impact of HIV infection on childhood health programs. *Focus: A Guide to AIDS Research* 2:12:1-2.

Villarreal, S.F. 1987. AIDS and young children: emerging issues. Testimony before U.S. House of Representatives.

In the Classroom:

Students Need to Know

In the Classroom: Students Need to Know

Kathleen Middleton, MS

T he AIDS crisis calls upon all members of the community to work together to prevent the further spread of this deadly disease. It requires that schools take a hard look at current instruction for health and family life, at the quality of staff in-service, at systems to involve community members in critical instructional decisions, and at related policies and guidelines. AIDS presents one of the biggest challenges educators have ever faced, the challenge of helping to save the lives of their students.

Today's adults did not learn about AIDS or its prevention in school. Nor have the vast majority of the nation's teachers had the opportunity to learn how to teach about AIDS prevention in preparation for their chosen profession. Needless to say, educators are anxious about their role and responsibility, especially since prevention education is, to date, the only deterrent. Certainly teachers recognize the importance of early and effective educational measures to help stop the spread of all diseases, but the fact that AIDS prevention requires education about sexuality and drug use as well, makes many administrators and teachers uneasy. The Centers for Disease Control recommends that teachers need to be trained, communities need to be involved, and classroom time needs to be provided at *each* grade level to assure that students acquire essential knowledge appropriate for that grade level. This is truly a task that calls upon schools and communities to work together to reach common goals. It requires that teachers, administrators, parents, community leaders, religious leaders, public health and medical professionals come together to plan the appropriate approach for integrating AIDS education into the school curriculum.

The authors contributing to this section all agree that education about AIDS should be taught within the context of a comprehensive school health and family life education program. School districts will be better able to deal effectively with the integration of AIDS education in a timely manner if they already have in place:

- articulated curricula for health and family life instruction
- established qualifications for teachers and requirements for teacher training
- systems to appropriately involve the community.

As Quackenbush points out, much of the conceptual foundation for understanding AIDS and HIV infection, and thus how to prevent its spread, does not include information about the disease. This is particularly true in the primary grades where instruction can focus on the difference between illness and wellness; understanding of communicable diseases and their prevention; cognizance of common health practices that help stop the spread of disease in general; and awareness that sick people need empathetic care and medical attention. A foundation of basic health and family life instruction allows for depth and breadth of instruction to become more AIDS specific as students progress up the grade levels. However, teachers in all grades and in all subjects need to have a level of understanding about AIDS—its transmission and its prevention—to handle the inevitable questions that will arise in the classroom. And, as more and more persons with AIDS appear in classrooms, teachers will need to know how to deal skillfully and sensitively with students' questions and concerns.

Ideally, education for health starts very early and continues throughout life. Pollock contends, "Health instruction begun and continued throughout elementary school years has the advantage of timelessness. Decisions and actions that affect the individual's health do not wait for physical, social or legal maturity" (M. Pollock and K. Middleton, *Elementary School Health Instruction*, Times Mirror Mosby, in press.). School districts that embrace this philosophy and value quality health and family life education are poised and ready to face the challenge of AIDS education.

12

AIDS Education in School Settings: Preschool-Grade 3

Marcia Quackenbush, MS

A mong the many proposals made to provide AIDS education to young people and children, surely one of the most
controversial is the suggestion that we should prepare ourselves
to talk about AIDS with very young children. How, critics ask,
can anyone reasonably contend that children five or six years
old should hear about a disease that raises topics like sexual
intercourse, death, condoms, homosexuality, and intravenous
drug use? These are reasonable questions, yet there are persuasive reasons to consider AIDS education for young children in
classroom and other settings. The suggestion being made here
needs elaboration, but it can be stated simply: AIDS has become a significant issue in this country; young children quite
naturally have questions and anxiety about AIDS; and adults
will want to provide age-appropriate information to young children to answer their questions, assuage their anxiety, and help
them protect themselves.

Much of what we advocate as "AIDS education" for the young child does not directly involve AIDS at all. Its purpose is to help provide the framework for a better understanding of AIDS and other diseases at a later time. For young children, we would not suggest that special units focused exclusively on AIDS be presented. The proper place for AIDS education will usually be in the context of other lessons on health. By integrating AIDS information into the normal classroom curriculum, we can offer the lessons in an age-appropriate manner. We will also demonstrate to students that, while any concerns they may have about AIDS are reasonable and understandable, they do not need to feel overwhelmed or fearful about the disease.

Already in this book and elsewhere, you have read about the seriousness and magnitude of this epidemic. Children are beginning to share this awareness with us. AIDS is mentioned on television news and talk shows, radio programs, and in conversations among adults. As children begin to read, they see the word printed in newspaper headlines and on magazine covers. As more and more communities are touched by the AIDS epidemic, more children will have parents, other relatives, friends or acquaintances affected by the disease. They hear comments about AIDS in the school yard, from older children and from peers. The simple fact is that the AIDS epidemic is a major event, and it has become, in one way or another, a part of each of our lives.

Because of all they hear, young children are naturally curious, and sometimes anxious, about AIDS. Careful planning of classroom lessons about health, privacy and human relationships can lay a foundation which allows children to state the questions they have, and for teachers and parents to answer them.

Preschool Settings

The preschool child will generally be best served by a willingness on the part of adults to answer questions as they arise and set appropriate standards for good health and safety practices. Personal hygiene habits are being established, and rules are set about matters like crossing streets and talking to strangers. The child, both at home and in a preschool or daycare setting, is also learning about family roles, the distinction between men and women, and other social relationships. Specific questions about AIDS are not common in such young children, but curiosity about physiology, genital function and some aspects of sexuality is normal. Answering questions honestly and positively, using proper terms for genitals and other body parts, might be considered a "preliminary" AIDS education for young children.

Kindergarten

The child's understanding of these lessons and sense of how receptive to questions adults are will lay the groundwork for later education about many concerns related to AIDS, and about AIDS specifically. In kindergarten, the material can become just slightly more complex. At this age, children often first become interested in, and anxious about, death, and they may associate death with serious illness or malevolent criminals. Social relationships become more sophisticated and independence is greater. The best course, again, is for schools and parents to continue to teach children health and safety skills and to respond to questions and fears children have.

First and Second Grades

The child in first or second grade should begin health education lessons on preventing drug abuse and child sexual abuse (teaching children about their right to privacy, different kinds of touch, how to avoid molestation, etc.). These health lessons offer two important tools to help children avoid exposure to HIV. They can decrease the likelihood of later use of IV drugs and decrease the possibility of HIV infection through sexual molestation. We hope these lessons will become part of a comprehensive health education program that is started early and continued throughout the course of a student's school career.

More sophisticated considerations of human relationships are also appropriate at this age—talking, for example, about how one relates differently to one's parents, one's friends, a stranger and so forth. The health education curriculum can also communicate some important concepts about health and disease. What does it mean to be healthy? What is it like to be sick? Are some diseases easy to pass and some hard to pass? (Colds and flus are easy to pass, AIDS is hard to pass, and children do not need to worry about getting AIDS in their interactions with others at school.)

Germs and their role in disease can be explained simply, along with a description of places germs are found: in the mouths of people with colds and flu (which is why you don't share cups with someone who has a cold); for some diseases the germs are in blood (so you should always call a teacher or grown-up for help if a schoolmate or friend is injured and bleeding, and not touch the blood yourself); some germs are in feces or urine (which is why people should wash their hands after going to the bathroom); and some germs might be on the street (so you should not eat a piece of candy you find on the ground).

172

Third Grade

Third graders will be interested in health and disease, in death, in sex, and in human relationships. They understand that marriage is a special relationship between two people who care very much for one another. They are interested in and can understand simple explanations of mammalian reproduction, perhaps using family pets as examples (a female dog has to mate with a male dog before she can have puppies). Most schools do not teach more detailed information about human sexuality at this age, but it is important for educators to expect that individual children may raise some fairly specific questions. If a third grader has been exposed to the concepts mentioned above, answers to other questions, should they arise, can follow in a matter-of-fact, age-appropriate manner. It could be stated simply, for example, that people also have sex, that some diseases can be passed sexually, and that AIDS is one of those diseases.

Values

The question of values naturally arises in education involving human sexuality. Parents will have more influence on children's values than schools, and public schools certainly should not take on the task of determining the personal morals of their students. There are, however, some important values underlying school programs. First, we do not want to teach in a manner that could cause children to feel badly about themselves or negatively about human intimacy and sexuality. Second, though most people, including children, have sexual feelings and this is quite natural, sexual activities like intercourse are not appropriate for children. Third, curiosity is natural and questions are healthy. We want children to ask questions and especially encourage them to discuss their thoughts with their parents. Fourth, comprehensive health education including lessons on health and wellness, human relationships, sexuality and AIDS should be offered in a manner that is consistent with community values, and parents must be involved in their development and have an opportunity to review materials to be used.

While these recommendations for educating young children may seem controversial to some, we think for most educators and parents they are not. We are not advocating that explicit information about the sexual transmission of AIDS be discussed in early elementary classes. We are encouraging teachers and administrators to think about the kind of foundation they are providing their students. Will they have the necessary tools to understand AIDS transmission and prevention at the appropriate time?

Exceptional Circumstances

There will be two circumstances in which more specific AIDS education will be necessary for very young children. The first is when a child has a parent, relative or close friend ill with HIV infection. In this circumstance, the child may have particular and understandable anxieties and concerns. The child may need individual attention and assistance understanding the disease. It is also possible that other children will learn of the illness and harass or ostracize the child. In such a case, education for schoolmates would be called for, along with strong interventions to protect the child from further negative attentions. This education might include discussions of how serious the disease is (though one should try to avoid the idea that AIDS is invariably fatal—neither the child nor his/her family

174

may see it that way); some suggestions about what makes people feel better when they or someone they know is ill (obviously, being harassed is not helpful); reassurances that this is not a casually transmitted infection; and explanations as to why people (the students themselves) might act negatively when they know someone's parent (relative, friend) is ill.

The other exception will be the classroom or school with a known HIV-infected child in attendance. Though the future may see greater tolerance of such children in our school systems, at present these situations often lead to public controversy and draw media attention. It is most responsible, therefore, to address these issues with students and respond to their concerns. A classroom teacher might set aside time to talk with students, first asking what they have heard or what they know about the situation, and then addressing the fears or concerns the children have. It will be important to acknowledge that HIV infection is very serious, which is why people are alarmed, and then to explain that there is no real risk of children in the school becoming infected through the presence of an infected student. If local AIDS education specialists are available, ask them to consult with the school in planning this kind of program.

Parent education would be an essential part of the response as well. Unless parents are well-convinced that their children are not at risk, our efforts with the children themselves will probably fail.

Parents

With young children, parents are the primary educators about sexuality, relationships and personal values. Parents, much more than schools, can help instill in children the self-esteem and thoughtfulness they will need to follow through on

175

commitments to care for their own health and well-being. For the seven- or eight-year-old child, this may be played out in the struggle of how many cookies one should eat, trying to be nice to one's friends, or what it means not to brush one's teeth. If these skills are nurtured in the young child, however, the 14 or 16 year old will have a less difficult time saying no to the lure— and risk—of illicit drugs and early sexual activity.

Parents and schools in partnership can build the foundation our children today need to help them avoid exposure to HIV in the future.

13

AIDS Education in School Settings: Grades 4-6

Jory Post, MA

Anyone having the opportunity to observe a current events discussion in an upper elementary classroom today will be in for a surprise. The level of sophistication and access to information is much greater than one would imagine. A high percentage of topics discussed often lean towards the sensational or even morbid: accidents, rape, murder, death, and now, AIDS.

AIDS is everywhere—and kids know it. They are barraged by it in the media in all its forms: TV news, TV specials, radio, magazines, and newspapers. Their families talk about AIDS at the dinner table and their friends talk about it at school.

While fourth to sixth grade students have a continual flow of information regarding AIDS, they don't always have the ability to translate and interpret that information accurately. When this happens, facts become distorted and myths begin to form and crystallize. Some of these myths are based on misinformation that can lead to the spread of the disease. Others can lead to unwarranted bigotry and prejudice.

It is the role of society to provide accurate information to its citizens, especially when their health and welfare are at stake. When a disease like AIDS begins to carve its way through a population, society is responsible for designing, implementing, and disseminating programs that will increase everybody's awareness. There should be no allowance for political or economic barriers to stifle the flow of information to any who have a life or a friend's life to lose. Neither should there be allowance for personal prejudice to falsify information or misrepresent the truth.

While researchers across the world are working frantically to solve the mysteries of HIV, it will probably be a long time, if ever, before we see either a vaccination or cure. Therefore, our only reasonable course of action is to educate all segments of our society in how to prevent its spread.

It has never been enough to tell people that their behavior could lead to an early death. The abuse of tobacco, alcohol and other drugs persists even though people continue to die from their effects. The same will also be true with the prevention of AIDS. Those people who are already used to a behavior will not give it up easily, even at risk of death. We must reach our impressionable youth before they have created habits which could lead to their deaths.

Unsafe sexual practices and shared IV needles are the two major transmitters of AIDS. Given that these behaviors are beginning as early as elementary school in many places, information about preventing AIDS must be shared with students as early as possible. If we wait until grades 7-12 it could be too late for many.

Context

While AIDS education must begin at the earliest grade levels, it should not become its own course of study. AIDS is scary business, with plenty of rational fears attached, but there is a danger of creating irrational fears as well. In order to prevent kids from growing into sexually dysfunctional adults, much care must be given to the integration of AIDS education into already existing curricula.

AIDS issues fit under many headings including family life education, drug education and health education. An individual school's choice will depend on its own curricular goals and on community standards. In some cases, schools will need to analyze and revise current curriculum design to meet the more pressing societal needs.

An ideal context for AIDS education with upper elementary students (4-6) would be as an extension of a family life education class within a comprehensive health education program. Such a program would begin with lessons addressing self-esteem, family and friends, peer pressure, decision-making and refusal skills. Those issues would be continued into the upper grades where students would also begin looking at human growth, reproduction, heredity, sexuality, and finally, AIDS and other sexually transmitted diseases.

Content

The current level of sophistication in music, videos and movies has created an informed and inquisitive group of upper elementary students. Many have also had access to the Playboy and pornographic television channels. There is little they haven't seen or heard. There is a strong need to deal with sexuality in an open, honest and sensitive way. AIDS as a consequence of sexuality must also be addressed openly and honestly.

AIDS education can begin by taking inventory of what students know, including what they have heard, what they have seen, and what they think they know. A curriculum can then be adjusted to be relevant to a specific audience. All future lessons will prove, disprove and/or expand what they already know.

Rather than expect that students will learn everything they need to know about AIDS within a classroom setting, we should begin in grades 4-6 teaching them about available resources so they may develop personal learning and research skills. They should be taught how to look for articles dealing with AIDS in both newspapers and periodicals. They should also be taught how to classify AIDS-related issues into subcategories such as politics, economics, human rights and statistics.

The vocabulary of AIDS should be increased extensively in the upper elementary grade levels. Students' foundation of future understanding around AIDS issues will be affected by the strength and depth of their vocabulary. By the sixth grade, students should have come in contact with most major terms related to AIDS.

After finding out what students know, teaching them basic research techniques, and familiarizing them with definitions, teachers can help students grapple with the greater reality of AIDS.

As stated earlier, it is assumed here that AIDS should be addressed as one part of a larger health education and family life curriculum, therefore its natural first occurrence is in conjunction with other sexually transmitted diseases (STDs). Students should be aware that sexual beings have responsibilities to themselves and others. One of those responsibilities is understanding the nature and causes of STDs. Students should be able to compare a variety of STDs as to their incidence, transmission, symptoms and prevention. If time permits, it is also a good idea to precede this lesson with a similar comparison of diseases in general such as chicken pox, smallpox and the common cold.

While studying diseases and STDs, the concept of epidemics will certainly arise. The understanding that AIDS is an epidemic can be made more relevant by discussing and analyzing epidemics throughout history.

Students at these grade levels are fascinated with what makes the body work. It is important for students to begin to have a general understanding of healthy immune systems. (What does it mean to have a healthy immune system and how can it be kept healthy?) It is a good idea to introduce the word 'efficient' to describe the healthy immune system, so that an easy transition can be made to the understanding of a deficient immune system.

While students will probably not thoroughly grasp a detailed explanation of HIV, the concept should be introduced. This discussion should include a description of other diseases that derail the immune system as well, so commonalties can be observed.

The transmission of AIDS is one of the most important concepts to develop at this grade level. Students are beginning to experience puberty and they are curious about sexuality and drugs and other things that are new to them. Students need to know how AIDS is and isn't transmitted. This information must be clear and straightforward. (You definitely can get AIDS through sexual contact, you definitely can't get AIDS through hugging and dry kissing, and nobody knows for sure if you can get AIDS through wet kissing, although there have been no known cases to date.) This lesson should separate information into what is fact and what is myth.

Once students are clear about the ways AIDS can and can't be transmitted, prevention can be addressed. If they know how to get AIDS, they should be able to understand how to prevent it. The best prevention for AIDS, without question, is abstinence: abstain from IV drug use and abstain from sexual activity until ready for a monogamous relationship. Most people feel that this is the only rational suggestion for prevention at this age level. The difficulty with this as the only method is that not all students at this age level are involved in rational decisions and behaviors. There are students who are either already experimenting with sex and drugs or will be in the near future. Those students cannot be ignored and left prey to a deadly disease because they make uninformed, risky choices. They must be taught to understand what is meant by safer sex. They must be told about condoms, nonoxynol-9, and other methods that help protect them from contact with the AIDS virus. They must understand the increased risk of multiple partners. There can be no secrets about the transmission of AIDS. Withholding information because of moral dilemmas must give way to the right to live.

Students in grades 4-6 will have a natural interest in treatments for those who already have AIDS. They will want to reassure themselves that problems have solutions. The lack of available treatments will be a valuable lesson in itself. They need to know that there are no long range treatments, no cures, and no vaccinations. In the larger picture, they will be learning a hard but important lesson for us all—we cannot always repair the consequences of our behaviors.

At these grade levels, students not only have the ability to discuss and debate issues, they enjoy it and gain more from it than most other activities. Having been given a solid content background about AIDS, students will want to have a forum in which their own views can be presented. This should be facilitated by teachers, allowing students to give their own opinions and express the opinions of others regarding a variety of AIDS-related issues. Such issues might include public policy, civil rights, employment, insurance and health care, antibody testing, and persons with AIDS in schools.

Students also enjoy predicting the future and being asked for their input regarding solutions to problems. Students should be asked to map out their own solutions to critical aspects of the AIDS issue. Some will be made mostly of fantasy; others may be seeds of future discoveries.

By the time students have completed the sixth grade, they should have an accurate and complete understanding of the problems related to AIDS, taking with them to higher grade levels an understanding of how to avoid contact with the AIDS virus, as well as an ability to offer meaningful insight and suggestions based on sound information.

AIDS Education in School Settings: Grades 7-9

Cheri Pies, MSW, MPH

What is especially noteworthy about young people between the ages of 13 and 15 is the broad spectrum of developmental stages they reflect. They are not quite adolescents, yet they are no longer preteens. Their bodies are changing and developing. They are constantly adjusting and readjusting to fit in to the current norms or fads, and, at the same time, they are becoming more defined in their person and place in the world. It is a rich and puzzling time.

All this internal and external commotion has made it challenging to design and select curricula on AIDS for young people in this age group. A number of thoughtful curricula have been written for junior and senior high youth (see references). All review the basic information about AIDS, some offer a special emphasis on STDs, others highlight communicable diseases, and a few have a mixture of both along with activities on decision-making and communications skills. Most outline learning objectives, lesson plans and specific activities. For the most part, these curricula provide a generic plan for AIDS education, thus leaving room for input from parents, teachers, other school personnel and community leaders to insure that the lessons accurately reflect the values of the community.

Despite the availability of already prepared lessons and information, utilization of such materials is spotty. School boards may not be prepared to introduce AIDS education into the curricula. Some parents or community groups may feel middle school youth are too young to hear this information. And, critics of any education addressing issues of sexuality or drugs may contend that talking about them will encourage children to engage in these behaviors. This being the case, it is essential that we have a clear and practical understanding of why we must teach our youngest teens about AIDS, what the learning message should be, and how to present information in dynamic and creative ways.

Why Is It Important?

It may be too late if we wait to tell young people about AIDS and high-risk behaviors until they are 16 or 17 or 18. Youth of today are repeatedly bombarded with messages about sexuality, drugs, AIDS and more by music, magazines, television, movies and their peers. This constant flow of information draws attention to these issues, stimulates curiosity, creates confusion and prompts questions. Young people need a place where they can be assured of getting accurate, nonjudgmental, honest answers to their questions and accompanying concerns. Too often they think they have only their peers to turn to for information. Too often the information they get from peers is incorrect.

Teens need a supportive environment in which to practice their decision-making and communication skills. It is not enough to teach young people to "just say no" or to know when to say when. Young people can't be expected to learn appropriate behaviors on their own when there is a question of life and death. As adults, it is our responsibility to provide them with learning opportunities to practice effective and successful behaviors for living healthy lives.

AIDS is certainly the epidemic of our lifetime. It is a disease that has created fear among many segments of the population. The middle school child may have concerns about causal contagion and inaccurate information about prevention. Some may be engaging in high-risk behaviors, or they may have friends who are. Others may be victims of sexual abuse. Certainly, many early teens are under an enormous amount of pressure to conform and to participate in certain behavioral "tests," any number of which include drug and sexual experimentation. Having the facts about AIDS could save their lives.

Adolescence is a time for developing a sexual identity, a task that begins in these early teen years. Teens are also struggling with their individual identity. Questions like "Who am I?" "What do I like to do?" "Where do I start and my parents end?" are paramount. These questions, like the need to conform, can lead to experimentation, which in turn, can lead to risky behaviors. They need the information and they need to get it early enough so that they have time to think about it, ask questions, and begin practicing how to respond in certain situations.

Young teens don't give the same emotional charge to sex and sexuality that adults do. In fact, this age may be the best for conveying information, instilling values and encouraging critical thinking. It is often at this time that embarrassment and squeamishness about sensitive issues such as sex and sexually transmitted diseases develop. Their energy is high, their confusion rampant. What better time could there be to focus this energy on a frank and thoughtful discussion of sex, sexuality, drugs and AIDS?

AIDS touches the lives of young people in countless ways. One may have a parent or relative with AIDS. Perhaps another knows someone with HIV infection or ARC. Another may know someone who has died from this disease. Whatever their experience with HIV, early adolescents must have access to age appropriate information and know that there are people to whom they can turn for honest answers, responsible advice and thoughtful support.

Once we have determined the logical and rational reasons for teaching young teens about AIDS, we need to clarify what the specific content and messages should be and how the content and messages are different from what they have learned in elementary school.

How Is the Message Different?

Younger children require basic information about disease, health and values, presented within the context of their concrete experience. They must be given the opportunity to learn about basic human biology, sound health practices, communicable disease prevention, decision-making and communication skills. As they get older and their world broadens, the young teen needs repetition of this information, with examples from their current world view. The lessons for students age 13-15 must address the realities of their day-to-day lives.

The extreme ranges of emotional, physical and social development typical of the 13 to 15 year old create confusion and stress. Lessons on self-esteem, important in the elementary years continue to be critical now. Such lessons instill self-awareness, self-confidence and personal pride, while reassuring young teens that the changes they are experiencing are normal.

Facts and information about health issues such as AIDS must be direct and specific. Young teens are only beginning to develop skills in abstract thinking. At the moment they are consumed with the facts. They need to have an understanding of communicable diseases and recognize that AIDS is one of them. The message must be frank and concrete. Young teens need to be told, "If you get AIDS, chances are you will die."

This age group understands the concept of risk, even if they don't believe that it is something they have to worry about. We can give examples of using a seatbelt in an automobile to protect oneself in the event of an accident or not smoking to avoid getting cancer. Many are sophisticated enough to identify those at risk for any number of outcomes, including pregnancy and sexually transmitted diseases. Whether they are engaging in risky behaviors, young teens can comprehend the need for avoiding risk and can undoubtedly identify ways to avoid risk for behaviors in which they and their friends engage. Again, because of the concrete nature of their curiosity, a spectrum of risk education behaviors would be appropriate and useful.

What Should the Messages and Specific Concepts Be?

Five specific concepts should be covered when teaching students in grades 7-9 about AIDS.

Students need a general and basic overview including a clear description of how AIDS is transmitted, how AIDS is not transmitted, why it's important to learn about AIDS now, and ways in which AIDS can touch one's life. Also essential is factual information about how they can protect themselves from the AIDS virus, as well as a discussion of all aspects of this disease, not just transmission and prevention.

Students need guidelines and suggestions for healthful behavior choices with appropriate activities to practice those behaviors. Such activities must address decision-making skills, communication skills, assertiveness training and self-esteem building.

Students need an understanding of risk, risk behaviors, risk reduction and prevention, including a continuum of risk behaviors and risk reduction techniques. Pros and cons of risky behaviors need exploration in conjunction with discussion of family and community values.

Students need descriptive information about the ways AIDS is affecting their community, the United States, and the world. Such information must be up-to-date, identify risk behaviors not risk groups, clarify populations most affected to date, and explore the financial and human costs of AIDS.

Students need to learn where to turn for advice, help and support in the event they have further questions or service needs related to AIDS. Teens need to know how to find resource and referral information in the phone book, or from local community sources. Students need an opportunity to practice locating key resources and having specific questions answered.

The messages about AIDS for this age group simply need to be clear, concise and direct. Listed below are a few key messages.

- Everyone needs to know about AIDS.
- Avoid IV needle sharing and sexual intercourse; this is known as abstinence.
- It is okay to avoid sexual activity until you are ready.
- If you are already engaging in sexual and drug-using be-

haviors, you can stop if you want, you can seek help, you can protect yourself from infection (condom use, other safer sex strategies, limit your sexual partners).

- Know your personal values and learn to recognize when something does not feel right to you.
- Know when to say when.
- Education about AIDS is prohealth and antidisease, not antisex.
- If you are going to have a future to plan and live for, you must know how to stay healthy.
- It is okay to ask any question so that you will have all the information you need.
- You don't have to make decisions alone. If you are puzzled, confused, there are people whom you can turn to for help.

Knowing why and what to teach to early teens about AIDS is not enough. Knowing how to teach this information is pivotal. Perhaps the most essential element in educating middle school youth about AIDS is the deliberate and sensitive preparation of teachers from all disciplines. Teachers must be well-versed in AIDS information so they can develop innovative and nonthreatening lessons to introduce the information into an already existing curriculum. They must have an opportunity to explore their own concerns about sexuality and drugs, practice effective communication techniques, identify successful communication and decision-making skills, and take time to understand the complex nature of the AIDS epidemic.

Information about AIDS is best presented in an integrated curriculum offered over a period of time. This provides students with an opportunity to put AIDS in its proper perspective as well as time to integrate the complexity of issues and feelings. In addition to health education courses, AIDS education units can be logically and practically integrated into courses on math, English, social studies, current affairs and geography. Such units should follow lessons that cover communication skills, decision-making, drug use prevention, and sexuality. Young teens cannot be expected to learn about AIDS without some foundation on which to base the discussions that inevitably follow.

References

AIDS Council of Northeastern New York. 1986. *Teaching about AIDS*. Albany, NY: Author.

Minnesota Department of Education. 1980. *Sexual health and responsibility selos* [some essential learner outcomes] (Curriculum Bulletin #60). St. Paul, MN: Author.

Minnesota Department of Health. 1986. *Sexually transmitted diseases, a junior and senior high school health education curriculum*. St. Paul, MN: Author.

New York City Board of Education. 1986. *Family Life including sex education, supplementary materials related to AIDS*. NY: Author.

Ohio State Department of Health. 1986. *AIDS virus information package*. Columbus, OH: Author.

Pies, C. and Stoller, L. 1987. *Teacher's curriculum guide on AIDS*. San Francisco, CA: San Francisco Department of Public Health and San Francisco Unified School District.

Quackenbush, M. and Sargent, P. 1988. *Teaching AIDS: A resource guide on acquired immune deficiency syndrome*. Rev. ed. Santa Cruz, CA: Network Publications.

Sroka, S. 1986. *Educator's guide to sexually transmitted diseases*, 2nd ed. Santa Cruz, CA: Network Publications.

Yarber, W. 1985. *STD: A guide for today's young adults*. Waldorf, MD: American Alliance Publications.

Yarber, W. 1987. *AIDS: What young adults should know*. Waldorf, MD: American Alliance Publications.

AIDS Education in School Settings: Grades 10-12

Marcia Quackenbush, MS

I n school settings today, we can provide AIDS education more easily to high school students than to any other age group. There are several reasons for this. First, the need for such education is widely accepted and AIDS education can easily be integrated into existing health and family life education courses. Second, high school students are developmentally mature enough to understand AIDS and related issues—drug use, death, sexuality—more easily than their younger counterparts. Third, materials are now readily available to help instructors and administrators in their efforts. Fourth, since many schools are following this course, there is a professional community of support that can share materials, policies, experiences and problem-solving ideas.

Rationales

Other reports have reviewed the need for teen AIDS education in some detail (DiClemente, Zorn and Temoshok, 1987; Haffner, 1987; Quackenbush, 1987). We know that teen sexual activity is quite high—about half of U.S. high school students are sexually active, and by age 17, 57 percent of teens have had sexual intercourse (Louis Harris Associates, 1986). Unprotected or unsafe sexual encounters are certainly common in this group. There are 1.2 million teen pregnancies in the U.S. annually (The Alan Guttmacher Institute, 1981), and reported rates of sexually transmitted diseases among teens continue to be alarming (Bell and Holmes, 1984; O'Reilly and Aral, 1985; Shafer, 1987). Drug use generally among teens is significant, and conservative estimates suggest over 1 percent of high school students have used heroin (Bachman, Johnston and O'Malley, 1987), and many more have used other drugs intravenously.

Even more disturbing are recent reports showing the presence of HIV infection among a significant percentage of the teen population in high incidence areas. In New York City, 1 in 50 young military recruits is testing positive for HIV antibody, and in the Washington, DC metropolitan area this figure is 1 in 100 (Centers for Disease Control, 1987). If this trend continues, the potential for the spread of HIV among teenagers is enormous and frightening.

In addition to these known risk factors, we find that teens are quite interested in learning about AIDS in classroom settings (DiClemente, Zorn and Temoshok, 1987; Strunin and Hingson, 1987).

Materials

A number of school districts and states have developed curricula and resource guides for classroom education, and these are usually available on request (see, for example, Alameda County AIDS Curriculum Task Force, 1987; Erickson et al., 1986; Webster, 1987). In addition, three independently produced curricula for high school students are currently available (Quackenbush and Sargent, 1988; Sroka, 1987; Yarber, 1987). Each of these curricula takes a different approach in teaching method, using factually sound materials as a basis. These resources together provide a wide range of lesson plans and materials, and by integrating selected portions of these and other resources, educators can tailor a program specifically for a particular community.

It is important to remember that it was not until well into 1986 that any of these materials was readily available. AIDS education is still a relatively new endeavor, and schools with sound programs in place are to be congratulated on their aggressive response to the issue.

Concepts

The concepts we want to teach high school students about AIDS do not differ from those we would teach a general adult audience. There are four important points to communicate:
- AIDS/HIV infection is caused by a virus, not a lifestyle. It is not a "gay" disease.
- AIDS/HIV is not casually transmitted. You will not contract HIV infection in the normal course of your daily contact with friends and acquaintances.
- Under the proper circumstances, anyone can contract

AIDS/HIV infection. Most typically, HIV is transmitted through sexual intercourse (vaginal, oral or anal), the sharing of needles in IV drug use, or from an infected woman to her fetus or newborn.

- You can protect yourself from AIDS or HIV infection. First, do not use drugs, and do not share needles for drug use, tattooing, ear piercing or any other reason. Second, abstain from sexual intercourse; or have intercourse with only one lifetime partner who does not use IV drugs and has had sex with no one but you; or, if you do choose to be sexually active, use safer sex techniques, including condoms, to avoid infection.

Students will need to understand that AIDS has a long incubation period and that most people presently infected have no signs or symptoms of illness. They should also understand the meaning of "safer sex" and the how-to's of condom use. If this material is too controversial for a classroom setting, educators should offer contact numbers for information hotlines, public health clinics, or other resources where students can learn more.

Messages

Information alone is not enough to persuade teenagers to act to protect themselves from HIV infection. In a 1986 Massachusetts survey of over 800 teenagers, 92 percent knew that HIV could be passed through sexual intercourse, but only 15 percent of those who were sexually active had changed some aspect of their behavior to protect themselves; and of that group, only 20 percent had taken effective measures (Strunin and Hingson, 1987).

At this point, the question we need to be asking is not,

"What do teens need to know about AIDS?" This is already well-enough established. Rather, we should be asking, "How can we get teens to act to protect themselves?" Support for formal evaluation projects has been slow in coming, so our present knowledge about how to effectively impact teens about AIDS prevention is based on generalizations from other areas of study, and the intuitive impressions and anecdotal experiences of educators. We review some suggestions below:

- *Students need to be convinced that AIDS is a real and serious personal threat.* In an early San Francisco study of gay men, those who personally knew someone diagnosed with AIDS were more likely to take measures to protect themselves (Research and Decisions Corporation, 1984). In school settings, providing students an opportunity to meet with someone who has AIDS may encourage them to see the disease as something real, serious and personal. A San Francisco project called "The Wedge" is currently under way in which trained teams consisting of a health educator, a medical professional, and a person with AIDS go to classrooms and answer students' questions (Cox, 1987).
- *Future plans for childbearing are important for many students, especially—but not only—young women.* An HIV-infected individual cannot biologically parent a child without grave danger to the child's health. For many teens, this is a persuasive argument for prevention.
- *Students respond better to lessons about their rights than their responsibilities.* To exercise one's rights, certain responsibilities must be met. If one wishes to guarantee one's right to have correct information, for example, there is a responsibility to ask questions about things that are not clear. A teenager has a right to become a parent only when he or she is ready to do so, and corresponding

with this is a responsibility to say no to sex if he/she is not ready. (For further development of these ideas and other rights and responsibilities, see Haffner, 1987, and Chapter 6).

- *Students who have something to look forward to are able to take more effective measures to prevent health complications.* In a 1986 Harris Poll for Planned Parenthood Federation, the students who were most likely to avoid pregnancy were those who felt they had a lot to lose by becoming pregnant. They were involved in school activities or athletics, or were preparing for college. The students who became pregnant were more likely to have poor grades or family problems and be economically disadvantaged (Louis Harris and Associates, 1986). Self-esteem and the ability to hope and plan for the future are precious commodities in youth. We should nurture and encourage them at every possible opportunity.

- *One of the developmental tasks of adolescence is to join and belong to a peer group.* We cannot expect teens to go against the inclinations of their peers ("just say no") without explicit and repeated exercises to help them develop skills in this regard. Classroom role plays and discussions of vignettes that present situations in which a young person is encouraged to try out a drug, to have unprotected sex, to drive a car after drinking, and so forth, can help students practice the assertiveness skills they will need when faced with real life risk situations.

- *We need to work to develop a peer ethic in the youth community that discourages risk activity and rewards healthy decisions.* Similar strategies have worked in antismoking (Telch et al., 1982; Perry, Killen and Slinkard, 1980) and antidrinking (McKnight and McPherson, 1986; Mann et al., 1986) campaigns. Perceived group leaders and important media personalities can offer teens persuasive positive messages. When the peer community honestly believes that drugs, teen sex and unsafe sex are not cool, we will see a remarkable drop in teen pregnancy, sexually transmitted diseases and the possibilities of HIV transmission.

These and other messages that will help the high school student choose health behaviors thoughtfully and well are not going to be delivered through AIDS education alone. Integrated programs in values clarification, decision making and assertiveness, along with efforts to promote teen self-esteem, will all contribute to a milieu in which information about AIDS can be applied skillfully throughout the student's teen and adult life.

References

Alameda County AIDS Curriculum Task Force. 1987. Alameda County AIDS information packet for 7th-12th grade students. Alameda County Office of Education.

The Alan Guttmacher Institute. 1981. *Teenage pregnancy: The problem that hasn't gone away.* New York: Author.

Bachman, J., Johnston, L. and O'Malley, P. 1987. *Monitoring the future: Questionnaire responses from the nation's high school seniors 1986.* Ann Arbor, MI: Institute for Social Research.

Bell, T. and Holmes, K. 1984. Age-specific risks of syphilis, gonorrhea, and hospitalized pelvic inflammatory disease in sexually experienced U.S. women. *Sex Trans Diseases* 11:291-295.

Centers for Disease Control. 1987. *Morbidity and Mortality Weekly Report* 36:18.

Cox, K. 1987. Personal communication.

DiClemente, R., Zorn, J. and Temoshok, L. 1986. Adolescents and AIDS: A survey of knowledge, attitudes and beliefs about AIDS in San Francisco. *American Journal of Public Health* 76:1443-1445.

Erickson, M. et al. 1986. *Preventing AIDS through education: Instructional resources for schools.* White Bear Lake, MN: Minnesota Department of Education.

Haffner, D. 1987. *AIDS and adolescents: The time for prevention is now.* Washington, DC: Center for Population Options.

Louis Harris and Associates. 1986. *American teens speak: Sex, myths, TV, and birth control.* New York: Planned Parenthood Federation of America.

McKnight, A.J. and McPherson, K. 1986. Evaluation of peer intervention training for high school alcohol safety education. *Accident Analysis and Prevention* 18:339-347.

Mann, R. et al. 1986. School-based programs for the prevention of drinking and driving: issues and results. *Accident Analysis and Prevention* 18:325-337.

O'Reilly, K. and Aral, S. 1985. Adolescence and sexual behavior: Trends and implications for sexually transmitted disease. *Journal of Adolescent Health Care* 6:262-272.

Perry, C., Kellen, J. and Slinkard, L. 1980. Peer teaching and smoking prevention among junior high students. *Adolescence* 15:277-281.

Quackenbush, M. 1987. Educating youth about AIDS. *Focus: A Review of AIDS Research* 2:3.

Quackenbush, M. and Sargent, P. 1988. *Teaching AIDS: A resource guide on acquired immune deficiency syndrome.* Santa Cruz, CA: Network Publications.

Research and Decisions Corporation. 1984. *A report on designing an effective AIDS prevention campaign strategy for San Francisco: Results from the first probability sample of an urban gay male community.* San Francisco: Author.

Shafer, M. 1986, June 16. Testimony before the Select Committee on Children, Youth and Families. Washington, DC: US House of Representatives.

Sroka, S. 1987. *Educator's guide to AIDS and other STDs.* Santa Cruz, CA: Network Publications.

Strunin, L. and Hingson, R. 1987. Acquired immunodeficiency syndrome and adolescents' knowledge, beliefs, attitudes and behaviors. *Pediatrics* 79:825-828.

Telch, M. et al. 1982. Long-term follow-up of a pilot project on smoking prevention with adolescents. *Journal of Behavioral Medicine* 5:1-8.

Webster, C. 1987. Teacher's guide—AIDS the preventable epidemic. Portland: Oregon State Health Division.

Yarber, W. 1987. *AIDS: What young adults should know.* Reston, VA: American Alliance for Health, Physical Education, Recreation and Dance.

The Religious Setting:

A Natural Place
for Learning

The Religious Setting: A Natural Place for Learning

Cathie Lyons

W hat role should churches and synagogues play in AIDS prevention education? How much influence should religious beliefs have on the content of AIDS education materials? By providing information about safer sex practices and condom use won't AIDS education programs promote behaviors which violate religious teachings? Human sexual conduct and illicit drug use have been overwhelmingly implicated in the transmission of AIDS. Doesn't that make AIDS primarily a moral issue rather than a medical issue? Isn't it really sinful behavior that causes AIDS, and isn't AIDS a sign of God's anger?

These questions, and the answers being given to them, are having an impact on AIDS prevention education in this country. From the United States Congress, to local school boards, to Hometown USA the scope and content of public health education about AIDS, and governmental funding for it, have been affected profoundly by the deep seated faith stances of religious leaders, lawmakers, educators, parents, and health workers.

One might expect a unified, clear voice of agreement from church and synagogue about the content and purpose of this nation's AIDS prevention education thrust. To be sure, for many persons of faith, AIDS does raise profound moral concerns about human behavior, sexuality and sinfulness. In addition, prohibitions against homosexuality, sexuality outside of marriage and substance abuse are found in Jewish, Catholic and Protestant teachings alike. And yet, the opinions being expressed by congregants and religious leaders about AIDS prevention education and the role of religious institutions as AIDS prevention educators are as diverse as the thinking and theological positions of those who have engaged themselves in the debate.

AIDS has not brought about unanimity of religious opinion. Rather, the urgent need to prevent the further spread of AIDS has fostered a spectrum of responses. At one extreme are the views of those who believe that the only effective way to stop the spread of AIDS is for persons to adhere to established religious teachings about human sexuality and abstinence from illicit drug use. At the other extreme are those religious leaders who believe that religious teachings and prohibitions about human sexuality and substance abuse are of utmost importance, but should be supplemented with explicit information and education about other potentially effective methods for reducing the risks of transmitting or contracting the human immunodeficiency virus, should a person choose not to abide by religious teachings.

When a few United States Catholic Bishops took a stance acknowledging that, at times, there is good reason to include accurate information about condom use in AIDS prevention education, they took a noticeable and controversial step which some of their colleagues felt went too far toward condoning condom use.

Other religious leaders have gone even further calling upon the religious, educational and public health sectors to cooperate fully to make scientifically sound and appropriate information available to every family and individual in this country. This latter strategy affirms how important it is for religious institutions to work cooperatively with health professionals and other educators to help persons understand the different things they can do to protect themselves from contracting or spreading the virus that causes AIDS.

In what follows, Jewish, Catholic and Protestant writers address AIDS prevention education from their own personal points of view within their faith traditions. Each is intimately concerned about AIDS, its prevention, and how their communities of faith can play a powerful and constructive role in stopping the spread of AIDS.

This nation is now several years into an AIDS epidemic, faced with a disease for which there is presently no medical means of prevention, cure or effective long-term treatment. One million to one and a half million persons are thought to be infected with the human immunodeficiency virus, which they can pass on to their sexual and intravenous drug use partners, and which mothers can transmit to their babies during pregnancy or childbirth. Though persons of all ages need to be informed fully about AIDS, there is a critical and urgent need for AIDS prevention education to reach the youth of this nation. Sexually active adolescents who are confronted daily with the availability of drugs and who experience peer pressure to engage in sex and use drugs make up a very special group of persons whose behaviors make them vulnerable and at risk for contracting or spreading the virus.

How have the churches and synagogues responded and

what might they do in the future? In many regards, religious communities have reacted slowly and hesitatingly to this nation's number one public health crisis. Some religious figures proclaimed initially that AIDS was a sign of God's wrath and a form of punishment inflicted upon homosexual persons. Though such statements continue to be expressed, persons of faith and religious groups are also responding with more compassionate words and deeds. Religious pronouncements are calling for the protection of the rights of persons with AIDS, and congregations and institutions are working together to develop direct service ministries with persons with AIDS. But the greatest challenge of AIDS has yet to be dealt with adequately by either church or state. AIDS can be prevented, and all sectors of society can work together to provide AIDS prevention information and education.

AIDS affects every sector of society and every sector is challenged to do its part to extend the reach and effectiveness of prevention education. Ecumenical and interfaith groups, churches and synagogues have unique roles to play and can bring much needed information to millions of people in congregations and communities large and small across the nation.

AIDS prevention education, in essence, is about life. It is about affirming one's own life and the lives of others. It is about protecting oneself from contracting or spreading the virus that causes AIDS. Churches and synagogues, working cooperatively with public health workers, educators and schools, have an important and powerful role to play in AIDS prevention education, and in affirming that the worth of a human life and the desire to protect it from unnecessary harm or danger are values central to religious teachings and to disease prevention.

16

AIDS Education in Religious Settings – A Catholic Response –

Catherine Pickerel

That education about AIDS is of the highest priority today cannot be denied. The simple facts that (1) AIDS kills and (2) we possess information that can prevent more deaths force admitting this truth. While having no difficulty acknowledging the reality of the AIDS crisis, many Catholic educators have faced hard questions about how to educate about AIDS. We learned that AIDS is transmitted through the exchange of body fluids in nonmonogamous sexual activity and by sharing contaminated needles in drug use. Both methods of transmission have been clearly identified in Catholic theology as being immoral. For a long time, the epidemic seemed to be confined primarily to the gay community in this country, a community living what the Catholic Church considers to be an immoral lifestyle. Eventually we learned that the proper use of condoms during sex and sterilized needles during drug use would help to prevent transmission of the AIDS virus. Again, the information received was about activities considered to be immoral.

There have been other morally disturbing facts to be considered, however. Under the guise of Christian righteousness, we heard that AIDS was a just punishment from God upon the "immoral" gay community. We also heard statements from our students that echoed that same sentiment. Cases of violence against gays increased, and we knew that to be a part of the fear and prejudice that was growing with the epidemic.

What were we to do? Were we to limit our educational efforts to programs about abstinence and the sanctity of sex in sacramental marriage? This is what Secretary of Education William Bennett would have all educators in the private and public sectors do. Catholic education certainly took this approach when I was in school. And Catholic teens were sexually active, got pregnant and contracted sexually transmitted diseases. Today, Catholic teens are sexually active, get pregnant, have abortions, contract STDs and do intravenous drugs. Are we then, in good conscience, to share information with Catholic teens that seems to endorse immoral practices—using condoms during nonmarital sex and sterilized needles during illicit drug use—in an effort to save them from the AIDS virus?

A key element in any discussion about morality is the notion that morality involves free choice, and that we do not always choose the highest, best, most loving, most Christian course of action. That being so, we must acknowledge the fact that not everyone will choose the value of sex within sacramental marriage only. But a choice of some other value for sexual activity should include knowledge of the possible consequences of that choice. Specifically, someone who chooses to have sex involving the exchange of body fluids without the use of a condom, and without an intimate and extensive knowledge of the sexual and drug history of the partner, must include as a possible consequence the transmission of the AIDS virus. We

212

cannot make moral decisions for our students. We cannot make any decisions for them. But it is our obligation as educators to give them as much information as possible to use when they do make their own decisions, or at least let them know how to obtain information. We can also encourage them to use a decision-making process that seeks to understand available alternatives, the consequences of those alternatives, how to discern the values underlying each alternative, and the Christian (for us, Catholic) values, ideals and teachings regarding those alternatives.

With regards to AIDS, I, as a Catholic educator, do want my students to know and understand the Church's value and teaching regarding sex within sacramental marriage only. I want them to know that the Surgeon General recommends abstinence outside of marriage as the only sure way to prevent the sexual transmission of AIDS. I also want them to know what consequences they might face if they choose some other value that would allow for and even encourage premarital or extramarital sexual activity.

I recall my own adolescence as a time of disagreeing—with my parents, with the Church, with the school administration, with adult patterns of behavior, with all kinds of things. Luckily, my parents, my Church, my school, my God, and seemingly the adult society that surrounded me all forgave me throughout that process. Never was I given a death sentence for any disagreement. Today an adolescent who disagrees with the Church's moral teachings about sex and drugs should not be handed a death sentence because we decide to withhold information about condoms and sterilized needles as means to prevent the transmission of the AIDS virus. We should also consider that an adolescent might engage in sex even though she or he does in fact believe in the value of sex within sacramental marriage. We all do sin from time to time, after all, even after emerging from the confusion of adolescence.

The recent statement of the Administrative Board of the National Conference of Catholic Bishops, "The Many Faces of AIDS: A Gospel Response," recognizes that some members of our pluralistic society will not agree with the Catholic understanding of human sexuality and will act accordingly. The bishops state, then, that educational programs rooted in a moral vision consistent with their own could provide accurate information about condoms and other practices recommended by medical experts as a means of preventing AIDS (i.e. sterilizing needles used in drug sharing). Certainly the same approach can be considered for the microcosm of our society found in Catholic high schools. While taking the responsibility to educate as creatively as possible for the values of sex within sacramental marriage, of abstinence and chastity, of living a drug-free lifestyle, we must also take responsibility for recognizing that our students may opt for other contradictory values. Within the context of our value-laden curriculum, we must also include information regarding the other choices that they might make or are already making.

The school community I serve took on the issue of AIDS education. I offer our experience as one model for other Catholic high schools. Let me begin with something we did not do, but perhaps should have done—staff education. If a school has not yet begun student education about AIDS, it is important to educate its administration and staff first. This will help accomplish three objectives. First, such education can help staff members deal with their own, perhaps misinformed fears and/or prejudices about AIDS and people with AIDS. It may also offer healing moments for staff who are dealing with the terrible reality of having a friend or family member with AIDS. Second, administrators and staff members will be united in an approach to AIDS and prevention education. Third, all staff members will be equipped with accurate information to answer questions about AIDS and people who have AIDS. We know that students do not limit asking such questions to the science or theology classroom. If a student feels close to a coach, a sewing teacher or the attendance secretary, that is the person who will receive the questions about AIDS.

The second step must, of course, be student education. At my high school we decided to have a school assembly on AIDS. AIDS education up to that point seemed to be at the discretion of individual teachers or department chairs, which is not a good way to assure that graduating students will have even a minimal level of information about the disease. The assembly, then, was a step in the right direction. We invited a panel to speak, each addressing a specific aspect of the disease. A representative of a local AIDS foundation spoke on the history of the disease and gave some basics on the virus. A member of a university-sponsored AIDS health project spoke about how AIDS is transmitted and how transmission can be prevented. A nurse from a local hospital helped us to focus on the personal and interpersonal aspects of AIDS with stories of her own patients and what she had learned from them. Finally, a man named Christian Haren spoke to us of his own experience as someone with AIDS. Each student and staff member also received an educational pamphlet that had been recommended for a high school audience.

If you should consider a similar type of assembly for your class or school, you might have some hesitation about inviting a person with AIDS to speak, based perhaps on fears of how your students might receive such a person. I know that the experience of just one school cannot be considered a standard for such things, but I offer you ours, primarily because meeting Christian Haren proved to be a turning point for our school.

Learning about AIDS is vital to stemming the tide of the

medical epidemic. But there is another tide to be stemmed, one that religious schools must attend to. AIDS education can help to stem the tide of prejudice and fear against people with AIDS and people who are homosexual. As the bishops emphasize in their statement, no matter what moral stance we take against homosexual or any other premarital sexual activity, we cannot condone any form of prejudice that can lead to violence or the abrogation of human rights for any segment of society. Furthermore, we must do whatever we can to eliminate such prejudice. Education can be a wonderful way to disarm prejudice and fear. Our AIDS assembly and meeting Christian Haren proved to be just such an educational moment at our school. Here was a man who would not let his audience deny that AIDS involves people. He told us that AIDS does happen, that it could happen to us. At the same time, he taught us about people with AIDS, about their needs, about the humanity that we share with them. Quite frankly, we came to love this man. We now have a personal interest in AIDS, and a personal interest in persons with AIDS.

We knew that we could not be satisfied to let our educational efforts end there. One assembly, meeting one man, did not satisfy the need. Follow-up is being done. For my purposes here, I will skip over a few of the more obvious possibilities for additional education—the science and health classrooms, the social studies courses that deal with current affairs—and focus on my department. I am a theology teacher, teaching a course on morality to sophomores, and an elective on death and dying to seniors.

The morality course addresses the evil of prejudice, with the text (*Understanding Christian Morality* by Ronald Wilkins. Dubuque, IA: W.C. Brown, 1982) highlighting racial prejudice that leads to violence. This provides an easy jumping-off point for a discussion about prejudice against homosexuals, and

216

about the fears, myths, misconceptions students might have about homosexuality and homosexual people. It also provides a good opportunity to clarify the Church's teaching against homosexual (and indeed all premarital sexual) activity as distinct from the misconception that the Church condemns homosexual persons in and of themselves. Most important, it provides a time to dispel the notion that AIDS is an exclusively gay disease, and to clarify the distinction between deciding the morality of an action and our call to respect the basic human dignity of all persons (underscored by Jesus' command to stay out of the business of judging others). All of this also allows me to restate or to clarify information about the transmission of AIDS and ways to prevent transmission.

Teaching about AIDS fits naturally into the course on death and dying. It did not take the death of a celebrity for our students to recognize the fact that AIDS kills. The general fear of AIDS often inspires students to talk about the disease in the death and dying classroom. Discussion about AIDS in this context can also inspire great compassion for persons with AIDS, especially when coupled with guest speakers who have AIDS or who serve people with AIDS.

Other theology courses offered at our school provide additional moments for education about AIDS. A course on Christian sexuality on the freshman level presents an obvious setting for such education. Even a junior level course on the sacraments offers such a possibility when it treats the Anointing of the Sick. When all of this is linked with science, health and social studies classes, and the occasional extracurricular conversations with students about movies or articles dealing with AIDS, we have the opportunity to assure that our students are well-informed and, we hope, compassionate in their response to AIDS.

Catholic and other religious schools can take a strong leadership role in our country's response to AIDS and in ongoing programs of education about AIDS. Christian Haren came to our school in 1986. The public schools in our area are only now (1988) at the point of allowing people with AIDS onto campuses to speak about the disease, to help break down the some of the prejudice our students have learned to have against them. We can talk readily and enthusiastically to our students about a gospel response to people with AIDS, and about gospel teachings against prejudice. We can certainly teach about the sanctity of sex within a sacramental marriage. And we can present information about condoms and sterilized needles in the most value-laden context possible. The bishops' statement about AIDS has already stirred up controversy in our Church, but it makes a point that cannot be ignored or disputed. We are called upon to make an effective and compassionate response to the AIDS epidemic in our society and world.

17

Educating for Life: AIDS and Teens in the Jewish Community

Andrew Rose, LCSW

Among the many laws and moral imperatives that have governed Jewish life for centuries there are a few that clearly stand out as guiding principles. Paramount among these is *Pikuach Nefesh*, "saving and sustaining life." Saving a life takes precedence over all other considerations, even if it means violating other honored commandments.

Pikuach Nefesh is the basis for AIDS prevention education in the Jewish community. We recognize that saving lives is what is at stake and takes precedence over other considerations, such as possible embarrassment when talking publicly about sexual behavior. AIDS prevention education has saved countless lives already and will continue to play an essential role for the foreseeable future. It gives us an opportunity to affirm life at this crucial time.

Clearly, it hasn't been that simple in religious settings or anywhere else. Questions about morality have continually been framed in ways that confused rather than clarified our values and responsibilities. That is an historical tragedy, but one that is not too late to transform.

I see religious settings as especially good places for AIDS education. In our congregations, youth groups and religious community organizations, we have the unique opportunity to frame our moral concerns in a way which deepens our compassion, our commitment and our overall understanding of how our ethics and core values do and should impact the AIDS crisis. That is the particular challenge of AIDS education in religious communities.

AIDS education is about much more than prevention. While baseline medical and epidemiological information will always be necessary, our efforts must also encompass the human reality of AIDS, our responsibility to transcend narrow self-interest ("All I want to know is how to keep that virus away from me!") in the midst of any social crisis, and our mandate to act. AIDS education also needs to enable and empower us to make difficult personal decisions about our own behavior, now and in the future.

This may sound like an overloaded, unrealistic agenda at a time when basic facts must be transmitted. I believe, however, that it is both possible and necessary, and will share some of our specific experience later in this chapter. First, I will discuss some of the specifically Jewish historical experiences and values, in addition to *Pikuach Nefesh*, which we draw on when developing AIDS education programs.

Drawing from Jewish Values and History

Jews have an historic commitment to education. We know the immeasurable value of knowledge, and we know the bitter danger of ignorance. We have too often seen that ignorance is destructive and can take on a life of its own.

Jews have been scapegoated during epidemics, as well as other times, becoming a convenient and vulnerable target for the fears of the majority. We have often suffered the consequences of people's inability to find an explanation, reaching instead for someone to blame. And we know that this process of blaming and scapegoating has been a tragedy not only for us, but ultimately for everyone.

So it is with AIDS. AIDS is frightening. It can be confusing, especially when misinformation abounds. AIDS makes people feel uncomfortable and angry, evoking the feeling that if only blame can be fixed and certain people isolated, the problem will be solved.

That is a framework of fear, not morality. It appears not only as overt discrimination, but also as more subtle "them -vs.-us" assumptions—that AIDS is out there somewhere but could not possibly be touching the "good people." Every human being can be sensitive to the dangers of separating out the "other" and viewing them as contaminated. As Jews, we are particularly sensitive. AIDS education, which reminds us of our own history, reinforces that sensitivity and clarifies where we need to stand.

As mentioned earlier, Jewish life has been sustained by many guiding principles. Some are called *mitzvot*, meaning "commandments" or "righteous deeds." Among the most well-known and respected *mitzvot* is *Bikkur Cholim*, literally meaning "visiting the sick." But the full meaning encompasses a much broader scope that no one who is sick or disabled should be isolated from the community.

AIDS education has offered an opportunity to enhance our whole community's understanding of this fuller meaning. For example, *Bikkur Cholim* impels us to advocate for sufficient home and hospice care resources, giving people support and comfort rather than isolation at home or unnecessary hospitalization. *Bikkur Cholim* also moves us to protest the discrimination that isolates people with AIDS and their families. The point is, AIDS education is not a moral problem. It is an opportunity to deepen our sense of morality, and to transmit that to our young people.

Recent Trends and Special Considerations

1987 saw a burst of activity in the Jewish community's level of involvement in AIDS education. AIDS education outreach programs have emerged in San Francisco, Los Angeles, Miami and Chicago. Both the B'nai Brith Youth Organization and the National Federation of Temple Youth have focused programming efforts on AIDS, reaching widely throughout the United States and Canada. And individual congregations and teachers in many cities have begun to see to it that their young people are given accurate information about the disease, its prevention and appropriate Jewish responses to it.

In our work in San Francisco, we have learned to be flexible in the face of teens' changing level of knowledge. The general education videos that were effective a year ago tend to have a lesser impact now. There is a growing familiarity with basic medical and epidemiological information, but it is usually sprinkled with misconceptions and areas of lingering confusion. The opportunity to ask questions is still essential.

Acknowledging the level of sexual activity among teenagers is an issue in many arenas, but it is a particularly sensitive one in religious settings. We have found it very important to communicate that no one at any age, at any time, should feel pressured to be sexually active if he or she does not feel ready.

We do not assume that the teens we speak with are currently sexually active. But they *will* need this information at some point, and are likely to know others who do.

At the same time, we see this as an especially frightening time to come of age sexually, and our objective is not to make young people phobic about sexuality. It is more important than ever to affirm sexuality as a positive part of human experience, and to link it with respect for oneself and genuine caring for others. And while we discuss specific behaviors in terms of transmission, risk and prevention, we put forward a view of sexuality as much more than a list of things you can or can't do. Sexuality is intertwined with intimacy, affection, commitment and pleasure, and needs to be considered in its fullness.

Part of acknowledging the whole spectrum of sexual expression is the assumption that in any group of young people, some will grow to be lesbians and gay men. Thus, we steer clear of the erroneous belief that teens will only be heterosexually active. We also discuss that even though AIDS is clearly not a gay disease, people's feelings and attitudes about homosexuality have a lot to do with the ways they have responded to it. Misinformation, fear and discomfort about homosexuality become especially dangerous when they create barriers to becoming informed about AIDS.

This is a frightening coming-of-age time not only for young people, but also for their parents. Yet another advantage of religious settings is that AIDS education programs can include parents, providing information, answering questions, discussing concerns, and giving families the opportunity to support each other. We have made presentations to parents and teens together, then divided them into separate groups for questions and discussion. Other formats have kept parents and teens in one group, encouraging them to write their questions down rather than feel constrained by having to ask them out loud.

Some sessions have separated into small groups of parents together with other people's children. Whatever the format, I
have repeatedly heard parents express their gratitude for their
children getting AIDS information, even while wishing it were
not necessary, or while shaking their heads that these topics
have become part of public discourse. Again, the imperative to
preserve life takes precedence over people's comfort. And over
time, it gets less uncomfortable.

Bringing Our Agenda to Life

In addition to reinforcing basic AIDS information, providing a context for questions, and offering an affirmative framework for sexuality, our AIDS education agenda (mentioned
earlier in this chapter) endeavors to:
- bring home the human reality of AIDS
- assist youth in making thoughtful personal decisions
  about their behavior
- enhance young people's sense of social responsibility.

Our strategies for these three objectives, respectively, have
involved hearing directly from Jewish people with AIDS and
their families, acting out role plays, and brainstorming about
possible action strategies. All are based on understanding Jewish values mentioned previously along with *Tikkun Olam*, the
mandate to bring justice and healing to the world.

It has been tremendously moving to see the effects of
people with AIDS talking with young people about the personal reality of being diagnosed. They discuss telling one's
family, living with hope and uncertainty, coming to terms with
mortality, and so many other aspects of living with AIDS. I
have seen it have a deep and positive impact on a group's level
of understanding and compassion—AIDS is no longer a bar-

rage of statistics or "somewhere out there." It is present with a living, breathing, likable human being. And in addition to raising the level of compassion, it also has a sobering effect. AIDS is suddenly not so remote or impossible to get, and the sense of invincibility so many youth carry, and which so often stymies AIDS educators, gets shaken up a bit.

Role plays are especially effective in dealing with issues of personal decision making. As in other settings, our role plays have participants talking with a reluctant sexual partner about using a condom, talking with a friend at school he or she knows is engaging in unsafe sexual or drug-taking behavior, or dealing with a teacher being diagnosed with AIDS. The advantage is that in religious settings, we are not constrained by prohibitions on discussing values. This lends itself to deep and helpful discussions of the role plays, sometimes difficult to achieve in public educational settings.

Drawing from Jewish values and historical experiences in order to act responsibly in the present requires a review and discussion of precepts already mentioned here, leading to plans of action. Additionally, we are developing a program which shows AIDS-related discrimination in comparison with anti-Semitism, linking our need to remember those who have suffered before with our mandate to learn from their experience and honor their memory.

Finally, we have developed suggestions for education, protection and action using the framework of the famous three-part quote from Rabbi Hillel:

- "If I am not for myself, who will be for me?" highlights the importance of learning the facts about AIDS and taking measures to protect oneself.
- "If I am only for myself, what am I?" points toward educating others, volunteering for AIDS organizations, organizing food drives, raising funds, writing letters to

public officials, or participating in interfaith programs. It might also mean finding ways to be supportive of young people whose parents, brothers, sisters, or friends are diagnosed with AIDS or ARC, or who are diagnosed themselves.

- "If not now, when?" speaks for itself.

There is no reason, and no time, to wait.

18

– AIDS –
Contemporary Challenge to the Protestant Churches

Claudia L. Webster

Lyle L. Loder died of AIDS at the age of 36. He had begun his professional career as a United States two-year home missionary serving from 1973 to 1975. Throughout his life, he contributed immensely to the church community. But perhaps his best, most cherished role was as a member of the planning committee for the United Methodist National Consultation on AIDS Ministries held in San Francisco in November 1987. It was then that I first met Lyle. I was moved by his enthusiasm for the Consultation, and by his dedication. Most of the day he would rest in order to conserve his energy for the panel discussions and presentations in which he was to take part. I sat on his bed, and in the short time we had together, we became friends. With Lyle, that was easy to do. He was loving and friendly; in a very real sense, he personified the Protestant tradition of deep concern for others.

Two and one half weeks after the National Consultation on

AIDS, Lyle Loder died.

He was but one of many dynamic church people who have succumbed to AIDS. This terrible disease has claimed ministers, church workers, lay leaders, a bishop, and many, many church and family members. It will claim more. The impact of the losses has rippled out to touch thousands of others, and to present Protestants with a challenge that has never been equaled. We must face realistically the ways this epidemic affects youth in the church as well.

Historically, Protestants have been known for their programs of social concern, responding with Christian love to sufferers of such diseases as leprosy, tuberculosis and mental illness. The church has been in the forefront of the fight for human understanding and help for those in need. Now, the arrival of AIDS will require the churches to put into practice all the social love and concern at their disposal.

The dilemmas presented by AIDS permeate every belief system. Churches find themselves dealing with questions which they've never had to confront before. Denominations are being forced to consider complex issues of human sexuality and, especially, homosexuality. Other issues include those concerning notions of intimacy, outreach to alcoholics and people addicted to other substances, the changing social world as it relates to the church, and even the sexual expressions of clergy and church employees. No church congregation will remain untouched as the AIDS epidemic continues its spread. The time to prepare a rational Christian response is now.

In keeping with the Protestant heritage, that response should be based on unquestioning love for others. That means programs based in love for all those infected with the human immunodeficiency virus (HIV), those diagnosed with AIDS related complex (ARC), and those with AIDS itself. People need to be kept within the life of the church community, whatever their illness. Furthermore, it is in trying times that the families of patients most need the support and counseling of their spiritual leaders. This is the church's special and historic role. Such programs and such an attitude will surely test the commitment of every denomination, but that is what gives a church strength.

Practical steps for preparing churches to face the AIDS issue, with specific focus on youth concerns, follow.

Written Policies for Dealing with AIDS, ARC, HIV

Each church should prepare written policies on HIV infection for the church community. These can address such issues as employees who are HIV-infected, workplace guidelines for employees generally, procedures in rituals such as communion (is a common cup shared? how is communion to be served to those who lack energy to walk to the front of the church?) and funerals (if the deceased is survived by a same-sex partner, is he or she treated the same way a bereaved spouse would be?), and so forth.

Special policies will apply particularly to youth. Policies should be adopted concerning the attendance of HIV infected students in the church day schools or Sunday school programs. We believe such students should not be hindered in any way from participating fully in the life of the church. Camping or other family or youth field trips should also be open to any HIV infected adolescent. The adults in charge of such activities, or personnel in the church and camping setting, should be familiar with infection-control guidelines concerning disposal of any sanitary or waste products, first aid responses, and guidelines which protect the health of the infected individual as well (seeing that eating utensils and dishes are thoroughly cleansed, that raw-milk food products are not used and that food is protected from spoilage, etc.). If campsite bathrooms are cleaned by campers, proper instruction must be provided for the use of disinfectants and gloves.

Education of the Church Community

Once policies have been written, the next step is education of the various segments of the church community. This should encompass denominational agency staffs and volunteers, including child care agencies, community centers, residences, hospitals, colleges and universities, juvenile homes and community meal services.

Church members, including adults, teens and primary and middle school age groups also need education. To help encourage family communication on the AIDS issue, parents and children can be educated together for a part of the program. A critical issue that many churches are discovering is the need for human sexuality education before effective and responsible AIDS education can be presented. Many denominations have developed such programs at a national level. If a curriculum is not in place, we recommend one be developed.

Education Implementation

Subjects that need to be addressed are the same as by any AIDS education program: HIV and transmission of the virus as the first stage in the disease; a clear definition of the difference between asymptomatic infection, ARC and AIDS; the ways the disease is transmitted and is not transmitted, with emphasis on the fact that it is not transmitted by casual contact; and the needs of the persons infected with HIV. Personal stories from denominational families affected by the epidemic will bring the reality of AIDS home to the congregation.

Churches will also discover the need to address a number of related, often highly sensitive issues. These include: the role of abstinence, monogamy, safer sex practices including use of a condom, and, since sharing needles is a prime method of spreading HIV, the abuse of intravenous drugs. Has your denomination a clear and practical statement on these issues? This should bring about some lively and controversial discussion.

Any number of approaches can be successful in a church's educational efforts. Presentations can be made at the regular meetings of various church groups, including church school and youth groups. Special workshops on AIDS and related issues can be organized, these have proven extremely successful for a number of churches. Ecumenical workshops are also useful, employing the expertise of outside experts and/or collaborating with other denominations in a community. One denomination sponsored a weekend camp for their entire area, with education sessions focusing on Christian belief about human sexuality and family life, responsible sexual behavior, AIDS and other sexually transmitted diseases.

A Successful Child/Parent Education Format

Child/parent programs are an especially powerful way to teach about AIDS and the moral concerns of the church regarding AIDS and related topics. One successful approach used in this kind of program is described below.

An educational planning committee was organized for the specific purpose of setting up an AIDS education program for middle and high school youth in the church. Parents and ministry were represented on the committee, and they met with an AIDS education professional from the Oregon State Health Division. Questions and concerns about the need for such a program were discussed, along with ideas about how to carry out the program most effectively and consistently within the ideology of the church.

Four educational sessions were scheduled. The first was a meeting for parents. Then three meetings for youth themselves were set up. This program was promoted in the church bulletin, during regular church services and in the youth groups and teen Sunday school classes.

At the parent session, the need for AIDS education for teens was presented. The materials for the youth sessions were reviewed with the parents. (Materials included: *AIDS: The Preventable Epidemic*, a school curriculum; HIV and AIDS slide set; *Using a Condom*, a pamphlet. These materials are available from the AIDS Education Program, Oregon Health Division, PO Box 231 Portland, OR 97207. A video was also used, *A Letter from Brian*, produced by The American Red Cross and available from local chapters. Local health departments can also provide literature.) They watched the video that would be used with their children and received copies of the handouts for the classes, along with outlines for each youth session. The discussion addressed parents' reactions to the video, the content of the youth sessions, and the issue of talking with teens about sexuality. One parent group requested that the third youth session include a demonstration of proper condom use.

The student sessions, planned with the help of the AIDS education professional, covered the basics about AIDS—what it is, how it is transmitted and how it can be prevented. Discussions were also held on the moral and ethical issues raised by AIDS. The youth participants were encouraged to see not only their own possible risk and their need to practice prevention, but the broader concern of an appropriate Christian response to the epidemic, and particularly to their peers at school and elsewhere who might be at risk. Discussion topics to be shared with parents were suggested at the end of each session. The parents, having been prepared for this in their own sessions, were ready to have these talks with their children.

These parents and youth, working together within the context of the church to achieve a clearer understanding of the AIDS epidemic, are now better prepared to deal with the challenges that certainly face them in the future. The program has been measured a success. We are confident that these youth will make better choices for themselves concerning risks in the future, that both parents and youth will respond with compassion to those within and outside the church affected by HIV illness, and that a foundation for ongoing parent-child discussions about sexuality, love, morality and AIDS has been well-established.

Service for Patients and Their Families Following Education

"In our country and around the world, people who are ill have been cared for compassionately, especially during the past 50 years, as we have seen the hospice movement offer care to patients and their families. In bleak contrast, the majority of people who have AIDS and ARC are not receiving the same care and compassion."

–from a sermon on AIDS by
Dr. William Sloane Coffin
Senior Minister, Riverside Church, NYC

The need for service is great in all communities, and is going to increase at an alarming rate during the foreseeable future. Churches should be the bulwark of decency, moving away from recrimination to Christian concern. In many areas, a more adequate level of care can be easily met by expanding the current services of church-related nursing and convalescent homes to care for persons with AIDS or ARC. The need for patient care is extreme in some locations. Cases have been documented of hospitalized patients who no longer need hospital care, but cannot find a nursing home to take them.

The church is well known for providing day-to-day support to its members during times of stress. Now, that service must be extended to persons with AIDS or ARC. They face many ordinary daily tasks that must be performed, and that can make all the difference in their ability to stay in their homes as long as possible. The simple preparation of a meal, even a trip to the grocery store, is often more than a person with AIDS can manage. Just having someone stop by, to talk or perform a task that the rest of us find easy to do, is a great need and greatly appreciated. These are roles the church communities can perform so well. Many of these tasks are well within the capabilities of church youth, and we think encouraging youth participation in this kind of program offers them a remarkable opportunity to learn more about the rewards of compassion and service.

Other Areas of Support and Education

The AIDS epidemic threatens to be so overwhelming that no one agency, church or school will be able to provide adequate services and education. All need to join together in cooperative projects that unite sectarian and church communities. One effective way that churches can speak to the wider community is through support for public school education programs on sexually transmitted diseases and AIDS.

Sermons are also an important vehicle through which church communities and the community at large can be educated about the realistic risks of AIDS and the path of compassion for those affected. Emphasis can be directed to the Biblical basis for a church's response to the epidemic. The story of the Good Samaritan is one that comes readily to mind as a call to help others wherever and however we can. The way we care for those in our midst who suffer has been the subject of countless sermons. In his time Jesus went with lepers and prostitutes. Today he would certainly go with persons with AIDS and their families.

By speaking these words from the pulpit, and by teaching these lessons in youth and adult Sunday school classes, ministers and other church teachers can help disempower the word "AIDS," alleviating the silence it sometimes imposes because of our fears, apprehensions and discomfort. If a minister can talk about AIDS in the sanctuary, surely we can discuss it at home with our family. If we can discuss it with our family, we may also be able to discuss it with our neighbors, our friends and our greater community. The possibilities for prevention reach a long, long way.

Conclusion

There is no doubt that AIDS presents a severe challenge to the Protestant church. But the church has long been a pioneer in education, health and social care. Now, this threat sends a call for the church to stand up and lead again. We worry, understandably, that our young people may be at risk, that members of the church may become infected, that tragedy may strike.

This is why we must be energetic in our efforts to teach prevention through the powerful voice of the church. We know, too, that despite our best efforts, individuals in our community, and perhaps in our church, are already infected and will become ill. Grieving deeply for those touched by the epidemic, we see the time has come once more to put the Protestant ethic, the Protestant heritage of love and concern, to work for the world in which we live.

References

Oregon Health Service. *Oregon Health Division guidelines for AIDS in the workplace.* Portland, OR: Oregon Health Service. AIDS Education Program.

U.S. Department of Health and Human Services. *Your rights as a person with AIDS or related conditions.* Washington, DC: Office of Civil Rights.

Facing the Issues:

Controversy and AIDS Education

Facing the Issues:
Controversy and
AIDS Education

AIDS education is essential and important, but it is not without controversy. Decisions must be made and stands taken, and whether the decision is to provide AIDS education prominently, to do so negligibly, or not to provide it at all, controversies will arise. Similarly, policies about participation of HIV-infected youth in schools or other programs are likely to inspire difficult responses regardless of what policy is chosen.

Schools, churches and community programs must deal now as never before with difficult issues such as IV drug use and sexual practices. There is a need to discuss these matters at an explicit level beyond what was once considered appropriate. This is unfamiliar territory for many. We are challenged, and sometimes pushed, to discover new boundaries and define new guidelines.

We believe the best course is to plan our approaches accordingly. We cannot avoid controversy, but we can prepare ourselves to meet it and do our best to see it is put into a nonsensationalist context. We can use community support and sound information as allies as we proceed.

For the sake of better AIDS education, and thus for the welfare of youth, it is important that a stand be taken to offer this information clearly, appropriately and explicitly. Young people's developmental capabilities to understand materials must be carefully considered, without, however, underestimating these capabilities. "Do we really need to tell 15 year olds about oral and anal sex?" someone asks. "Can we afford *not* to?" we counter.

19

Controversial Issues in the Classroom

Mary Lee Tatum, MEd

T he controversial issues in AIDS education are controversial for many reasons. Most obvious, of course, is the necessity of discussing AIDS in the context of human sexuality, a topic that has been troublesome for many schools for a long time. In addition, we must talk quite specifically about intravenous drug use as a risk behavior. Non-IV drug or alcohol use must also be mentioned in AIDS prevention education because anyone under the influence of substances is more likely to make careless decisions about risk activities.

Other controversies arise as well. We are talking about a disease that causes terrible disability, is sometimes grossly disfiguring, and generally leads to death. These are disturbing topics for young people whose energies more traditionally focus on the vigor of living and who are, in large part, healthy. We also find ourselves talking about fear and death in the context of sexual behaviors—not a very positive way of looking at sexuality! When we mention that the majority of Americans diagnosed with AIDS are gay or bisexual men, young people may respond with homophobic or discriminatory remarks. When we point out that Blacks and Latinos represent some 40 percent of U.S. AIDS cases (and about 80 percent of cases among women and children), there is a potential for young people to perceive this information in a racist context. When we talk in a clinical way about "AIDS as a universally fatal disease," or we say, "Many researchers believe everyone infected with the AIDS virus will progress to AIDS and die," we may not know whether we are describing someone close to one of our students—a parent, brother, aunt or friend who is HIV infected or ill. And, because AIDS inspires strong reactions from many people, including parents, teachers and young people themselves, we may find ourselves struggling with differences in values that have the potential to create divisiveness and conflict especially around the issue of sexual transmission. This means communities must arrive at some consensus about what should be taught, how it should be taught, and at what grade levels.

Teaching about AIDS in school classrooms will remain controversial for some time, no matter how mildly it is presented. If AIDS were caused by dirty hands, we would promote a noncontroversial curriculum to help young people decide to wash their hands frequently. As it is, we often find ourselves making decisions based on what is most "practical," most "acceptable" or most "realistic." The problem is that in our considerations of practicality, acceptability or realism, we may lose sight of what will be most effective in encouraging young people to protect themselves from risk. There is little controversy when the mandate for AIDS education includes only a video, lecture and question-and-answer period. It is possible that those who oppose sexuality education of any kind in public

schools intuitively know this brief exposure is ineffective—
that it will make little difference, therefore they let it pass.
Truly effective education in any subject area includes repetition
at different grade levels, age-appropriately.

A Consideration of the Issues

The most difficult conflict within school settings is not
apparently about the subject matter of AIDS, but about the
philosophy of education. Will we acknowledge that young
people wrestle with and make decisions about their own behavior, or will we simply "tell" young people what behavior is
acceptable, imply what behavior is not, and assume that in
"telling" them we have done our job?

The idea that we can "tell" young people shows lack of
understanding of the developmental stage of adolescence. The
search for identity begins in earnest at this time. It includes a
need for a nurturing family that communicates its values by
word and by deed. It also leads young people to look for independence and to rely on adults who understand this. They are
looking for input about themselves in their relationships. This
often leads them to stand outside the "group" and say, "What
do I have to do to belong?" We call this peer pressure—the
pressure a young person puts upon him or herself while contemplating what behaviors he or she would be willing to adopt
to belong to the group.

The affirmation the group gives to a young person is important and sought after. Therefore, although adult reflections
of wisdom and value are very important to young people, there
is usually some difficulty created when adult admonitions conflict with what is being said in the peer culture. We cannot offer
effective AIDS or other health education to adolescents without

remembering that young people have many sources of information that influence their attitudes and behaviors. What public schools can do is present, in a well-facilitated classroom discussion, the peer issues with which teens live every day.

We must, while we reinforce the importance of abstinence from sexual intercourse and drug use, also reflect our understanding that adolescents are, after all, free to make their own decisions. If we fail to include that in our approach to them, we lose their attention and their respect for our understanding of the dilemmas they face. Once we have established this respect, we can talk about decisions to have intercourse or use drugs. This is behavior that is clearly chosen by some young people. Consequences, possible protection and risks can be presented by both students and teachers. Given the developmental needs of adolescents, they are more likely to think through and internalize information presented in this context than if we simply tell them what to do and expect them to obey.

Another controversial issue is the idea that children are sexual. Innocence is seen as the opposite of knowledge about one's sexuality or the sexuality of others. It is also seen as the opposite of childhood experimentation or curiosity. The important thing to remember is that sexuality in childhood is just that: childhood sexuality. It involves feelings, both physical and emotional. It involves experimentation with perceived adult behavior.

Adolescent sexuality is also just that: adolescent sexuality. It carries with it all those developmental feelings and tasks of adolescence. They cannot be "protected" from knowledge. The question is only where will they get their knowledge? their attitudes? Where will they see behavior modeled? Who will talk with them about all of this to enable them to develop self-preserving wisdom?

AIDS education, unfortunately, carries with it the genuinely antisexual nature of our culture. Dirty jokes and pornography are constant reminders that we do not cherish and honor the nature of our sexual selves. Sex-to-sell in advertising, innuendo and suggestion in media programming are consistently a part of the message heard from early childhood through adulthood. It is, indeed, a fallacy to think that one can grow up hearing what the family, religious communities and schools have to say, and that the incredible media blitz will have little or no effect.

Genuinely prosexual attitudes have a difficult time in all of this. The message should be that our sexual nature—maleness, femaleness—is a priceless gift. It is to be honored. Our behavior is not controlled by intrusive or irresistible behaviors outside of ourselves. Our brains are in charge of our behavior from earliest times. This is the message educators have to give to teens: deliberate decision making, and the positive life experiences or dangers that can result.

The confusion lies in treating all sexual issues as if they were pornographic, or at best, not topics for polite conversation. In that atmosphere, it is very difficult to talk about positive decisions about a beautiful and wonderful part of life. The very existence of sexually transmitted disease and AIDS reinforces the idea that human sexuality itself has to do with dysfunction, discomfort, illness, and even death. It is actually specific sexual behaviors, not sexual feelings, or sexual awareness or attraction that get us into problematic situations. We have to delineate and define what it is we are talking about when we discuss any aspect of human sexuality. All concerns and interests surrounding human sexuality are not the same. Most importantly, there is no data to show that sexuality/AIDS education encourages teenagers to engage in sexual intercourse.

Suggested Approaches

As educators, we must recognize our interplay with our students' families and with their peer culture. When we remember and respect these influences on young people's lives, we have much greater likelihood of success.

The family should always be encouraged to do what it does effectively: teach about respect, sex roles, love, caring, life focus. In addition, when parents are involved in the development or review of the AIDS curriculum, a strong voice from the family is implicit. Homework lessons that involve parents establish a sense of collaboration between family and school, as well as providing parents an opportunity to discuss family values. Young people, for example, can ask their parents about what sorts of peer pressures they experienced as teenagers, and report back in classes on some of the differences and similarities between "then and now."

Another strategy is "continuum teaching." (This approach is in itself controversial because it focuses on the aforementioned possibility of internal decisions made by a teenager to guide his or her own behavior.) To facilitate this, the teacher develops a continuum of behaviors on a long paper arrow pointing in both directions. Behaviors that keep one completely risk free—no sexual intercourse, no IV drug use—can be listed at one end of the arrow. Behaviors that put one at highest risk—unprotected intercourse, sharing needles—can be listed at the other end. In between, behaviors that go from slight to moderate to serious risk are positioned. (The teacher can list behaviors before class to be sure only the things that are judged appropriate for the classroom in his or her district are on it. Or the class can come up with the behaviors to be listed and discuss where they should be placed on the arrow.) The arrow should be a light or no-color at the safe end and become a progressively deeper color. As the teacher talks about each behavior activity he or she can move physically from one end of the arrow to the other. This exercise gives a comprehensive, sobering, visual and verbal confrontation with behavior, consequences, and the obvious questions: where do you want to place yourself on the continuum? what do your behaviors have to be to keep yourself there?

Training peer leaders in health as well as in family life education can also help us in facing the controversies raised by AIDS education. When young people hear about prevention from peers, the messages in our classroom lessons are strengthened. If the peer group looks down on drug use or being sexually active, or supports the use of condoms for those who are sexually active, our own statements in this regard seem more reasonable. This resonance leads to less conflict between peer values, family values and classroom education. Peers can also be helpful in monitoring homophobic or racist responses—when peer leaders speak out against racism and homophobia, the impact will be felt in the youth community.

Integrating AIDS education into a full and comprehensive health and/or family life education program can help avoid controversy. AIDS prevention reasonably fits into lessons on drug prevention and human sexuality, including topics such as sexually transmitted diseases and sexual decision making. Comprehensive health programs lay a foundation of knowledge and understanding for students, so that a thorough discussion of AIDS risks is easier for students to accept and appreciate. If they have already heard about human sexuality in a general context that acknowledges that sexuality is a natural, healthy element in our lives, AIDS education will not lead to a permanent association of sex with death and fear. If all students have had this comprehensive background, teachers of other subjects—history, social studies, psychology, biology, and so forth—will be able to teach lessons involving AIDS-related issues (civil liberties vs. public welfare, for example) more easily as well.

Teachers talking about AIDS will want to establish ground-rules generally acceptable for classroom discussion in family life education programs. These should include a student's (or teacher's) right to pass, to decline to answer questions concerning personal opinions, and not asking intimate questions about personal sexual practices or personal family behaviors. There may also be rules about language used in class (for example, that while teachers will help students understand the meaning of slang terms for sexual anatomy or activities, correct terms will be used in classroom discussions), confidentiality and so forth.

In the classroom, educators can be careful in their own choice of language and clear in their communication of concepts. "Yes, Blacks and Latinos are greatly affected by AIDS. This is not because it is any easier for a Black person to contract AIDS, but because there is a greater problem with IV drug use in poor, urban communities, and a disproportionate number of urban poor in our country are Black or Latino." Such comments can help avert misunderstandings or the promotion of racist ideas. Similar care in language can help divert homophobic responses. And, when we speak respectfully about persons who are HIV-infected, students acquainted with such individuals can feel supported.

Educators can also be prepared for difficult or controversial topics to be raised by students themselves. Challenging discussions of death and disability have developed in many classrooms addressing AIDS. A variety of strong opinions is often expressed. New and sometimes unpleasant information may be shared with students—perhaps that IV drug users actually draw blood into their syringes to make sure they have reached the vein before injecting their drug; or that some people with AIDS may have violent, chronic diarrhea; or that people practice sexual activities the students might not have known existed. Such knowledge can lead to powerful emotional reactions by students. The skilled educator will be ready to acknowledge these issues and facilitate productive discussions—"Yes," we can tell our students, "AIDS is an emotional topic. We need to realize what our feelings are so we can better understand our own responses to and responsibilities in the epidemic." Teachers may want to make themselves available to expand upon or discuss questions asked on an "after class" basis.

Conclusion

Teaching about AIDS in the classroom of public schools will remain controversial for some time and will continue to include some or all of the following considerations:

- Shall we "tell" young people what to do and emphasize fear, or shall we respect their ability to process information and develop decision-making skills for themselves with our input?
- How will we meet the resistance to comprehensive family life/sexuality education programs that include AIDS?
- Will we define sexuality more clearly and help young people sort out behaviors that do and do not put them at risk?
- Can we convince the public that sexuality information will not encourage adolescents to have sexual intercourse?
- Will we encourage abstinence, but not to the exclusion of other decisions people might make?
- How will we confront AIDS and put it in the context of

251

sexuality as a cherished and respected aspect of human life?

Schools have traditionally been committed to public health. Education is our most important weapon in the fight against the AIDS epidemic. We want young people to stay at the lowest possible risk. It is important for them to know that, armed with adequate knowledge, they are, in fact, in charge of their own behavior and can protect themselves from danger by exercising their decision-making and assertiveness skills in a healthy way. By facing the controversies squarely so that we may educate young people thoroughly and responsibly, and by demonstrating productive approaches to conflict and controversy in our own classrooms, we will best be able to help them in this task.

References

Howard, M., Mitchell, M.E. and Pollard, B. 1984. *Postponing sexual involvement*. Atlanta, GA: Grady Memorial Hospital.

Mast, C.K. 1986. *Sex respect*. Bradley, IL: Respect for Sexuality.

Quackenbush, M. and Sargent, P. 1988. *Teaching AIDS*. Revised Edition. Santa Cruz, CA: Network Publications.

Yarber, W.L. 1987. *AIDS: What young people should know: Instructor's guide*. Reston, VA: American Alliance for Health, Physical Education, Recreation and Dance.

Adolescents and AIDS: Legal and Ethical Questions Multiply

Abigail English, JD

T he AIDS epidemic is receiving virtually constant attention
in the media, and for good reason. According to U.S. Surgeon General C. Everett Koop, the AIDS crisis is presenting
legal, ethical, social and economic dilemmas that will be at
least as difficult to solve, if not more so, than the medical
conundrums presented by the disease.[1] While the vast majority
of the attention given thus far to the AIDS crisis has focused on
the problems affecting the adult population, pediatric AIDS is
becoming a matter of increasing concern.[2]

Curiously, there has been little mention of adolescents in all
the public attention being given to AIDS, at least until very
recently. This is beginning to change, however, as awareness
grows that some segments of the adolescent population may be
at high risk for contracting the disease, or at least for becoming
infected with the virus. Indicative of the growing concern over
adolescents and AIDS, in May of 1987, the first major article

appeared in a medical journal addressing AIDS and adolescents,[3] and in June the House Select Committee on Children, Youth, and Families, held a hearing on AIDS and teen-agers.[4]

A multitude of legal issues concerning AIDS and adolescents has already arisen. Can an adolescent independently consent to an HIV antibody test, without parental permission? What is the scope of the confidentiality protection of an institutionalized adolescent known to be infected with the virus? Who, if anyone, is liable if disclosure of an adolescent's antibody status results in discrimination or other harm to the adolescent? Conversely, who, if anyone, is liable if an adolescent suffering from AIDS engages in sexual activity, or shares needles with a drug using companion, while in a group placement under public agency supervision? Can educational or social services programs legally refuse to serve infected youth? These are only a few of the *legal* questions. Some of them do not yet have clear answers, and the answers to others may change rapidly in the coming months and years.

These legal questions are matched by equally difficult ethical questions now confronting those in the fields of medicine, law, social services, juvenile justice, and public health who work with the adolescent population. These individuals are struggling to balance what often appear to be conflicting ethical duties—to the infected youth or youth with an AIDS diagnosis, to the high-risk youth, to other adolescents under their care, to themselves, and to the general public.

Epidemiology of AIDS

The human immunodeficiency virus (HIV) has been identified as the causal agent of AIDS and is often referred to as "the

256

AIDS virus." Although there is no definitive "AIDS test," blood tests can show whether an individual has developed antibodies to HIV, and therefore is likely to be infected with the virus. It is estimated that there are between 500,000 and 1,750,000 HIV-infected individuals in the United States who do not yet show symptoms of AIDS.[5] How many of these individuals will go on to develop AIDS-related complex (ARC) or full-blown clinical AIDS is unknown. Although drug treatments that have shown some success in arresting the progress of the disease have recently become available, no cure currently exists. AIDS is considered invariably fatal, often within a year or two of diagnosis.

According to the Centers for Disease Control, as of November 9, 1987 there were 189 cases of AIDS among 13-19 year olds, a 28 percent increase in five months. The total number of AIDS cases as of November 9, 1987 was 45,436. Of the teenagers diagnosed with AIDS, 46 percent are White, 34 percent are Black, 17 percent are Latino, and 3 percent are all other races. 7,687 cases of AIDS have been reported among 20-29 year olds, 21 percent of the total reported AIDS cases. Because of the long incubation period for this disease, many of the individuals who developed symptoms of illness in their twenties probably became infected as teenagers.[6] At least one small study in New York suggested that significant numbers of adolescents are infected. Blood samples from 200 apparently healthy adolescents were screened, and nine of the samples, or 4 1/2 percent, showed the presence of HIV antibodies.[7]

"High-Risk" Adolescents

The degree to which adolescents are in danger of becoming infected with the HIV virus depends on the extent to which they engage in activities referred to as "high-risk behavior"[8]— unprotected sexual intercourse (or other forms of "unsafe sex") or sharing needles—or the frequency with which they are exposed through other means such as blood transfusions.[9] The incidence of sexual activity among adolescents is high.[10] Only 20 percent of sexually active 15-19-year-old girls report use of condoms the last time they had sexual intercourse.[11] It is estimated that one in seven teenagers currently has a sexually transmitted disease (STD).[12] Testifying recently before the House Select Committee on Children, Youth, and Families, one adolescent medicine expert asserted that demographic changes, including increasing numbers of families living at or below the poverty line, will place even more teenagers at risk for STDs, including AIDS. In addition to the direct risk to teenagers themselves, those who become pregnant and are infected either prior to or during pregnancy also risk exposing their babies before birth.[13]

Although intravenous (IV) drug use is not common among adolescents generally, in a 1986 study more than 1 percent of high school seniors reported that they had used heroin.[14] It is likely that the proportion is higher among high school dropouts. Moreover, drug use is not the only context in which teenagers may share needles. Teenage girls often pierce each other's ears, with several using the same needle. Tattooing may also involve the sharing of needles.

Despite the high incidence of sexual activity and sexually transmitted disease among adolescents, it cannot be assumed that all of the affected adolescents are equally at risk for HIV infection or AIDS. Particular subgroups, such as teens with a high number of sexual partners, minority youth who use intravenous (IV) drugs, and homeless youth who engage in street prostitution and/or IV drug use, may be at greater risk, particularly when these young people are in geographic areas where the incidence of AIDS and HIV infection is high.[15]

Testing

The testing of adolescents for HIV infection is being proposed with increasing frequency in a wide variety of settings, including juvenile detention and correctional facilities, the foster care system, and teenage pregnancy programs. Testing is also being sought in connection with epidemiological research studies to determine the prevalence rates of HIV infection among adolescents or in subgroups of the adolescent population. The wisdom of testing adolescents, either on an individual basis or as part of a more widespread "screening" program, remains to be determined and is a matter of current controversy. Those opposed to the practice point out that, since only the presence of HIV antibodies, and not the disease itself, can be revealed, and since the disease is generally fatal, with no treatment available for asymptomatic infection, testing for AIDS is fundamentally different than testing for infectious diseases that can be treated or cured. Moreover, they contend that little consideration is given to what action to take if test results are positive.

One of the first groups of experts to consider the issue, the Adolescent AIDS Task Force of the San Francisco Department of Public Health, has recommended against routine testing, even of "high risk" adolescents who are incarcerated, and has sanctioned testing based only on clinical symptoms, for individual youth who strongly desire to be tested on a voluntary basis, or for pregnant adolescents.[16] In contrast, the Los Angeles County Grand Jury has called for testing of youth admitted to the county juvenile hall or probation department camps.[17]

In the absence of research studies or published clinical reports, the full implications of testing adolescents are not yet known. Potential disadvantages include the possibility that notification of a positive test result might provoke serious mental health problems or even suicide attempts among adolescents. There is also the risk, particularly in the absence of appropriate counseling and other support services, that some adolescents learning of a positive test result might, as a gesture of despair or defiance, engage in increased high-risk behavior. Moreover, adolescents identified as infected are likely to experience stigmatization and discrimination, including denial of services and efforts to isolate them from their peers.

Nonetheless, some public health officials suggest that if testing is done on a strictly voluntary basis, and appropriate individualized counseling is made available to test subjects, testing can be an educational tool forming a significant part of an overall prevention strategy. Thus for some adolescents, voluntary testing[18] based on individual clinical criteria may provide valuable information to motivate the teenager to modify his or her future behavior—to stay free of AIDS if the test result is negative, or to protect others from infection, in the case of a positive test result—or to make important decisions about pregnancy. Moreover, testing for epidemiological purposes, to determine the rates at which HIV antibodies are present in the adolescent population by age, sex, race, geographic area, sexual preference, or other factors, may be appropriate. Such data could provide a basis for essential service planning and for advocacy on behalf of adolescents in an era of intense competition for scarce resources. For whatever purpose testing is undertaken, legal and ethical requirements of consent and confidentiality should be carefully observed.

Consent for Testing

While ordinary parental consent is required for medical care of a minor, almost every state has enacted laws permitting adolescents to give their own consent for diagnosis and treatment of sexually transmitted (sometimes termed "venereal") diseases or contagious diseases.[19] In states where AIDS, or HIV infection, has been determined by statute, regulation, or case law to be a contagious or a sexually transmitted disease, adolescents would be able to give independent consent for testing.[20] Even in the absence of an explicit determination by statute or otherwise, medical data clearly support the argument that AIDS is a sexually transmitted disease,[21] and thus that minors may consent to their own tests or treatment. Federal regulations governing consent for participation in medical research would also seem to permit adolescents to consent to their own HIV antibody test as part of a research study if they could legally consent to the test under state law.[22]

Under both state laws and federal regulations, in order to give independent consent, an adolescent must be capable of giving an informed consent—in other words, of understanding an explanation of the nature and consequences, including the risks, of the procedure. In view of the uncertain prognosis currently associated with a positive HIV antibody test result, determining whether an adolescent's consent is truly "informed" may be somewhat more complex than with equally simple procedures which have less serious implications. In all cases, the adolescent should be screened for suicidality and should be carefully counseled, both before and after the testing.

A more difficult question is whether an adolescent can be required to submit to an HIV test involuntarily. Some experts have suggested generally that where an adolescent has the legal right to consent to care, that right includes the authority to refuse the care.[23] In some states, special statutes or regulations govern consent for HIV antibody testing. In California, for example, an HIV antibody test may be administered only with the "written consent of the subject to the test." [24] In the event of such a requirement, only the adolescent himself or herself could consent to a test. California law permits another person to consent on behalf of the subject of the test only if the subject is not competent to consent, and minors under the age of 12 are deemed incompetent. For an incompetent minor, the parent, guardian, or "other person lawfully authorized to make health care decisions" may consent to the test, but only when necessary to render appropriate care or to practice preventive measures. Under the California statute a judge may consent only for minors who have been adjudged dependents of the court.[25] In Kentucky, however, interim policies recently developed by the Cabinet for Human Resources authorize testing of adolescents over age 10 in state custody who fit a broad profile of "high-risk." These policies permit either the court (for children in temporary custody) or the state social services agency (for committed minors) to consent to tests for minors who have "a. experimented with or used intravenous drugs; or b. been sexually active and had sexual contact with members of risk groups, or with a known carrier, or [have] a history of sexual promiscuity." [26]

Confidentiality

Apart from the potentially negative consequences for the mental health of individual adolescents who are tested, the primary concern about testing of youth stems from the significant likelihood of stigmatization and discrimination against those identified as infected. If strict confidentiality of test results can be maintained, this risk may be somewhat alleviated, although maintaining confidentiality of highly sensitive information is difficult at best.

Although adolescents generally want to be assured that

health professionals will not disclose the information revealed in the course of a medical interview, the teenagers often do not realize the consequences that may result if they themselves disclose sensitive information to friends or others, as they often do. Some adolescent medicine experts have suggested that it is important for health professionals to counsel infected adolescents about the risks of disclosure, keeping in mind, however, their need to share information with someone to avoid a damaging sense of isolation.

A few states have enacted laws specifically guaranteeing the confidentiality of HIV antibody test results and/or prohibiting their use for discriminatory purposes.[27] The California statute permits disclosure of test results only by the test subject or the person authorized to consent to a test for an incompetent: each separate disclosure requires a written authorization; and stiff financial penalties are imposed for any unauthorized disclosure.[28] Not all states have enacted strict protections for confidentiality of test results; and even in those states which do have strong protections, adherence to the confidentiality requirements is not always consistent.

Pressing arguments are raised that a range of professionals and service providers—foster parents, social workers, probation officers—have a "need to know" the antibody status of high-risk adolescents with whom they work. Claims are made that this knowledge is essential both for the benefit of the adolescent tested and for the protection of other youth and staff. However, in view of the potential damage that may occur from identification of an adolescent as infected, these claims must be carefully evaluated in light of the medical facts and whether revealing test results would actually result in greater protection for the adolescent in question or for others. While in rare instances disclosure to one or more of these professionals might be justified, in many cases the reasons for confidentiality will outweigh the need to know.

Many experts urge that policies which carry the least risk of individual stigmatization or discrimination should be preferred. For example, utilization of appropriate infection control procedures in case of blood spills can adequately protect staff in detention facilities even if they do not know a youth's antibody status. Similarly, counseling and education regarding modes of transmission and avoidance of high-risk behavior should be targeted at all adolescents, especially those at high risk, regardless of their antibody status, as the San Francisco Adolescents AIDS Task Force recommended in its guidelines.[29]

Some professionals and others working with high-risk adolescents worry about their potential liability. For example, should a counselor in a group home warn the sexual partner of a teenager known to have tested positive? This question presents a true dilemma, because the counselor may have conflicting ethical duties—to maintain confidentiality for the individual patient and to prevent serious harm to another—and may also run the risk of conflicting legal liability—for breach of confidentiality and for failure to warn. There are no cases at this time imposing a legal duty to warn in the AIDS/HIV context, and there is conflicting legal authority in the case of other infectious diseases, such as hepatitis B. Legal developments in this area should be carefully watched.[30]

Access to Services

Those adolescents who may be at higher risk—homeless or street youth, homosexual youth, IV drug users, sexually active adolescents with high rates of sexually transmitted disease, and the sexual partners or needle-sharing companions of any of these adolescents—are subgroups of the adolescent population who are also at high risk of discrimination. To the extent that these young people become known as possible or actual carriers of the AIDS virus, this risk of discrimination might be enhanced. Homeless youth, particularly when they are from out-of-county or out-of-state, are an unpopular group in many cities, viewed as "someone else's problem" but nevertheless a drain on local resources. Homosexual youth are already subject to ostracism and discrimination in many communities. IV drug-using adolescents, already victimized by the scarcity of resources to address their drug problems, may be doubly victimized by discrimination or lack of resources for their AIDS-related problems. And, with the highest rates of sexually transmitted disease among poor minority youth, the problems of racial discrimination and poverty may be compounded by discrimination based on AIDS carrier status.

There have already been numerous attempts to deny HIV-infected children, or those suffering from AIDS, access to elementary and secondary schools. Proposals are surfacing to require testing of high-risk adolescents prior to placement in foster care or juvenile detention or correctional facilities. While the intended result of the proposed testing is not always clear, the high level of fear of contagion that prevails—often without regard to the actual means of transmission—increases the likelihood that identification of infected or high-risk youth will result, directly or indirectly, in their inability to obtain services ordinarily accessible to teenagers. They may also be subject to attempts to isolate or segregate them from other youth in the delivery of those services. Two recent cases illustrate these problems:

> In a recent situation a 14-year-old girl who had used drugs and was sexually active had been accepted by a residential program for disturbed

youth. While she was awaiting placement, her mother, concerned about her health status, had her tested for the HIV antibody. When she tested positive, her mother, thinking that knowledge of the test result might help the program treat her appropriately, disclosed the result. Thereafter, on their fourth or fifth review of the girl's file, the program staff concluded that her history of drug use, which they had known all along, made her an inappropriate candidate for their services.[31]

A 15-year-old boy attempted suicide after he was notified of a positive HIV antibody test result. A local judge "quarantined" the boy in an adult psychiatric hospital because he allegedly had engaged in street prostitution, even though he expressly stated his intention to refrain from sexual activity. The boy was subsequently released at the request of the state health agency.[32]

Moreover, high risk and HIV-infected youth and adolescent AIDS patients may experience extreme difficulty in obtaining the specialized services they need. Medical care for AIDS patients is costly, and adolescents, particularly if they are not living with their families, often encounter substantial difficulties in obtaining public or private insurance coverage or in locating other sources of free care. Mental health services for the adolescent population are already extremely limited, and few specialized services appropriate to the adolescent population suffering from, or at high risk for, AIDS have been developed.[33] If the existing limitations on adolescents' access to health care generally are exacerbated by HIV-infected status, high risk adolescents may find it extraordinarily difficult to obtain the medical care and mental health services they need.

Legal Protections

There are some encouraging signs in the efforts to protect against AIDS-based discrimination. For example, efforts to exclude children with AIDS from school have been successfully challenged in the courts.[34] In these cases, the courts have relied heavily on the medical data demonstrating that AIDS is not transmitted through casual contact.

Some cities and states have enacted ordinances or statutes prohibiting discrimination on the basis of AIDS. San Francisco, for example, has enacted an ordinance explicitly prohibiting discrimination based on AIDS, ARC, or HIV infection in any city services. Recently the United States Supreme Court decided that a contagious disease—tuberculosis—is a handicap within the meaning of Section 504 of the Rehabilitation Act, the federal statute which prohibits discrimination on the basis of handicap.[35] The decision has been heralded as an indication that a similar analysis should apply to AIDS, thereby providing protection for AIDS patients and infected individuals in federally funded programs. This expectation was borne out recently by a decision of the U.S. Court of Appeals for the Ninth Circuit which ordered a school system to permit a teacher with AIDS to return to the classroom.[36]

There are, however, some special problems with respect to preventing discrimination against minors. First, most AIDS anti-discrimination laws enacted thus far have focused on employment or insurance and do not speak to the specific settings which pose the greatest danger of discrimination for minors: the juvenile justice system, schools, and the foster care system. Second, while children and adolescents are entitled to protection of their constitutional rights, the courts have applied different, in some cases less stringent, standards in evaluating burdens on the constitutional rights of minors, both because of their vulnerability and immaturity, and because of the presumption that their parents, or the state acting *in loco parentis,* will act in their best interests.[37] Third, adolescents have more limited ability to advocate for themselves than adults do, and far more limited access to attorneys and other advocates. For these reasons, it is essential that advocates for adolescents, in whatever profession, maintain an intensive vigilance to ensure that in this AIDS crisis the individual rights of youth are not unnecessarily sacrificed.

Conclusion

Protecting adolescents from the adverse affects of the AIDS epidemic requires a dual strategy of prevention. The first aspect of this strategy must be preventing the spread of infection: enabling those who are not infected to avoid becoming so; and enabling those who are infected to avoid communicating the virus to others. Education is critical in this regard. The second part of the strategy is to prevent limitations on access to necessary services or discrimination against adolescents based on infection or perceived high-risk status. Within this framework, it is possible to evaluate the myriad of statutes, regulations, and policies being developed in response to the AIDS epidemic to determine the extent to which they would further either of these two purposes, and thus their likelihood of furthering the protection of adolescents.

Notes

1. "Doctors Who Shun AIDS Patients Are Assailed by Surgeon General." *New York Times*, September 10, 1987, p.1.

2. See, e.g., "Kids with AIDS," the cover story in the 1987 edition of *Newsweek*, Sept. 7, 1987.

3. Hein, "AIDS in Adolescents: A Rationale for Concern," May 1987 *N.Y. State Journal of Medicine* 290.

4. House Select Committee on Children, Youth, and Families, Hearing entitled "AIDS and Teenagers: Emerging Issues," June 18, 1987, Washington, D.C. (hereafter House Select Committee Hearing).

5. Barry, Cleary, and Fineberg, "Screening for HIV Infection: Risks, Benefits, and the Burden of Proof," 14 *Law, Medicine and Health Care* 259 (1986).

6. House Select Committee on Children, Youth, and Families, "Fact Sheet: AIDS and Teenagers," (June 18, 1987) (hereafter House Select Committee Fact Sheet).

7. See D. Haffner, *AIDS and Adolescents: The Time for Prevention Is Now*. Washington, DC: Center for Population Options (1987).

8. The definition of risk has been changed to encompass the notion of risk behavior rather than risk groups. Hein, *supra* note 3, at 290.

9. Approximately 11 percent of all hemophilia-related AIDS cases are among adolescents. House Select Committee Fact Sheet.

10. 70 percent of girls and 80 percent of boys have engaged in sexual intercourse at least once before age 20. National Research Council, *Risking the Future: Adolescent Sexuality, Pregnancy, and Childbearing* 41 (1987). More than half of teenagers interviewed in a recent poll reported having sexual intercourse by age 17. Louis Harris and Associates, Inc. *American Teens Speak: Sex, Myths, TV, and Birth Control* 13 (1986).

11. Testimony of Mary Ann Shafer, MD, at House Select Committee Hearing.

12. House Select Committee Hearing.

13. There are approximately one million pregnancies among teenagers each year. National Research Council, *supra* note 10, at 51.

14. Bachman, Johnston, and O'Malley, *Monitoring the Future:*

Questionnaire Responses from the Nation's High School Seniors 1986, Institute for Social Research, Ann Arbor, MI (1987).

15. Hein, *supra* note 3, at 295.

16. Adolescent AIDS Task Force, Perinatal and Pediatric AIDS Advisory Committee, San Francisco Department of Public Health, "Guidelines for the Control of Human Immunodeficiency Virus in Adolescents" (1987).

17. "Test Young Inmates for AIDS, Jury Urges," *Los Angeles Times*, July 29, 1987.

18. For a discussion of the risks and disadvantages of involuntary testing, see, e.g., Gostin and Curran, "AIDS Screening, Confidentiality, and The Duty to Warn," 77 *American Journal of Public Health* 361 (1987).

19. See, e.g., J. Morrissey, A. Hoffman, J. Thrope, *Consent and Confidentiality in the Health Care of Adolescents: A Legal Guide Appendix: State-by-State Table* (1986).

20. See, e.g., California Civil Code §34.7; California Health and Safety Code §1603.1(d).

21. See, e.g., Mueller, "The Epidemiology of the Human Immunodeficiency Virus Infection," 14 *Law, Medicine, & Health Care* 250, 256 (1987).

22. 45 CFR §46.402(a)(1986).

23. See, e.g., A.R. Holder, *Legal Issues in Pediatrics and Adolescent Medicine*, 2d ed., 247 (1985).

24. California Health and Safety Code §199.22.

25. California Health and Safety Code §199.27.

26. Kentucky Cabinet for Human Resource, Division of Family Services, "Interim Protocol Governing Service to Children with Acquired Immune Deficiency Syndrome."

27. See, e.g., Gostin and Ziegler, "A Review of AIDS-Related Legislative and Regulatory Policy in the United States," 15 *Law, Medicine, & Health Care* 5, 13-14 (1987).

28. California Health and Safety Code §199.21 and §199.22.

29. Adolescent AIDS Task Force, *supra* note 16.

30. Gostin and Curran, *supra* note 18.

31. Author's discussion with attorney regarding case.

32. "Boy Put in Psychiatric Ward as AIDS Suspect," *New York Times*, June 12, 1987, p.11.

33. Hein, *supra* note 3.

34. *Board of Education v. Cooperman*, 507 A.2d 253 (N.J. Su-

per A.D. 1986); *District 27 Community School Board v. Board of Education*, 502 N.Y.S.2d 325 (N.Y. Sup. Ct. 1986); *Thomas v. Atascadero Unified School Dist.*, 662 F. Supp. 376 (C.D. Cal. 1987).

35. *School Board of Nassau County v. Airline, 107 S. Ct. 1123* (1987).

36. *Chalk v. U.S. District Court Central District of CA*, No. 87-6418 (9th Cir. Nov. 18, 1987).

37. See, e.g., *Parham v. J.R.*, 99 S.Ct. 2493 (1979); *Bellotti v. Baird*, 99 S. Ct. 3035 (1979).

21

AIDS and IV Drug Use: Prevention Strategies for Youth

Jack B. Stein, LCSW,
with Sally Jo Jones and Glen Fischer

T he distribution of transmission risks associated with reported AIDS cases has remained remarkably consistent
since 1981. Prevention efforts require attention to those populations most directly affected and those thought potentially to
be. With the publication of the Surgeon General's widely-ac-
claimed report on AIDS in 1986 came a strong call to action to
target adolescents as the next likely "at risk" population in need
of education. With this sanctioning of prevention efforts targeted at youth came a flurry of activity as to how best to
achieve such a task amidst the diversity of viewpoints held.

Although HIV is known to be an infectious agent spread
through several well-documented modes, the strong association with sexual activity has led to AIDS being referred to by
many as a sexually transmitted disease. Although sexual transmission is considered to be the primary mode of transmission
nationally and globally, a comprehensive prevention effort

might best refer to HIV as "behaviorally transmitted." The rapidly growing numbers of individuals now being reported infected with HIV as a result of sharing IV drug needles or "works" (equipment used to inject drugs) clearly speaks to this need.

When we turn our attention to the concerns of youth as a population targeted for AIDS prevention it is understandable why such an emphasis must be placed on the sexual activity component of HIV transmission. Reported high levels of sexual activity (much of it very risky) is well-documented within this population. However, as with adults at-risk, effective prevention among youth cannot be achieved unless we aggressively attend to the strong relationship between drug use and HIV transmission and pose realistic options for risk reduction.

Responding to the myriad of sensitive issues faced in prevention efforts is significantly challenged when our target population is young. Yet we have little choice but to take on this challenge—the alternatives may be nothing less than fatal.

To properly respond to this challenge, a full understanding of the unique issues surrounding AIDS and substance abuse must be achieved. To do so, this chapter will address the following major areas:

- HIV transmission: the substance abuse connection
- Substance abuse and youth: reasons for concern
- A prevention model
- Strategy design to target youth

HIV Transmission: The Substance Abuse Connection

In a forceful report issued in February 1988, Admiral James Watkins, chair of the presidential AIDS commission, urged a significant increase in annual public spending and the hiring of thousands of additional workers to fight the spread of HIV among active IV drug users (Davidson, 1988). The report, based on the testimony of hundreds, was a clear recognition of the impact of drug use on the continued spread of HIV. Such a recognition was based on the following major issues of concern.

One of Every Four AIDS Cases to Date Has Been an Intravenous Drug User

IV drug use is the second largest transmission category for AIDS in the United States, representing a consistent 17 percent of the diagnosed cases nationally. In addition, when the drug using habits of gay and bisexual males with AIDS are examined, 7 to 11 percent of these individuals also have a history of IV drug use. This means at least one quarter of all AIDS cases to date have been IV drug users (Centers for Disease Control, 1988).

Contaminated Needles and/or Works Are Now, Directly or Indirectly, the Major Source of AIDS Among Women, Newborns, Prisoners and Minorities

Over half of all women diagnosed with AIDS have been IV drug users (Centers for Disease Control, 1988). More than half of the children diagnosed in the United States have a parent who is an IV drug user, while more than 90 percent of all AIDS cases in state, federal and county prisons and jails were found to be among IV drug users (National Institute on Drug Abuse, 1987).

Demographically, AIDS has taken a disproportionately heavy toll in our Black and Latino populations. In fact, these two groups are three times more likely to have AIDS than Whites overall, and are even more at risk if they are IV drug users. Nationally, 81 percent of people who have contracted AIDS exclusively through IV works-sharing are Black or Latino; a relatively smaller 29 percent of cases attributed exclusively to male-male sex are from these groups (Centers for Disease Control, 1988).

AIDS Cases Linked to IV Drug Use Are Now Spreading Rapidly Throughout the Nation

The relative proportion of needle-linked AIDS cases compared to gay or bisexual cases is beginning to rise particularly in several northeast states. Retrospective studies of blood samples from New York City drug users suggest large increases in HIV seropositivity rates over the ten-year period from 1977 to 1987 (from 50 percent in 1985 to 61 percent in 1986-87 in one study). A seropositivity study of Baltimore drug addicts in 1987 showed a 29 percent level, which approximates that of New York in 1979. In several northeast states, IV drug use is now considered the predominate risk factor in new AIDS cases reported (National Institute on Drug Abuse, 1987b).

The Potential for These Numbers to Increase Even More Is Real

Infected drug users are the greatest single threat to potentially widespread infection with HIV in the heterosexual population. This link is through heterosexual partners and offspring. In fact, four out of every five exclusively heterosexual cases among native-born Americans are the sexual partners of IV drug users.

IV Drug Users Are Extremely Difficult to Reach With AIDS Prevention Messages

A number of barriers exist in effectively reaching drug users both from an individual and environmental perspective.

These include:
- lack of awareness of personal risk
- incomplete information about risk
- lack of knowledge of risk reduction
- lack of awareness of drugs as a cofactor
- mistrust of health authorities
- denial
- fatalism
- fear of peer/spouse rejection
- addictive nature of risk behaviors
- the impairment of judgment, effect and behavior caused by drug usage
- the presence of laws that encourage works-sharing
- the absence of prevention messages tailored to the needs of drug users
- lack of space in treatment programs
- socioeconomic disempowerment of high-risk persons

In summary, IV drug users are a population alienated from society, and frequently from their families. Because of their inability to organize and advocate for themselves as a group, they are the least likely to receive adequate attention with respect to both prevention and support services. As HIV continues to spread, their access to already overtaxed healthcare facilities, financial assistance, housing, psychological services, support and educational groups, and legal advice will be extremely limited unless immediate interventions occur.

Substance Abuse and Youth: Reasons for Concern

As we make a transition from the general concerns of HIV transmission and IV drug abuse to those particularly pertinent to an adolescent population, a few major issues need to be highlighted.

Substance Abuse, Including Intravenous Use, Is Widely Practiced by Young People

Estimates indicate there are several million recreational/ regular users of cocaine and heroin, and a significant number are under the age of 21. In surveys conducted, for example, over one percent of high school seniors report having used heroin. Of individuals who seek treatment for a drug problem, more than 80 percent report administering drugs to themselves intravenously during the year before treatment. Of these, nearly 10 percent are under the age of 21 (Nurco, Cisnin and Balter, 1982).

Youth Begin to Experiment with Drugs at an Early Age

Reports indicate that the median age for first use of drugs other than alcohol and cigarettes in a population of young males is between 17 and 22. In a treated population of narcotic addicts, the median age for first nonopiate drug use was 15.6 years. The belief is firmly held that such early drug use is often a significant factor eventually leading to IV drug use. At a minimum, this level of drug use activity at such an age could likely contribute to a weakened immune system and/or impaired judgment during sexual activity (Nurco, Cisnin and Balter, 1982).

Polydrug Use Among Adolescents Is Reported to Be High

A recent study conducted by 800-COCAINE, a nonprofit drug information and treatment referral service in New Jersey, reported that of 100 teen calls, 100 percent reported use of more than one drug and 89 percent used more than two drugs simultaneously. Again, concerns exist as to the level of immune suppression concurrent with such drug use in addition to impaired judgment leading to unnecessary high-risk activities (Hospital and Community Psychiatry, 1986).

Most IV Drug-Using Youth Will Be Initiated into
Needle Use After Dropping Out of School
In this respect, those most at risk for HIV transmission through sharing works will not benefit from newly-instituted school-based AIDS prevention initiatives (Des Jarlais and Friedman, 1986).

One Million Teens Run Away Each Year
Of these, nearly 75 percent become involved in drug use, trafficking, and/or prostitution. Again, opportunities to reach this at-risk population through traditional educational methods are unlikely to be successful (Haffner, 1987).

Parents' and Adolescents' Use
of Substances Are Closely Related
Generally, youth are more likely to use alcohol and drugs if their parents are consumers or if they perceive them to be so (New Jersey Women's Resource Panel on Substance Abuse, 1986).

Barriers to Changing Youth's Drug-Using Behaviors

Clearly, HIV transmission has now become yet another critical reason why substance abuse among adolescents must be curtailed. However, many barriers exist in effecting the necessary changes in behavior among youth with respect to drug use in general, and these are complicated by the advent of HIV.

279

Only through a careful analysis of some of these major barriers can we move to developing an effective strategy of intervention.

Peer Pressures Are Strong Among Youth

The pressure to conform to cultural fads that exist among youth is an extremely powerful and difficult deflector of behavior changes required to prevent HIV transmission.

Adolescents Are Frequently Known for Their Impulsive and Risk-Taking Behavior

A feeling of invulnerability often pervades among youth. "That can't happen to me" is a commonly quoted phrase regardless of the dangers inherent. For example, 10 percent of the driving population in the 16-25 age group is responsible for 25 percent of fatal auto accidents (Korcock, 1987).

Lack of Information Is Relatively High Among Youth

Many adolescents may simply not be informed of the risks involved with drug use and HIV transmission. Youth-oriented educational programs are relatively recent and still nonexistent in some parts of the nation. In addition, much of the focus has been on sexual activity as a risk factor, leaving the correlation to drug use still unacknowledged.

Traditional Educational Settings May Not Adequately Reach At-Risk Youth

Although teenage students report their school as the single most reliable source of information about drug use, those youth most at-risk will probably not be reached through this setting (Koop, 1987). Even highly visible media campaigns may not fully reach a more "on-the-fringe" adolescent population such as runaways.

Parental Attitudes/Ignorance May Severely Limit
the Level of Information Conveyed to Youth

Although 83 percent of parents polled expressed their support of AIDS education in public schools (Korcock, 1987), disagreement prevails among various factions as to the nature of the prevention messages to be conveyed. High levels of specificity are required in developing safer sex messages for adolescents. This is equally the case with drug-related messages. However, frank explanations to youth of the risks involved in sharing IV needles, or of methods for needle disinfection, will probably be met with extreme resistance.

A Prevention Model

As we reflect on the numerous barriers that exist in educating a drug using population, both adult and teen, the ability to effectively intervene seems limited. Yet, many opportunities do exist to effect change. Designing these prevention strategies requires not only a clear identification of the existing barriers, but a sound understanding of the key elements of prevention education. A description of a model for health education as it relates to HIV prevention follows. This model will then be used as a framework to discuss strategy design to address the drug-related issues associated with HIV transmission and youth.

Unfortunately, knowledge alone does not seem to be a sufficient motivator to eradicate risk behavior among drug abusers. Initial research in the New York City area, shortly after epidemic spread of the virus among intravenous drug users was recognized, provided optimistic data about behavioral changes stemming from information about the disease. Clients in drug treatment and addicts still on the street were aware of and concerned about AIDS, realized some transmission dangers, and were spontaneously attempting to decrease risk behavior— primarily by reducing works sharing, purchasing sterile needles for drug injection, or trying to clean works between users (Selwyn et al., 1985).

However, even in the face of accurate information about AIDS and clear evidence of the HIV infection threat, not all drug users demonstrate a decrease in high risk activities. This has led to a closer look at exactly what "drives" behavior changes in the face of the HIV epidemic.

Three domains basic to all human learning require attention when addressing prevention education: (1) cognitive, (2) attitudinal, and (3) behavioral. As shown in figure 1, these domains may be visualized as interlocking gears. In addition, we must also recognize that we do not live in a vacuum. Our knowledge, attitudes and behaviors are supported by and/or developed in reaction to a number of normative environmental elements as noted (National Institute on Drug Abuse, 1988a).

However, changes in one's understanding of the facts of HIV transmission (the cognitive domain), for example, will not necessarily drive automatic changes in risk-related attitudes or behaviors (figure 2). Similarly, attempts to induce risk-reducing behavioral changes will be thwarted if the individual's related factual understanding and beliefs are ignored. Any learning gains achieved in such isolation will tend to fade under the influence of unaffected domains. Hence, prevention is the result of multifaceted interventions as depicted in figure 3.

Strategy Design to Target Youth

The "gear model" for health education is a convenient template to assist in the design of an effective prevention strategy to target youth. The following steps provide a framework in

ELEMENTS CONTRIBUTING TO A
PERSON'S LIFESTYLE & HEALTH STATUS

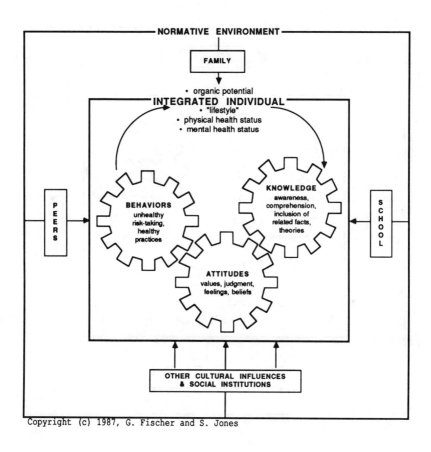

Figure 1

"RETOOLING" ONE ELEMENT DOES NOT NECESSARILY DRIVE CHANGES IN OTHER ELEMENTS

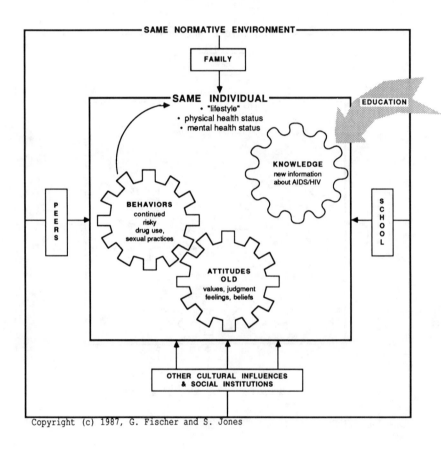

Figure 2

284

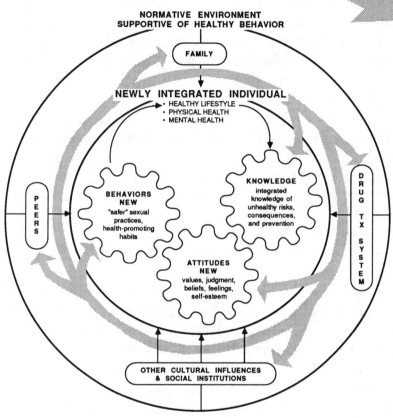

Figure 3

285

which to work (National Institute on Drug Abuse, 1988a).

Step 1. *Specify Target Population.* As in any prevention program, it is essential that the target audience be clearly identified. "IV drug using youth," although specific, is still too broad to create a program with the desired impact. For example, what might clearly be effective for adolescents in treatment may be extremely inappropriate for an incarcerated youth population. The first step of any such program design requires delimiting characteristics of the particular subset within the population you wish to focus on.

Step 2. *Determine Elements of the Individual and His/Her Environment on Which to Focus.* Our model for health education becomes extremely helpful at this point. Based on an assessment of the youth population targeted, interventions may have a strong attitudinal focus, for example, if informational levels are already high. In addition, a peer-oriented focus might be ideal if this environmental factor has been identified as a significant force amenable to intervention.

Step 3. *Specify the Design of the Intervention.* This entails identifying features of the design including activities to be conducted, materials required and locations targeted.

Step 4. *Identify Resources to Carry Out the Strategies.* Depending on the program needs, resources will vary greatly ranging from administrative support to funding allocation.

Step 5. *Determine How Program's Impact Will Be Evaluated.* In early years of AIDS prevention education, limited resources and experience created somewhat of a "fly-by-the-seat-of-the-pants" approach to program design. Subsequently, many early interventions had few/no evaluation components to justify any impact. Devoting attention to this important facet of program design is critical and cannot be overlooked.

Based on this five step approach, let us now focus our attention to some of the more relevant issues and strategies around youth and drug use. Note that this discussion is structured according to the three major domains of learning—cognitive, attitudinal and behavioral—that make up the core of our prevention model.

Issues and Strategies

AIDS Awareness and Education (Cognitive Domain): Stimulating Awareness

WHAT MEDIA/APPROACHES ARE EFFECTIVE
IN REACHING AT-RISK YOUTH?

Keep awareness messages simple, striking and clear. Use multiple communications channels simultaneously to saturate a target area and make certain the message is "heard." Posters, ads, public service announcements, comics, jingles, buttons, decals and hand-outs can be effective. Insist on high-quality, accurate, timely and attractive materials that stimulate interest without causing overload.

Find innovative ways to disseminate the message. Outreach workers have proven extremely efficient in some locations (YES Project in San Francisco; HERO in Baltimore) while mobile vans with public address systems have been tried in states such as New Jersey. All of these techniques are excellent opportunities for information to be distributed. In most of these programs, condoms and bleach are used as attention-grabbers, as well as practical tools for prevention.

Language used requires critical attention in view of subcultural differences, illiteracy rates, and non-English speaking needs.

WHERE/WHEN SHOULD THESE MESSAGES
BE COMMUNICATED?

Communicate in natural settings where the target group

congregates: inner city playgrounds, malls, neighborhood shops and businesses, newsstands, churches, community centers, family planning and STD clinics, favorite radio and TV stations.

Insert prevention messages into special events that the target group is likely to attend: health fairs, contests (e.g. Rap 'N Down STDs Drugs and AIDS in San Francisco, "A Letter to My Friend" essay contest in Baltimore), ethnic festivals.

Use credible messengers who are sensitive to cultural barriers and other resistances in communication. Peers and respected leaders of the community are often more believable than "experts." Teen hotline operators (HERO in Maryland) have proven effective in reaching at-risk youth as have local or national celebrities such as Ray Dawn Chong's narration of the video "Sex, Drugs, and AIDS."

WHAT MESSAGE SHOULD BE CONVEYED TO CAPTURE ATTENTION?

Most research indicates that messages of fear do not work well alone. The death threat of AIDS can be powerful and arousing, but may also be counterproductive and desensitizing or contribute to stress-avoiding denial—especially in a population where the impact of HIV is still perceived as somewhat distant.

WHAT COMMON MISCONCEPTIONS ABOUT AIDS NEED TO BE OVERCOME?

Most adult drug users appear to know about the dangers of AIDS and HIV transmission by needle-sharing. Adolescents, however, may still be shielded from access to this information. Minority drug-using youth in particular are still in need of basic information regarding risks and nonrisks of transmission to themselves and others.

WHAT SPECIAL SUBGROUPS OF YOUTH
POPULATIONS NEED TO BE ALERTED?

Sexually active teens prone to IV drug experimentation are clearly most at-risk for HIV infection. In particular, those who are either school truants or dropouts and therefore not able to benefit from more traditional means of health education should be targeted. Runaways and incarcerated youth are critical target groups for prevention efforts.

Personal Motivation (Attitudinal Domain)

Emotional commitment and personal empowerment seem to be key prerequisites in motivating youth to assimilate AIDS/ HIV information and personally resolve to practice risk reduction. The following strategies have been suggested to enlist motivation and foster attitudinal change supportive of risk reduction.

Vicarious exposure to the experience of persons with AIDS who are seen as either peers or role models—through films/ plays/soap operas if personal experience is lacking. This does not necessarily have to take an approach of "this will happen to you if you don't behave properly," but as a means to provide a more personal connection to the impact of HIV on the target audience. Youth-identified community outreach workers who are comfortable discussing their former at-risk behaviors when they were younger has been shown to be a powerful motivator to teens currently at risk.

Personalized risk assessment and an individual estimation of the consequences of different behavior options. This is often accomplished during individual counseling in treatment settings but may also take place among friends/peers or during a street outreach worker's interaction.

Groups of family members and/or significant others have proven powerfully persuasive in sharing feelings about and pointing out the undesirable consequences of such addiction problems as substance abuse. Their confrontations, mixed with caring, concern and support, can be instrumental in encouraging personal responsibility for change—entering treatment or stopping IV drug use—but probably not for the more intimate sexual and works-sharing behaviors, especially among a youth population where much secrecy around such issues prevails.

Innovative invitations/opportunities for drug treatment have been offered to some high-risk IV drug users as a means of risk reduction motivation—with varying degrees of success. For example, a coupon program in New Jersey offers free and expedited service for outpatient detoxification. More than three quarters of the coupons were redeemed within four months. However, such incentives for youth may not be as successful. Offering treatment to teens in general requires a very special focus, especially as a means to promote AIDS prevention. Since many of these potential clients are being taught life and coping skills for the first time, a more intensive process is recommended by many youth specialists. Additional treatment options are now being suggested for teen drug users, with programs providing more staff skilled in youth-specific concerns and allowing more time per client.

Peer groups: it is theorized that AIDS prevention may be amenable to self-help/mutual support concepts that are effective components in a myriad of circumstances. This technique applied to youth could be a powerful motivator. Opportunities for such group work are probably limited to treatment settings or interventions within the criminal justice system.

Voluntary antibody testing: following risk assessment and personal counseling about the validity of the tests, the meaning of different test results and the potential for different reactions, antibody testing is viewed by many as a powerful motivator to make required changes for prevention of HIV transmission.

However, limited information is available regarding the long-range impact of HIV antibody testing to sustain behavioral changes among drug abusers. Some studies indicate an eventual increase in usage despite knowledge of test results. Controversy in this area still prevails and leads us to view this option with extreme caution, especially when addressing the concerns of a highly vulnerable teen population.

Behavioral Changes (Behavioral Domain)

Careful tailoring of risk reduction recommendations to the conditions/needs of the target group seems to increase compliance behavior. For example, admonitions to change works-sharing practices must take into account the actual circumstance and perceived needs of the drug user subgroup. When sharing is deeply embedded in traditions and reinforced by the realities of paraphernalia and syringe-purchase regulations, works-cleaning may be successfully introduced—especially if regular "flushing" of works with water is already practiced to keep them unjammed. However, any new method needs to be quick, safe, effective, cheap and simple. Programs in San Francisco, Newark and Baltimore discovered that boiling is seldom practical as a disinfecting technique due to the time required as well as the potential to destroy plastic syringes. The YES Project in San Francisco has found, through careful behavioral analysis, that local IV drug users will carry and use small bottles of household bleach, labeled with simple instructions to "flush twice" in that solution and then in water.

In summary, risk reduction practices must be acceptable to and do-able by the target group.

Environmental Support for Sustaining Healthy Lifestyles

Risk reduction behavior, to be effective, must be practiced continuously and become part of the accepted lifestyle of the individual. AIDS prevention efforts have tried to do either of the following:

- encourage a "critical mass" of positive support for the desired behavior(s) in one's social network that reinforces the new lifestyle as normative and acceptable;
- change the larger environment's reaction to "undesirable" risk behavior—by more or less tolerance of the recognized activity—in the hope of reducing costs/risks to the larger group.

Successful examples of the first approach have been demonstrated nationwide within the gay community, by increasing the public commitment to reduce risk behavior and modeling social change. Such efforts are limited among a drug abusing population for a number of reasons discussed earlier. When we focus upon achieving such a shift among at-risk youth, the challenge is clear. However, perhaps to our advantage is the very characteristic of this population that makes them unique— their youth.

While still in their development stage, youth are often more easily influenced to change a behavior than adults. In addition to making use of positive reinforcement from peers, opportunities abound to create the level of support needed to sustain change through targeted interventions in other areas of an adolescent's normative environment including family, schools and other cultural influences and social institutions.

Changing the larger environment's level of tolerance to certain behaviors among this population may be a greater challenge due to the very youth of the population in question. As they are in a formative stage of development, there is undoubtedly less willingness on the part of society to allow such behaviors to continue if they are able to be reshaped.

In some locations where drug use is rampant and treatment services overflowing with waiting lists for admission, some prevention specialists advocate for legislation making clean syringes more available and decriminalizing syringe purchase or carrying. Although rarely specified, these hotly-debated issues traditionally have been waged within the framework applied to consenting adults. We can only assume they will prompt even more debate and controversy when applied to a population under 21.

Conclusion

AIDS prevention efforts targeted to youth present a challenge unlike any other this nation has faced. Sensitive issues abound and often result in enormous delays in taking action.

The IV drug component of HIV transmission among youth is a very real one. Prevention efforts with a focus on this mode of transmission are essential to reduce viral spread. Efforts undoubtedly must be undertaken by schools as an important setting in which to reach youth. However, message content will be limited primarily to drug abstinence in spite of active drug use (and viral transmission) continuing.

Aggressive, targeted outreach efforts conducted outside of traditional educational settings will probably be more effective in reaching youth most at-risk. Through these less traditional educational methods, more opportunities may be available to address the immediate concerns of viral transmission.

Interventions must be designed in a well-planned and target-specific fashion. Recognition of the ways in which learning and behaviors are shaped, influenced, changed and sustained is critical in this process. And as no one individual, adult or teen, operates in a vacuum, we must constantly look towards the environment in which we live as both a barrier and a promoter of the changes required to successfully reduce the further introduction and transmission of HIV within an adolescent population.

References

Davidson, J. 1988. AIDS panel chairman urges increase in spending, hiring to fight epidemic. *Wall Street Journal*. February 25.

Centers for Disease Control. 1988. *AIDS Weekly Surveillance Report*. February 8.

Des Jarlais, D.C. and Friedman, S. 1986. *AIDS among intravenous drug users: Current research in epidemiology, natural history and prevention strategies*. Prepared for the Committee on a National Strategy for AIDS, Institute of Medicine, National Academy of Sciences.

Haffner, D. 1987. *AIDS and adolescents: The time for prevention is now*. Washington, DC: Center for Population Options.

Koop, C.E. 1987. Statement before the Select Committee on Children, Youth and Families, United States House of Representatives. June 18.

Korcock, M. 1987. Teen's needs different. *The U.S. Journal of Drug and Alcohol Dependency* 11(5).

National Institute on Drug Abuse. 1987. *Unit I: The Challenge of AIDS. AIDS and the IV drug user: A training program for drug abuse counselors*. Washington, DC: Author.

National Institute on Drug Abuse. 1988a. *A model for AIDS prevention. AIDS and the IV Drug User: A Training Program for Drug Abuse Program Administrators*. Washington, DC: Author.

National Institute on Drug Abuse. 1988b. *Issues and strategies in AIDS prevention. AIDS and the IV drug user: A training program for drug abuse program administrators*. Washington, DC: Author.

New Jersey Women's Resource Panel on Substance Abuse. 1986. *Facts on children of substance abusers*. Trenton, NJ: Division of Narcotics and Drug Abuse Control.

Nurco, D., Cisnin, I. and Balter, M. 1982. Trends on the age of onset of narcotic addiction. *Chemical Dependencies: Behavior and Biomedical Issues* 4(3):221-228.

Selwyn, P., Cox, C., Feiner, C., Lipschutz, C. and Cohen, R. 1985. *Knowledge about AIDS and high-risk behavior among IV drug abusers in New York City*. Presented at the annual meeting of the American Public Health Association, Washington, DC.

22

HIV-Infected Students and Schools

An Interview with David L. Kirp, JD

Editors' Note:

Dr. Kirp's book in process, *The Kingdom Where Nobody Dies: Stories of AIDS and America's Children*, recounts how communities have responded to HIV-infected children in the public schools. The communities include Swansea, MA; New York, NY; Ocilla, GA; Atascadero, CA; Kokomo, IN; Wilmette, IL and Chicago, IL. The book examines how communities make decisions, and how leadership roles and community history affect the outcome.

Your book focuses on some of the different experiences communities have had in coping with HIV-infected children of school age. Why did you decide to focus on this aspect of the AIDS issue?

Kirp: In the fall of 1985 a high school student diagnosed with AIDS was admitted to school in Swansea, MA. This was one of the first times that had happened. A month earlier, Kokomo, IN had made headline news when it barred 13-year-old Ryan White from school. Swansea not only admitted the student; townspeople formed a group to help the boy's family deal with this issue.

I had been trying to understand how communities were coming to terms with AIDS. So I flew out to this town and spent ten days in Swansea, to see for myself why this town had invited this boy—this family—in.

It's not as if this was the perfect town—it isn't that there wasn't homophobia, or everyday petty jealousies going on. But this was a place where ordinary people were much better than they had to be.

What I saw in Swansea was a superintendent, Jack Mc-Carthy, whose reaction was not to panic, but to learn and try to shape the story, and eventually trust the community enough to open the issue up for discussion. What I saw was a community that could deal with its own panic and that had enough trust in the superintendent to cope with this.

The boy with AIDS, Mark (his last name wasn't revealed outside the community until his death), was a softball player, well-liked in town. And that fact—that you've got a real person you're talking about—affected how the town responded.

I was struck by how this small town school board—many of them were high school dropouts—stood up some months later and told panicky school board members from other Massachusetts towns that there was no reason to worry about having a child with AIDS in their schools.

The experience in Swansea led me to write the book: I wanted to learn something about what makes certain communities open their arms and others lift the drawbridge in these situations.

How many communities did you study?

Kirp: Seven. In geographic terms, they range from Swansea to Atascadero, CA, from Chicago and Wilmette, IL to Ocilla, GA. They begin with Kokomo and Swansea in 1985, an early point in most people's understanding of AIDS. This was the summer Rock Hudson was diagnosed with AIDS and for millions of people, the first time they learned about AIDS.

In contrast to Swansea's positive experience, were there communities that had a negative experience?

Kirp: There was Kokomo, IN, which kept Ryan White out of school and fought in the courts for nearly a year to keep him out. And there was Ocilla, GA. This little rural south Georgia town kept a child out of school for four months, and then admitted him only after considerable state pressure, fears of a lawsuit, and on condition that the child live apart from his mother. His mother carried the AIDS virus, but the boy himself didn't. So here is a town so panicked it can't even distinguish between having AIDS and carrying the virus, or living in a family where someone is infected.

When the superintendent there asked for advice, a public health doctor in Ocilla told him, "You want simple answers? I'll give you simple answers. If you don't have the AIDS virus, you can't give it to somebody." But that very simple message just didn't get through. Eventually, pressure—from the media and the state—got the child back in school. But the child is separated from his mother and family members are treated as outcasts.

So the town really won.

Kirp: Yes. And that raises what I think is a crucial factor here . What the school does when it announces it is admitting a student with AIDS matters much less than that the school be enthusiastic that this child is in school. If school officials are not supportive, there's trouble for the family, the child and the town. In cases where families have to "win" from the community in the courts, they obtain admission to school but they still haven't won acceptance. They're still isolated in the community.

Which is what happened in Arcadia, FL?

Kirp: Most dramatically in Arcadia. There, the Ray family sued to have their three elementary school age boys—all of whom have hemophilia and are HIV positive—admitted to school. The family's house was burned to the ground shortly after a U.S. District judge ordered the boys returned to school, and there is evidence of arson.

A similar thing happened in Kokomo, IN where Ryan White was admitted to school only after the family won a court case. A year later, the atmosphere was still so hostile that Ryan said, "I want to get out because I don't want to die in Kokomo." The family moved in the fall of 1987 to a town that has gone out of its way to welcome them.

In Atascadero, five-year-old Ryan Thomas returned to kindergarten only after the ACLU filed suit on his behalf against the school district and won. Life is so difficult that the family wants badly to leave, but can't afford to.

So legal victories aren't necessarily real victories?

Kirp: That's right. In a town where panic has taken over, for whatever reason, it's a blessing that we have a system of laws that people can rely on. But courts can't settle the human issues.

You don't win people over by forcing them to admit a child to school through the courts. And this really is a concern: you're asking people to take a minuscule but nonetheless real chance with their children's lives. It's hard to find a substitute for talking through an issue that's so serious.

Otherwise, parents who don't want the child in question to attend school and then lose in court feel that matters have been taken out of their hands, decided by strangers for reasons they don't understand. There's a degree of resentment and truculence. The community doesn't participate in the court case; the people who lose say "Okay, but..."

In places where people have a chance to talk out their concerns, those who are uncomfortable with enrolling a youngster usually come around when they learn the facts. When a community decides to make a gift of its own trust and openness to this child, what follows is not only acceptance, but fund drives and cake sales; people turn around completely. The experience allows their passion to find an outlet.

What explains the range of responses to AIDS in the different communities—why does one community succeed in working together to resolve the issue while another becomes embroiled in a struggle?

Kirp: One thing I've learned is that stereotypes don't apply. The issue isn't liberal/conservative, it isn't black/white, it isn't rich/poor, it isn't north/south. What's crucial is the leadership, how medical knowledge gets communicated, and how the community has dealt with sensitive issues in the past—its history.

So you find a superintendent in liberal Carmel, CA persuading a family to keep their nine-year-old son out of school on the implausible theory that the other kids are going to turn on him. And you have Swansea, which is far from a liberal community, going way beyond just admitting a child to school to building a network of care, a group called "Friends of Mark" to raise money, take food to the family, and the like. What this really comes down to is an issue of community, of taking care of their own.

You mentioned leadership as a pivotal issue. Would that quality come from those already involved with the schools—superintendents, parents, teachers, principals, board members?

Kirp: The most obvious leader is the superintendent. He or she shapes the agenda to an extraordinary extent. Particularly if a relationship of trust has been built up, people in the community can be won over by the example set by the superintendent.

The superintendent can marshal the evidence to help people work through their fears, choose which doctors will present the medical picture, deal with the media, meet with people in the community, win over teachers, talk to church groups. All these things wind up being crucial.

Is this what happened in Swansea?

Kirp: Swansea's a good example. The town was small enough that everybody knew Superintendent Jack McCarthy. They'd had him as a coach; they'd had him as an English teacher; they'd known him, some of them, for thirty years. And he told the community: "Let's stay on the high road if we can."

Is there a another community where this model has been effective?

Kirp: Wilmette, IL in 1987 offers a textbook example of how leadership can work. (See page 309 for the strategies recommended by Wilmette's Superintendent.) In Wilmette the child was much younger. The community is different—it's an upper middle class Chicago suburb, very WASP-y, liberal Republican in its politics. Its public schools are the pride and joy of the community.

What distinguishes Wilmette is how spectacularly well-organized school officials—the board and the administrators—were. They had developed an AIDS policy beforehand. When the parents of a child who was HIV-positive notified the principal, the principal notified the superintendent and the system went into action. School officials immediately set up an AIDS hotline. AIDS information materials were pretested: a packet was sent to all parents, but only after a group of teachers and administrators reviewed the information. Even the experts who would meet with parents were prescreened.

The planning and implementation were extraordinary: everything was orchestrated, from the media contacts to discussions with pastors in town, who delivered sermons on AIDS the

Sunday after the story went public. They also got the benefit of some unplanned, "dumb-luck" things: one of the experts who talked at the public meetings was a doctor who was eight-months pregnant. Her presence implicitly said to parents, "How much of a risk could this be, if I am willing to be here?"

Wilmette also protected the privacy of the child and the family. Officials could say, "This family is really very brave because they came forward," and that was important, too—that the family had a sense of trust in the community.

So you believe the process will be more successful if the superintendent takes a leadership role, supporting and endorsing the presence of the student in school?

Kirp: Yes. Supportive leadership is not only morally wise and medically sound, it's also politically smart. If I were going to present a plan to a superintendent, I would suggest very strongly that those who have led in a way that allowed a child with HIV infection to remain in school are the ones who have succeeded—who afterwards have been praised by their constituents. And those who haven't wind up losing and feeling let down by the community they've led along and ultimately can't control.

Can you give an example?

Kirp: In Kokomo, the superintendent listened to all the parents around him saying, "No way." He took an "anti" position and got caught up in that popular sentiment—he basically abdicated to the mob.

What about not letting the community know there's an HIV infected child in school?

Kirp: Some administrators say, "We're not going to tell anyone about this, we're just going to do it." But that's hard, as a practical matter. If the strategy is going to work, the child's family has to keep it a secret, the child has to keep it a secret, anyone who knows or works with the child has to keep it a secret. This is asking a lot from people. Eventually, the secret is likely to slip out.

And I think people are entitled to know. They don't have a right to know the name of the child. But AIDS is so powerful and so new an issue that parents need to talk it through for themselves, so that they feel, in the end, that they've been part of something that really isn't just a routine bureaucratic decision. This isn't an issue where people are inclined to go along with whatever those in charge decide. It really becomes an issue of trust. And the best model of leadership is one that invites participation and shapes that participation to allow people to work through their fears—eventually to connect with their own feelings of compassion and caring.

If a community is forced by court order to admit a student, does that take some of the responsibility away from the district?

Kirp: Yes, and there are school boards in this legalistic age who want to be sued, because they believe it gets them off the hook on the liability issue. And some administrators believe a lawsuit is a "no lose" situation. If they win, they don't enroll the child. And if they lose in court, no one can blame school officials.

But those administrators are ignoring the impact of a lawsuit on a community. That's why "go ahead and sue us" is the antithesis of real leadership.

What about other people in leadership roles—what about the principal?

Kirp: The superintendent is the public figure who appears on TV, talks with the assembly. The principal is the personal link with the teachers and the staff—the people in the kitchen who wash the dishes, the janitors who mop up the vomit. The principal has to reassure the people he or she works with; and their help is needed in dealing with parents.

304

Kirp

The principal needs to be both a source of information and a source of caring—the person everyone can go to with their problems. The person who talks to classes if teachers want that, or arranges for an expert to talk. That's what happens when the principal is the leader among the cadre of teachers and staff— it's what happened in Wilmette and, later, in two Chicago city schools. The principal can also be a locus of trust for parents.

What about community organizers affiliated with the schools?

Kirp: In a politicized community, the schools are often at the heart of local politics. A principal in a such a community knows that to be effective he or she has to build a web of alliances with community leaders. And parents in a political community have probably cared about the schools and been involved for years. In this kind of situation, community organizers can call on that network of people who will naturally have a voice in the AIDS issue.

Community organizers play an important part because they are closer to parents than the superintendent. They're putting their credentials on the line in a very direct and personal way, making what becomes a really powerful statement. They're saying to parents, "Trust me, it's okay."

So which leadership roles are pivotal really depends on the community?

Kirp: The history of relationships in a community matters. You can't invent the sort of leadership we're talking about. In some places, the superintendent is the connection with the community, in some it's the principal. If there isn't a structured community organization, a good one isn't likely to be invented solely because of AIDS. The AIDS issue plays on existing histories—of the superintendent, of the principal—and in the process the real nature of the community emerges. And if there isn't a community—in the sense of people caring for one an-

305

other, that comes out too.

Could someone on a school board take a leadership position?

Kirp: If you want to understand almost anything about American institutions and how they behave, AIDS is a good place to look. School boards and superintendents have long histories. Sometimes the superintendent leads, the school board says yes. AIDS will probably be treated that way if that's the relationship that exists.

Elsewhere, there are ongoing struggles for leadership between the superintendent and the school board. And these tensions will probably surface in any situation having to do with AIDS.

Then there are school boards who work side by side with the superintendent to plan strategy and establish policy. That was certainly true in Wilmette: the chair of the board was a member of a public relations firm that does a lot of crisis management. That gave Wilmette access to his valuable professional experience when the AIDS crisis arose.

In most places, there is some give and take in the relationships among the key figures. The superintendent, for instance, can decide whether to play it safe or take a risk, or a school board chair can decide to push for an active role or sit back and let the superintendent take the lead. Community organizers or the PTA can opt to run meetings, speak out and encourage parents to participate, or they can absent themselves from the issue. The ideal situation is one in which all these groups and individuals are talking with one another and connecting, so there's a reinforcement of what's going on.

How is AIDS different from other issues?

Kirp: AIDS brings up powerful dilemmas. We're not used to that. Usually we go along with the decisions of school boards and administrators, leaving them a broad zone of discretion.

And then all of a sudden there's this issue that's just fraught with moral consequences. It's publicity and it's attention and it's anxiety—it's even life and death.

And the trick in these cases, I think, is for people to be in touch with their own feelings, to acknowledge their fears and push past them, so they can learn what the facts and myths are about AIDS.

Each person has to go through this process individually—to negotiate his or her fears, to become desensitized to phobias—then to begin to understand the need for compassion and want to help others. For any would-be leaders, it's really a two-step process: first deal with the fear, the "What's going to happen to me? What's going to happen to my kids?" Then look at, "What can I do to help?" This holds true at the community level as well.

What about the media's role? Is there a tendency for the media not to report the successful cases?

Kirp: Absolutely. What you hear about are burning houses. Asheville, NC admitted a child with ARC to school—peacefully and uneventfully—at exactly the same time the Ray family was driven out of Arcadia. Asheville got zero publicity outside North Carolina; Arcadia was reported all over the place. It's not that Arcadia doesn't matter, but it's not the entire story. The tales the media tell are going to affect how other towns cope in the future.

What kinds of things can school districts do in advance, even if they don't have HIV-infected students that they know of?

Kirp: Districts should realize that many of them now enroll HIV-infected students, even if they don't know who the students are. The issue isn't someone else's—it's theirs.

AIDS education means taking people through the steps of confronting fears, learning facts and understanding compassion. That means videos and discussions for parents and teachers. It means bringing in experts who can talk about the issues at a level people can understand and feel comfortable with. It means sending materials home with kids—ideally materials interesting enough that parents won't just toss them. And talking about AIDS in school makes it something that can be talked about—talk desensitizes it, demystifies it.

Education entails diminishing the element of dread associated with AIDS. At some point in the future, if such talking takes hold, AIDS can become just another disease—a taken-for-granted risk in our lives.

Suggested Strategies
for Public School Systems

William P. Gussner, PhD
Superintendent, Wilmette Public Schools
Wilmette, IL

Editors' Note:
In March of 1988, Dr. Gussner testified on the Wilmette experience before the Presidential Commission on the Human Immunodeficiency Virus Epidemic. The following recommendations are adapted from his testimony.

1. **Establish a district, board-developed policy for guiding the decision-making process *before* a case arises.** The policy should be general in nature, flexible and deal with all chronic communicable diseases. It should allow for the use of different strategies depending upon the unique nature of each case and the rapidly changing research, litigation and legislation.
2. **Respect the privacy rights of the student or employee who is infected.** Any policy should assure that once an employee or student with HIV infection notifies the school system, he or she is allowed to continue in the system to maintain individual confidentiality. Each case should be analyzed *thoroughly* prior to any decision regarding exclusion.
3. **Appoint an administrative committee** to review each case on an individual basis and serve as a decision-making committee.
4. **Select legal and medical consultants** who are known

within the community and are recognized experts in the field. If there are no AIDS experts in the community, use attorneys and medical doctors from the community with the authority to consult with experts in the field.

5. As soon as possible after notification, **identify those individuals who have a "need to know"** the identity of the student or employee with HIV infection. This group should consist only of those who work on a regular daily basis with the child or employee, and might include the principal, school nurse, primary teacher and social worker. This small "need to know" team should review decisions as they are being made.

6. **Develop, in advance, a system for informing members of the Board of Education** when a case comes up. It is preferable that the Board be notified face-to-face rather than by written memo.

7. In making decisions, **follow the best medical and legal advice available** and make sure decisions fall under the guidelines developed by the Centers for Disease Control (See Appendix B).

8. **Form a monitoring team** to meet on an ongoing basis after the Board decision to review all aspects of the case. (Wilmette's Monitoring Team meets once a month.) This team will keep apprised of any changes in legislation, litigation or medical research that could affect the decision.

9. **Develop communications that are sensitive to the individual involved and completely open and candid.** When developing communication strategies, involve the legal and medical consultants, the administrative committee, the Board of Education, the "need to know" team and the individual or family.

10. **Educate personnel on how the disease is transmitted.** Encourage them to express their concerns and anxieties and to

talk with key decision makers and experts.

11. **Offer support to all individuals involved**, whether employees, parents or children, who have difficulty with the decision. Support might include individual consultation and counseling, if required.

12. **Hold meetings to educate the community about Board decisions.** Include parents, public officials, clergy, pediatricians, students and media representatives.

13. **Develop and disseminate age-appropriate educational materials about the disease.** If possible, invite medical experts to explain the materials to students and answer questions.

14. **Credit all who contribute** as a team to successfully resolving the situation, particularly the family who had the courage to trust their problem to public officials.

15. **Protect all students and employees**, but especially the person with infection who is susceptible to other diseases, and make certain that parents or employees facing a similar problem in the future can have the confidence to ask the support of public officials.

Minority Populations:

AIDS Risks and Prevention

Minority Populations: AIDS Risks and Prevention

Gilberto R. Gerald

AIDS is disproportionately affecting People of Color, particularly in the Black and Hispanic communities. New studies continue to underline this issue with the passage of time. Native American and Asian communities are at a disadvantage in quantifying and analyzing the incidence of AIDS because the statistics on cases from those communities are lumped into one statistical category of "other" by the Centers for Disease Control. But cases have been reported from these two population groups, indicating a need for prevention activities to stop the spread while the numbers are still low.

The Centers for Disease Control's *AIDS Weekly Surveillance Report* shows that while Blacks make up only 12 percent of the nation's population, they consistently comprise 25 percent of all people with AIDS. Similarly it shows that while Hispanics make up 8 percent of the general population, they represent 14 percent of all people with AIDS. More startling is the fact that Black and Hispanic children represent 76 percent of all children with AIDS, and that Black women constitute 52 percent of all women with AIDS.

The AIDS health crisis exacerbates the underlying poor health and poor socioeconomic conditions among America's racial and ethnic minorities. AIDS is not the only health issue inordinately impacting minority communities. The failure of the health system to close the gaps that exist generally between the health of Whites and that of Blacks and Hispanics is well documented.

The *Report of the Secretary's Task Force on Black and Minority Health,* in January 1986, indicated that there are an average of 60,000 annual excess deaths—deaths that should not occur—among Blacks, as compared to Whites, due to heart disease and stroke, homicide and accidents, cancer, infant mortality, cirrhosis, and diabetes. Clearly the design of AIDS prevention and education programs for minorities must consider the failure of disease prevention activities in general in minority communities.

In addressing the issue of AIDS prevention in the context of minority youth one must also consider the failures of institutions to address adequately the problems of higher teen pregnancy rates, alcohol and drug use, and alarmingly high rates of sexually transmitted diseases.

We can also see differences in the way the virus is being transmitted in different populations. The differences are attributed to socioeconomic, not genetic, factors, and they suggest the need for a greater variety of strategies to affect a range of behaviors that place people at risk in minority communities. For example, while 80 percent of the cases among Whites nationally occur among gay and bisexual men, this is true for only 39 percent of the Black cases and 48 percent of the Hispanic cases. Conversely only 6 percent of the White cases of AIDS occur among IV drug users compared to 36 percent among both Black and Hispanic AIDS cases. Educational messages in minority communities must therefore emphasize and address a broader set of risk behaviors.

Understanding what behaviors are placing minorities at risk for AIDS requires careful analysis at the local level. National statistics do not begin to explain fully where local priorities need to be placed. There are significant differences between one region or geographical location and another in the way the virus is being transmitted from one person to another. There is a tendency to equate AIDS education and prevention in minority populations only with efforts targeted at curbing IV drug use as a means of transmission. This is dangerous since it can occur at the expense of addressing sexual transmission of the virus, particularly if this requires acknowledging homosexuality.

Although the percentage of gay and bisexual cases of AIDS among Blacks and Hispanics is proportionately lower than it is for Whites, it is still significant. Programs must be designed to address the need to protect this group from infection. This reality is complicated by their invisibility and by the fact that many do not self-identify as gay or bisexual even though they may engage in sex with other males. Their sense of identity is often more closely tied to their race or ethnic grouping than it is to any particular sexual behavior. Messages targeted to individuals who are self-identified as gay or bisexual will tend to be ignored by many gay or bisexual minority men. But it would be wrong to assume that for minority youth the issue of safer sex behavior between males is not an issue.

It is preferable to speak only of risk behaviors and not of risk groups when engaging in AIDS prevention and education activities. The AIDS-causing virus, HIV, infects humans without regard to race, ethnic background or sexual preference. Specific sexual practices and needle-sharing behaviors put individuals at risk for contracting or transmitting the AIDS virus.

The more we emphasize the capacity each individual has for transmitting the virus because of specific risk behaviors, the less likely the battle against the disease will continue to be complicated by prejudice and discrimination directed at specific population groups, whether gay and bisexual, Black, Hispanic, Asian, or Native American. The object is to wage a winning campaign against the virus, not against groups of people.

It is important to recall this goal of focusing on risk behaviors rather than risk groups when addressing the issue of AIDS and ethnic minority populations. It is the potential added stigma of AIDS that preoccupies minorities in responding to the crisis. There is significant resistance within Black and Hispanic communities to terming AIDS a "Black" or "Hispanic" problem despite the relatively higher incidence of the disease in these communities. The concern is well founded. Even without AIDS, ethnic minority populations, because of racism and poverty, are at considerable risk for discrimination in the workplace, in housing, in places of public accommodation, in schools, and in health care. Religious values within minority communities also play a significant role in distancing communities and institutions from an issue so closely associated with homosexuality.

Given this overall caveat of emphasizing risk behaviors, it is important in designing a prevention and information program that we recognize the diversity of American communities and target education and prevention not only in terms of addressing risk behaviors, but also in terms of racial, ethnic, socioeconomic groupings, and according to the age and level of education of the intended audience.

Everyone has an equal right to life-saving information about health care and disease prevention. But this information cannot be conveyed equally and effectively to everyone in the same way. The socioeconomic and cultural diversity of American communities requires that AIDS prevention and information be culturally sensitive and linguistically appropriate.

One of the most significant issues to be considered in developing prevention programs for minorities is having community control over the program messages. Having access to resources to develop prevention and education programs is a related concern. A glaring problem with many existing messages and images about AIDS is the invisibility of People of Color—they simply have been omitted from the picture. The impact of seeing a Person of Color with AIDS delivering an AIDS prevention message is rarely appreciated by someone outside the community.

Neither Black, nor Hispanic, nor Asian, nor Native American communities are monolithic. There is great diversity within each. Hispanics, for example, identify themselves by nationalities and by region of residence. There are significant colloquial differences between the language spoken by Puerto Ricans in the Northeast and Chicanos in the Southwest. Messages intended to impact members of Hispanic communities cannot be approached generically. A literal translation of English materials into Spanish can be irrelevant and ineffective for communicating to many Hispanics.

The best resources for developing prevention strategies in minority communities are members of the communities themselves. They, more than the best-intentioned outsider, understand the language and cultural norms that must be taken into account to effect behavior change in a specific community. The idea is not new with the AIDS crisis. White gay men have created effective messages precisely because of community control over those messages.

A reading of this section will underscore the need for utilizing human resources and talents from within minority populations in addressing the AIDS issue. Any approach to prevention that does not first recognize this need will be extremely deficient and uncaring from the start. Those approaches that do come forth from the communities themselves have a much greater chance of accomplishing our goal—the prevention of AIDS.

The Epidemiology of AIDS in Hispanic Adolescents

**Kenneth G. Castro, MD,
and Susan B. Manoff, MD**

I n the United States, the epidemic of acquired immunodeficiency syndrome (AIDS) is caused by a human retrovirus known as human immunodeficiency virus (HIV) (Fauci, 1988; Curran et al., 1988). This virus is transmitted from person to person through sexual contact, exposure to blood or blood components contaminated with HIV, and perinatally (Curran et al., 1988). The period between infection with HIV and development of AIDS is long and variable, with a predicted mean incubation estimated to be over 7 years (Curran et al., 1988).

Adolescence is a developmental stage characterized by concrete thinking, risk-taking behavior, and experimentation, particularly in the areas of sexual and drug use behavior. Adolescents are thus likely to be at risk for HIV infection and may respond to AIDS education messages differently than adults. This section will describe the epidemiology of AIDS in Hispanic adolescents and discuss areas for targeted or focused

Table 1
AIDS Cases and Cumulative Incidence (CI) per Million by Age Group, May 2, 1988

Age Group (years)	Hispanic		Other	
	No. Cases	CI/million	No. Cases	CI/million
<1-9	204	57.6	715	24.0
10-14	6	3.6	51	3.0
15-19	43	24.2	193	9.9
20-24	459	267.6	2254	114.2
≥25	7996	1068.1	48931	388.2
Total	8708	538.7	52144	246.0

HIV prevention programs.

Methods

Computerized AIDS case-report forms received at the Centers for Disease Control (CDC) through May 2, 1988 were analyzed. Demographic variables were reviewed to obtain the number of Hispanic adolescents and young adults with AIDS. We considered adolescents (15 to 19 years) and young adults (20 to 24 years) because of the long incubation for AIDS. Young adults aged 20 to 24 years at AIDS diagnosis probably became infected with HIV as adolescents. To calculate cumulative incidence, the number of persons with AIDS was divided by the corresponding population group obtained from the 1980 census. Age groups of persons with AIDS were arranged to conform to the 5-year age groups listed by the census.

Results

Through May 2, 1988, 60,852 persons with AIDS were reported to CDC. Of these 8,708 (14 percent) were Hispanics residing in the United States, for an AIDS cumulative incidence of 538.7 per million. This rate is 2.2 times higher than the 246.0 per million cumulative incidence for all other persons with AIDS (Table 1). Five hundred two AIDS cases were reported in Hispanics aged 15 to 24 years, for an estimated cumulative incidence of 143.8 per million, compared with 62.3 per million for other persons with AIDS in the same age group. The number of 15- to 24-year-old Hispanic persons with AIDS has increased continuously by year of diagnosis (Figure 1).

Of those 502 persons, 421 (84 percent) are male. Transmission categories are shown by gender in Table 2. The majority of

Table 2
Number and Percentage of AIDS Cases in Hispanics Age 15-24 Years, by Gender and Transmission Category May 2, 1988

Transmission Category	Male No. (%)		Female No. (%)		Total No. (%)	
Homosexual/bisexual male	217	(52)	0		217	(43)
Homosexual/bisexual male and IV-drug abuser	48	(11)	0		48	(10)
Heterosexual IV-drug abuser	119	(28)	42	(52)	161	(32)
Heterosexual contact with:						
IV-drug abuser	1	(<1)	22	(27)	23	(5)
Bisexual male	0		4	(5)	4	(<1)
Other*	2	(<1)	0		2	(<1)
Coagulation disorder	14	(3)	0		14	(3)
Recipient, blood transfusion	2	(<1)	6	(7)	8	(2)
Undetermined	18	(4)	7	(9)	25	(5)
Total	421	(100)	81	(100)	502	(101)**

*Includes sexual contact with AIDS patient and with person born in country where heterosexual HIV transmission plays a major role.

**Total not 100% due to rounding.

males (63 percent) were homosexual or bisexual, including 11 percent who also reported intravenous (IV)-drug abuse. Most (79 percent) of the adolescent and young adult female Hispanics with AIDS were IV-drug abusers or sex partners of male IV-drug abusers. A smaller proportion (5 percent) were sex partners of bisexual males. Compared with white non-Hispanic persons with AIDS in the same age group, a significantly larger proportion of heterosexual Hispanic persons with AIDS had used drugs intravenously (9 percent vs. 32 percent, P<0.001).

The geographic distribution and transmission categories of the 502 15- to 24-year-old Hispanic persons with AIDS are shown in Table 3. More than 72 percent of these resided in five states (California, Florida, New Jersey, New York and Texas). An additional 15 percent resided in Puerto Rico. In these states and territory, at least 76 percent of adolescent and young adult Hispanic persons with AIDS reported homosexuality, bisexuality, IV-drug abuse, or heterosexual contact with someone at risk for HIV infection. In New York and Puerto Rico, a significantly higher proportion of AIDS cases has been reported in heterosexual IV-drug abusers (43 percent and 58 percent, respectively), than in other states (P<0.001 in each). In contrast, there is a higher proportion of homosexual and bisexual males with AIDS among Hispanics aged 15 to 24 years in California, Florida and Texas. For 5 percent of the 502 patients, the mode of transmission was undetermined; however, 11 percent of the patients residing outside California, Florida, New Jersey, New York, Texas and Puerto Rico belonged to this group, which consisted of seven persons with incomplete or unobtainable information.

The proportion of AIDS cases in Hispanics that was attributable to sexual contact, IV-drug abuse, or transfusion of blood or blood products is summarized for two age groups in figure 2. In persons aged 15 to 19 years, 21 percent of HIV-1 infection

Table 3
Percentage of AIDS Cases in Hispanics Age 15-24 Years by Selected States/Territories and Transmission Category, May 2 1988

Percentage by State/Territory

Transmission Category	CALIFORNIA (N=86)	FLORIDA (N=19)	NEW JERSEY (N=29)	NEW YORK (N=191)	TEXAS (N=38)	PUERTO RICO (N=74)	ELSEWHERE (N=65)	TOTAL (N=502)
Homosexual/bisexual male	67	63	48	36	63	20	40	43
Homosexual/bisexual male and IV-drug abuser	15	16	0	5	13	16	9	10
Heterosexual IV-drug abuser	8	11	31	43	0	58	26	32
Heterosexual contact	0	0	14	9	0	3	8	6
Coagulation disorder	2	5	3	1	13	0	6	3
Recipient blood transfusion	3	0	0	1	8	0	0	2
Undetermined	3	5	3	5	3	3	11	5
TOTAL	98*	100	99*	100	100	100	100	101*

*Total not 100% due to rounding

and AIDS was probably due to transfusion of blood or blood products, while 74 percent were probably due to sexual contact or sharing contaminated needles during IV-drug use. Three percent of young adult persons with AIDS received transfusions of blood or blood products, while 92 percent probably were infected through sexual contact or during IV-drug abuse.

Comment

Compared to the proportion of the Hispanic population in the United States, AIDS has been disproportionately overrepresented in Hispanics, including Hispanic youth. The epidemiologic characteristics of these patients identify the main areas that must be addressed to prevent HIV infection in U.S. Hispanics. Specific knowledge of HIV transmission patterns and their geographic variation will help focus the prevention programs and strategies accordingly. In Puerto Rico and those northern states with many young Hispanic persons with AIDS, infection is mostly attributable to IV-drug abuse and heterosexual contact. In contrast, homosexual or bisexual contact seems to cause a larger proportion of AIDS in young Hispanics residing in California, Florida and Texas. Although most of the adolescent and young Hispanics with AIDS are male, the number of females with AIDS continues to increase. Those females who abuse IV-drugs or are the sex partners of male IV-drug abusers are at highest risk of contracting HIV infection and AIDS. Finally, although 5 percent of Hispanic persons with AIDS age 15 to 24 years did not fit the recognized transmission categories, most have incomplete or missing information. Our investigations of such cases demonstrate that when follow-up information is obtained, the majority of these persons represent likely instances of sexual and IV-drug-related HIV transmis-

Figure 1
Number of AIDS Cases in Hispanics Age 15-24 Years by Year of Diagnosis, 1981-1987

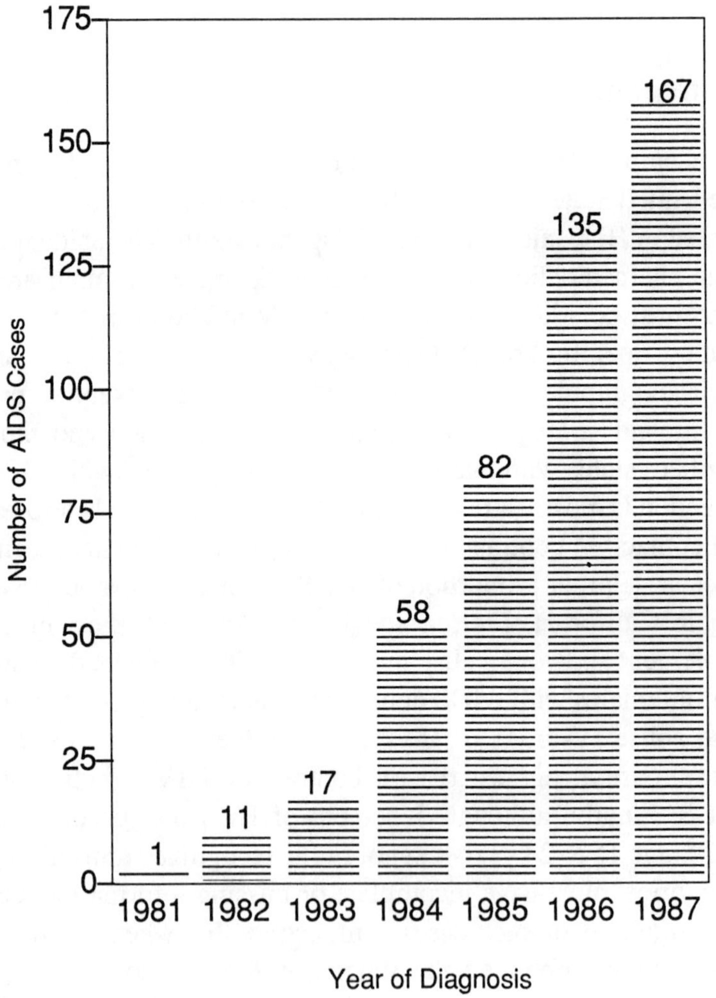

sion (Castro et al., 1988). Thus, the larger proportion of such cases occurring outside California, Florida, New Jersey, New York, Texas and Puerto Rico is likely to change once investigations are completed.

In general, existing programs aimed at preventing HIV transmission through transfusion of blood or blood products should significantly reduce new HIV infections. However, the impact of these programs in reducing the number of AIDS cases may not be noticeable for a number of years because of the long incubation period for AIDS. Anticipatedly, effective programs to prevent IV-drug-related and sexual transmission of HIV should reduce most of the AIDS-related morbidity and mortality in adolescent and young adult Hispanics. Thus, it is imperative that HIV and AIDS information and education be available to these youngsters by early adolescence.

Acknowledgments
We thank Dr. Martha Rogers for review of the manuscript, Dr. Richard Selik for assistance with the data analysis, Timothy J. Bush for assistance with the computer graphics, and Karen Foster for editorial assistance.

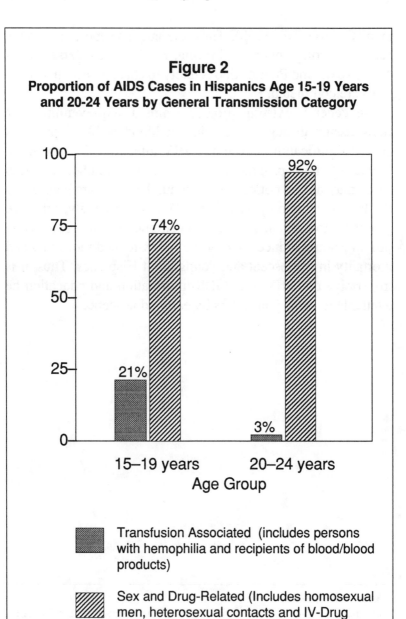

Figure 2
Proportion of AIDS Cases in Hispanics Age 15-19 Years and 20-24 Years by General Transmission Category

References

Castro, K.G., Lifson, A.R., White, C.R. et al. 1988. Investigations of AIDS patients with no previously identified risk factors. *Journal of the American Medical Association* 259:1338-1342.

Curran, J.W., Jaffe, H.W., Hardy, A.M., Morgan, W.M., Selik, R.M. and Dondero, T.J. 1988. Epidemiology of HIV infection and AIDS in the United States. *Science* 239:610-616.

Fauci, A.S. 1988. The human immunodeficiency virus: Infectivity and mechanisms of pathogenesis. *Science* 239:617-622.

24

Developing Innovative AIDS Prevention Programs for Latino Youth

Ana Consuelo Matiella, MA

A Personal Note

As I write this I cannot help but feel anger and remorse about the whole AIDS crisis and still find myself in the "Why us?" stage. So before I can be more positive and solution-oriented, allow me to vent some anger and say, "Here is another thing that we as Latinos have to worry about. Not only is it appalling that we disproportionately face some of the most serious, life-threatening health conditions in this country (i.e., diabetes, heart disease, drug abuse, hypertension) but we now also have to face up to the battle against AIDS! Ave Maria Purisima!"

I have been asked to write about how we are successfully educating our children about AIDS...our children. From the point of view of a Latina mother I take a painful look and acknowledge that a large number of our adolescent children are living in the streets, living on their wits, coping with life by engaging in high-risk behaviors.

In their chapter "The Epidemiology of AIDS in Hispanic Adolescents," Drs. Castro and Manoff of the Centers for Disease Control have provided a stark overview of the current situation: 502 Hispanic persons with AIDS ages 15-24 as of May 2, 1988. This is more than twice the rate for the general population. (See Chapter 23.)

There is obviously great concern among health professionals, educators and program planners as to how the AIDS virus will impact the adolescent population in the United States. There is unanimous agreement that, unfortunately, Latino and Black youth will be the most drastically affected.

Reaching high risk Latino and Black youth poses a special challenge because a significant percentage of minority youth are not in school nor in the job market, and often do not come in contact with traditional social systems until they are adjudicated and/or incarcerated.

This chapter will first explore some general cultural considerations that should be incorporated into the preliminary phases of planning education and prevention programs for Latinos; second it will summarize four innovative AIDS prevention programs targeting Latino high risk youth in four different cities in the United States; and third it will discuss the development of innovative educational materials using already established and accepted Latin American popular culture mediums.

Cultural Considerations

The Latino population in the United States is a diverse one. The population differs and the educational needs and motivators differ accordingly.

The Census Bureau and other government entities have grouped Latinos in the category of "Hispanic," for ease of access. There is resistance on the part of many Latinos to accept this label because, although it is a commendable attempt, the label overlooks the rich diversity of our separate cultures and (almost) denies our Indian and African ancestry. The term Latino will be used in this chapter because I believe this is the term that not only acknowledges our Spanish roots but also acknowledges our indigenous roots in the cultures of Latin America and Africa.

It is important to keep in mind that Latinos come from different economic and political realities, diverse geographic locations within the United States, and different countries of origin. We can be brown, black or white.

However, Latinos are bonded together by some *general* cultural traits that are worth mentioning: the use of the Spanish language for the monolingual and the continued desire and conscious decision to retain the use of Spanish for the bilingual; a strong Catholic tradition; conservative moral and social values; and traditional personal roles (Guernica and Kasperuk 1982).

The cultural issues surrounding the challenge of educating Latino adolescents about AIDS are very delicate in the context of the Latino family's values and beliefs. The family is the most important and most influential force in Latino life. In the best of all possible program plans, when designing a program targeting Latino youth, there should always be a family component in which family members are encouraged to participate in the planning and take part in the education process.

The concept of sexuality education in general is very gradually gaining acceptance among Latino families. Most Latino parents still consider information about such private matters as sex should be taught at home or not at all. It is especially difficult for young women to obtain reliable information. In an effort to protect young women from the "threats" of the outside world, young Latinas are shielded from sexuality information. For young men it may be somewhat easier, especially if the young man has an older brother, uncles, older cousins, or padrinos (godparents) that they can have "man-to-man" talks with.

School-based sexuality education programs are becoming more accepted among some Latino families but among more traditional families it may still be considered inappropriate. The importance of considering and incorporating Latino family values in the design and implementation of AIDS education efforts for Latino youth is again emphasized. The risks of not doing so are the alienation and further disempowerment of the Latino family in what should be considered an important community effort.

A word about homosexuality: homosexuality among many Latinos is generally considered something to be ashamed of. Because of this strong value, it is a taboo topic that is not discussed openly or is the object of jokes. A man who has sex with a man will probably not label himself as homosexual or bisexual. When targeting Latino young men in an education effort, therefore, it is advisable to address the high risk behavior. (For an interesting discussion on this subject, see "Latino Community Services," *NAN Multicultural Notes* 1:2, July 1987.)

In regards to designing effective educational materials, it is important that they be high interest, make maximum use of pictures and illustrations, and be developed at a low reading level. Translating English materials into Spanish is not enough. The information needs to be appropriate to the educational needs of the target population. Translations are considered by many Latino health professionals and consumers as ineffective short cuts. The task of educating already underserved Latinos about

AIDS is too important to merely translate existing materials that are most likely written at inappropriately high reading levels in English and then translated to equally as high or higher level Spanish. Simple pictorial materials with low readability will prove to be much more effective in reaching Latinos in general and Latino youth specifically.

There are two final and vital recommendations for designing effective and culturally appropriate prevention programs and resources. First, identify the specific group and high risk behaviors to be targeted in each community. Keep in mind that different urban regional areas have different needs and problems. A case in point from Drs. Castro and Manoff is data reflecting regional variations in how young people are being exposed to HIV. A larger number of young Latino AIDS cases in the northern states and Puerto Rico have been attributed to IV drug use and heterosexual contact, while in California, Texas and Florida there are more cases related to men having sex with men.

Second, include the target group in planning and implementation. It is of utmost importance that Latino youth education programs be designed and implemented with their direct involvement at the specific level in which the services are being provided.

Four Model Programs Targeting Latino Youth in the United States

The following four model programs were chosen because they involved Latino youth in planning and implementation and because they have met with documented and cost effective success.

The Pilsen Catholic Youth Center
AIDS Peer Education Project

The Pilsen Catholic Youth Center (PCYC) is located in the Pilsen section of Chicago, an area that is 85 percent Mexican American. The Center was originally founded to offer an alternative to youth gang activity, to assist the area's youth in achieving personal development, and to educate them on their responsibilities as citizens and Christians.

In October of 1987 the PCYC received one of five national grants from the U.S. Conference of Mayors to implement an AIDS Peer Education Project. The project targets high school age teens and their parents with a series of "talks" in schools, churches and community settings. Eight high school senior volunteers were initially trained as peer educators with AIDS prevention information. Although the project only started in November of 1987, by April of 1988, these eight teens had reached over 500 people.

The Pilsen project targets families of high risk teens by offering parent talks usually facilitated by one adult and one teen. Many of the parents that attend these talks are parents of youth who are out of school and already involved in gang activity. Because many of them realize the risks their sons and daughters are taking, they come so they can learn strategies for passing on AIDS information. One of the approaches the Pilsen Center staff and peer educators have found helpful is to have the information communicated in a language usually considered the sole domain of young people. Altagracia Perez, the Associate Director of PCYC states, "though some young people are surprised to hear this 'street talk' in an educational setting, we find that it is sometimes the only way to insure that the information is being understood." Ms. Perez reports that there has been resistance on the part of Latino parents to accept the street talk, but she contends that with young people who are not academically sophisticated and are involved in high risk behavior, it is still the most effective approach.

In addition to the peer education talks, the teens are involved in designing and writing their own promotional and educational materials. These resources are being developed for young people by young people and are expected to be culturally sensitive, appealing and effective.

At the time of this writing, the eight peer educators were conducting market research to find out from their friends, in school and out of school, what would be the best way to impart information. Besides conducting informal interviews and gathering opinions, they were collecting images, magazine pictures, fads, fashion items and other relevant information that would facilitate reaching their target group more effectively.

The East Los Angles Rape Crisis Center Teen TAP Program

The Teen Teatro AIDS Prevention Project—Teen Tapp— is a bilingual teen theater sponsored by the East Los Angeles Rape Crisis Center. The performers are five Latino students from the continuation education program in Lincoln High School in East LA. This part of Los Angeles has one of the most concentrated areas of Mexicans and Mexican Americans in the country. (Los Angeles is the second largest Mexican city in the world, second only to Mexico City.)

This innovative and educational program targets in and out of school Latino teens and their families through an entertaining play called, "AIDS: It Can Happen To You." The play is bilingual with every interaction that is spoken in Spanish repeated in English within the context of the dialog. The performers, in addition to receiving acting lessons from coach and program coordinator, Rosemary Romas, are also trained in AIDS education and are employed by the Rape Crisis Center as regular part-time employees. When they are not acting, their job consists of staffing the Spanish Language AIDS Hotline for the Center.

Teen Tapp has become increasingly popular in the high schools in Los Angeles and Southern California. Prior to doing the play on AIDS the students had been involved in performing plays on date rape and violence. Since many of the local high school students were already familiar with the group's work, they have received several requests for additional appearances and are well-received by their peers. The usual format of presentation is to perform the play first and then conduct a question-and-answer session. The question-and-answer period is often lengthy, interesting and emotionally charged.

In addition to performing in the Los Angles area, the group has performed in other cities in California and the Southwest. According to Ms. Ramos, what makes "AIDS: It Can Happen to You" so popular is that the play is based on real life possibilities that most young people can relate to. That coupled with talented and dedicated performers achieves results.

ACTT - El Teatro Juvenil De La Comunidad

McAllen, Texas is in the heart of "El Valle"—the Rio Grande Valley in Texas. This area of Texas has the largest population of migrant farmworkers in the United States. (NCAS)

ACTT - El Teatro Juvenil de la Comunidad does not deal exclusively with AIDS education. The bilingual skits written by Carlos Trevino of the Hidalgo County Planned Parenthood are on all different kinds of issues affecting Latino teens: Latino culture, peer pressure, teen suicide, drug abuse prevention, sexuality, and AIDS. Trevino is himself a former migrant worker and is now the director and writer of the ACTT project.

The performers are 18 volunteer high school students who have an interest in acting and community service. The program targets Latino parents and teens. They perform in a variety of settings including schools, detention centers, migrant parent education projects, churches and neighborhood centers.

The presentation is done in three phases. In Phase I the student performers act out a 3-5 minute unresolved skit. In Phase II the performers stay in their roles and take questions from the audience about their decisions. The audience challenges their decisions and becomes involved in creative problem solving. In Phase III the performers go back out to the audience, this time as their real selves and introduce themselves and tell why they are doing what they are doing. Phase III also includes background and content information on the topics that were presented.

"One of the reasons that ACTT has been so successful," Trevino states, "is that the audience finds their own solutions and prevention strategies and they do not feel like they have been lectured to." It is empowering to know that you hold the solution to your own problems.

The Latin American Youth Center

The Latin American Youth Center in Washington, DC uses a multiservice approach to reach minority youth engaging in high risk behaviors.

In addition to providing information and youth counseling services, they have successfully used several strategies involving young people in the implementation of innovative AIDS education programs. In the past year the Latin American Youth Center has coordinated an extensive campaign targeting Black and Latino youth in the Washington, DC area. The campaign has included wide distribution of condoms in matchbooks that read "Ser macho es usar condones" (It's macho to use condones) and "Por el amor y la vida, usa condones" (For love and for life, use condoms); bumperstickers using idioms that are used by the young people in the area, i.e., "AIDS Isn't Bumping—

Learn the Facts;" radio programs targeting youth; and an AIDS poster contest.

The most popular strategy has been the LatiNegro Theater Collective production of "AIDS: The Reality in the Dream" a 20-minute collage of movement, music, poetry and drama that explores how AIDS can realistically affect youth. The LatiNegro Theater collective was formed in 1986 by a group of Latino and Black youth. They perform on issues affecting Latino and Black communities in different settings including schools, jails, parks and community organizations. Summer productions have been performed in the streets of Washington, DC.

To add to this project's multiservice and comprehensive approach, the Latin American Youth Center's next step is to implement a peer counseling AIDS education project.

Innovative Resources and the Use of Popular Latin American Culture

The use of popular art forms to design education resources is both effective and entertaining. Latin American popular culture provides us with a wide range of choices and adaptations to meet the educational needs of the target groups.

Fotonovelas are an ideal example of a popular Latin American medium that can be used to educate. Fotonovelas are high interest, comic-book-type booklets that use photographs and a minimal amount of written material as dialog to convey messages. The visual impact and element of entertainment inherent in fotonovelas may attract adolescents who have a tendency to rebel against traditional modes of education. Similarly, comic books also offer an opportune educational medium. Several good comic books and one or two fotonovelas have been developed to address AIDS education in Latino communities.

One particular comic book directed towards teens is "Rappin': Teens, Sex and AIDS" produced by the Multicultural Prevention Resource Center in San Francisco. "Rappin" is a clever attempt at informing Black and Latina young women in the inner city about AIDS and safer sex measures. Plans are underway to produce its counterpart for young men.

Other forms of popular culture used with considerable success in Latino AIDS education efforts are videos in telenovela format such as "Ojos Que No Ven" (Eyes that Will Not See) produced by the Institute Familiar de la Raza in San Francisco; community theater efforts such as Teen Tapp and ACTT; radio programming targeting high risk teens with radio dramas and popular music; and the catchy Columbian tune that is often heard on Spanish radio stations, "La Cumbia del SIDA" (A Dance Tune About AIDS).

One last example of the use of popular culture in creating educational materials is the Mexican "Loteria" poster, designed by Herbert Sequenza of La Raza Graphics in San Francisco, produced by the Instituto Familiar de la Raza. The poster is a visually powerful use of the popular Mexican bingo game to communicate the message, "When you deal with AIDS you deal with death." All of the above examples show sensitive planning, an intimate knowledge of the specific Latino target groups, and commitment to quality AIDS education.

25

Delivering Difficult Messages: AIDS Prevention and Black Youth

Renetia Martin, MSW, LCSW,
and Florence Stroud, RN, MPH

Reflections: Being a Black Parent

I have just returned from an afternoon with my eleven-year-old daughter. It was filled with the usual amount of tension, intense energy (on her part) and pure enjoyment of just being together. The day was centered around her audition for a place in an acting company and we shared a lovely anticipation as we traveled to the meeting. Yet the director had clearly chosen someone before we arrived. Even my daughter could tell he barely had enough energy to sit through the first fifteen minutes of what was supposed to be a half-hour interview. She had had such high expectations and incredible excitement for the past two days looking forward to her possibilities for "real" stage performance. Her disappointment as we left was a descent into gloom, affecting her energy and mine to the point that I was angry with myself for even exposing her to the possibility and then the let down.

It occurred to me on the way home, as she was bouncing back over a huge cup of ice cream, that facing disappointment is not all bad in this day and time. There is so much for which she must be prepared. I reflected further on our recent experience seeing a movie together concerning love, seduction, sexuality, family relationships, class, and color, about the conflicts of a sweet fourteen-year-old—the amazing pull and power at that age of being in or out, being with it or being a stiff, open to the world or afraid to explore it, and most powerfully, to be loved or not to be loved, the key to all of our self-esteems.

In all of this I am reminded of what a wonderful and dreadful period adolescence was for me. The Hollywood version doesn't always address the torment of the pressure to belong and be accepted by one's peers while trying to define who you are, to experience all that is around you while trying not to look too conspicuous, to interpret the sexual energy and integrate the conflicting messages from family, school, friends and church. It is no small wonder that it was the bleakest and most depressing time of my life. It occurs to me, as we look at today's youth and pass on to them the traditional do's and don'ts, that we have forgotten how awful the first rejection feels, how hard it is to not be loved and to try to remember "to do what we are told."

I see my daughter and panic. The world is more complicated today than thirty years ago—we expect more of our children and they expect more from us. Are we letting each other down? Looking at my eleven-year-old soon-to-be-sixteen, and my co-author with her eighteen-year-old son, confuses me. What do we expect from our schools, our families, our friends, our children and their peers with their ever-present, newly-budding sexuality and the fear of AIDS piercing the thin line between being a rational parent and a hysterical frightened maniac? What do we expect of ourselves?

During these times of doubt I fall back on what I believe and what we say to others: you must believe our youth can be reached. We can create an environment for effective education and caring instruction. We can seize the teachable moment to talk about taboo issues that are hard for them and for us.

Black Youth, Black Parents

Our experience is based on being black, urban, and sometimes single parents. We clearly acknowledge that outside of urban areas and the Black community exist other cultures and very different issues, which are addressed elsewhere in this book. We will consider here some of the special concerns about AIDS-related risks in the Black community pertaining to youth.

The message we give to Black youth regarding sexual attitudes and behaviors is layered by the multiple burdens we bear as Black parents, educators and professional leaders in the community. AIDS is only one of the fatal diseases threatening the Black community. Hypertension, cancer, cardio-vascular disease, and homicide/suicide are the primary health threats. AIDS is yet another item on the long list about which we must say: "be cautious," "be careful" and "don't do."

The Current State of the Black Community and AIDS

The Black community has been struggling for years with difficult feelings about AIDS, and with good reason. We are tragically overrepresented in incidence reports of the disease. Though we make up only 12 percent of the total U.S. population, a full 25 percent of U.S. AIDS cases are among Blacks (Centers for Disease Control, 1986). We are told by experts that AIDS originated in Africa, and there seems to be an underlying message that somehow Blacks are responsible for the rise and spread of the epidemic. This is all too familiar. Once again, Blacks feel, some social problem (the incidence of syphilis and other STDs, the teen pregnancy rate, homicide, and drug use) is being blamed on us. There is often a feeling that we don't need to listen to this information because so much of what has been said on these issues before has been presented in racist terms. Millions of dollars are being spent on AIDS programs, but we see very little evidence of this in our local communities. It is not surprising to hear expressions of anger, suspicion and despair when Blacks talk about AIDS.

Homosexuality is also a complicated, difficult and taboo topic. Negative judgments are common. Many Black gay people identify more strongly with being Black than with being gay. Their presence in the Black community may be low-key because of the terrible risks associated with higher visibility: isolation from and rejection by peers and family, and ostracism from the Black community. It would almost be a "better" stigma to be an IV drug user, if one were able to make such a choice. The low visibility of Black gay people supports the notion that homosexuality belongs exclusively to the province of White Americans.

We lose the trust of our gay youth when we continue to hold such judgments, but these days we face other risks as well—the loss of young Black lives. During the teen years, youth experiment with sex regardless of race. They are impressionable and absorb from those around them attitudes to adopt and images to protect. In the Black community, this often means that while men may have sex with other men, they do not think of themselves as homosexuals. When we identify AIDS as a disease of homosexuals, these men do not consider themselves to be at risk.

This is quite a message to Black youth. We limit our ability to provide safe, realistic guidelines by denying that these high risk behaviors exist. We are telling gay youth that they will be isolated, lack support, and lack access to accurate information about AIDS and safer sex. We are telling all our sexually active youth that we do not need to worry about AIDS because men having sex with men is different than the existence of homosexuality in the larger community. Young Black men and women, whether or not they are sexually active, need and want clear direction and information about sexuality. It is incumbent on us to be direct and straightforward regarding AIDS transmission and high-risk behavior. We must say what it is and talk about how and why condoms must be an essential part of sexual expression.

On with the Facts...

The need for educational programs targeted for youth is a subject of national concern and considerable controversy. Differences of opinion exist as to the magnitude of the risk of transmission of HIV infection in youth and thus the need for a major educational effort. Sexuality issues including discussion of homosexuality, use of condoms (or other contraceptives in general), pregnancy and abortion—which have always been provocative—must be confronted again within the context of this lethal disease.

An examination of AIDS prevalence data among adolescents and young adults is compelling as a basis for developing targeted education programs (Schwarcz and Rutherford, 1988). When combined with other indicators, such programs become imperative. During the past 10 to 20 years, the average age of first sexual intercourse among adolescents has declined, while the overall percentage of sexually active teens has increased. As individuals progress though adolescence, their sexual activity increases. For example, at age 13, 10 percent of teens nationally have had sexual intercourse at least once, and by age 17 the proportion of those engaging in sexual intercourse has increased to 57 percent (Louis Harris Associates, 1986). By age 20, 70 percent of the females and 80 percent of the males have had sexual intercourse at least once. Black adolescents are almost twice as likely to have sexual intercourse as White or Latino youth (National Longitudinal Survey of Youth, 1983). An analysis of data derived from the National Survey of Young Women conducted in 1971, 1976 and 1979 shows that a greater proportion of Black adolescents between the ages of 15 and 19 were sexually active and had their first sexual experience earlier than White adolescents. Comparable data for adolescent males from the National Survey of Family Growth conducted in 1976, 1979 and 1982 indicate that Black males between the ages of 17 and 21 were more likely to be sexually active and to have had their first sexual experience at a younger age than White males (O'Reilly and Aral, 1985).

Drug use is also a concern for AIDS transmission among adolescents generally and Black youth specifically. We have no national figures on prevalence of IV drug use among adolescents, but we know that 1 percent of high school students report using heroin and several million have used cocaine, stimulants or other opiates (Johnston, O'Malley and Bachman, 1985) which can be injected. In addition, non-IV drug and alcohol use can lead to poor judgment and lack of resolve to follow safer sex practices. Rates of drug and alcohol use are generally higher among minority youth than the general population.

Education and Prevention

Current AIDS surveillance data shows a disproportionate burden of AIDS/ARC in the Black community. There is indication that the spread of the virus in these communities has accelerated. With the exception of a few communities strongly impacted by the disease (New York, Los Angeles, San Francisco, Miami), Black AIDS education and prevention programs are minimal or nonexistent. Some of the factors impeding the mobilization of these communities for effective education include (1) lack of awareness about the magnitude of the problem, (2) political and ideological constraints, (3) lack of appropriate recruitment efforts to staff such programs and (4) most importantly, lack of funds to initiate and maintain effective programs.

The Black community's beliefs and attitudes about AIDS and its receptivity to education and prevention programs are determined by culture, language and the stigma we and the larger society attach to identified at-risk groups. There is limited access to health care facilities and public health education programs in the Black community. Clients must often rely on publicly-funded clinics or county hospital health care services. Excess rates of premature mortality, teen pregnancy, sexually transmitted disease (STD) and substance abuse reflect deficits in the delivery of effective programs to these communities.

Both the larger society and some groups in the Black community look at such bleak conditions and despair of ever seeing positive changes in health status and services for Blacks. "Why bother," is the lament, "it will always be like this." Efforts lag, funding falls, programs fail. We cannot allow ourselves this sort of indulgence in the area of AIDS prevention. It simply is not accurate. The truth is, our youth can be reached and want to be, but no single approach will work. Our endeavors must be sustained and reinforced using multiple vehicles to get the information across. If, as a community we are able to listen, the kids will tell us what we need to know to help them. If, as a community, we are successful with AIDS education, the payoff will be greater than just prevention of the spread of the epidemic. It will mobilize the resources in the community to confront the on-going problems of unwanted pregnancy, STDs and drug abuse. For the first time in the Black community, we will be able to help youth struggling with issues of sexual orientation by giving them the support they need to explore their sexuality in a safe and nurturing environment.

Approaches that Work

One of the recommendations on public education made by the National Academy of Sciences reads as follows:

> ...special educational efforts must be addressed to teenagers, who are often beginning sexual activity and also may experiment with illicit drugs. Sex education in the schools is no longer only advice about reproductive choice, but has now become advice about a life-or-death matter. Schools have an obligation to provide sex and health education, including facts about AIDS, in terms that teenagers can understand (Institute of Medicine, 1986).

It is the spirit and substance of this recommendation that has guided and informed our educational efforts with youth in San Francisco. We would like to describe three projects designed to educate both in-school and out-of-school youth about

352

AIDS, and discuss their particular relevance to the educational needs of Black youth.

School-based Education, San Francisco

In the fall of 1985, a survey was conducted among high school students in our public school system to determine their knowledge, attitudes and beliefs about AIDS. The results revealed that students had a lot of misinformation about AIDS, that they wanted accurate information and that they believed it ought to be a part of the curriculum (DiClemente, Zorn and Temoshok, 1986). Of special concern was the finding that Black and Latino students had a poorer knowledge base about AIDS than their White counterparts. For example, Black and Latino students were approximately twice as likely as White students to believe that AIDS could be transmitted through touching, kissing or being near someone with AIDS (DiClemente, Boyer and Morales, 1988).

In San Francisco, a joint task force including teachers, parents, Health Department staff, and school administrators was formed to develop a policy and plan for educating students. This policy was adopted by the School Board and Health Commission. The program that grew from this joint policy had a short-term and long-term strategy.

The short-term strategy required that during the spring of 1986, students would have at least one class session on AIDS. Students' response to this session was gratifying. Students wanted information and, after some initial uneasiness, asked excellent questions. Parents were given the opportunity to review materials and to attend special evening meetings to discuss the classes.

The longer-term strategy required the development of a curriculum on AIDS for middle and high school students. Special trainings were set up for teachers who would present these materials in classrooms. Mentor teachers were identified at different campuses, and they received in-depth training on AIDS and communicable diseases. This is an ongoing process and, as further needs are identified, attempts will be made to respond appropriately. Currently the curriculum materials are being expanded to reach to the fifth grade level. Ultimately, AIDS education will be offered for students from grade 5 through grade 12.

San Francisco is a multicultural city. It is essential that educational materials in this and similar locales be culturally appropriate and respect the diversity of the student population. There is an effort to develop materials that are, in one sense, culturally *neutral*—that no cultural standards are violated in what is presented. In a general approach such as this, we are confident we can impart important knowledge to a broad spectrum of youth. We also believe there is a need to further emphasize our prevention messages for minority youth in a more culturally focused medium.

Rap Music Contest

A second program we initiated, therefore, was the "Rap'n down AIDS" contest geared to youth from 13 to 19 years of age. Since rap'n is a contemporary form of communication among Black adolescents, we felt it would be an effective medium motivating youth to educate peers about ways to protect themselves from AIDS and to prevent its spread. This program enlisted youth who were in school as well as those who were not. Cash prizes were offered to authors of winning entries, and topics to be included in the raps (i.e., modes of transmission and methods of prevention) were specified in contest rules. The contest was followed by a series of meetings with those who participated so we could learn what they learned and determine whether it modified their behavior or helped them to think more critically about the consequences of certain sexual behaviors and the use of drugs. The winning raps have been developed as television and radio public service announcements. Staff from the Department of Public Health and several community-based agencies continue their work with the diverse youth in our community to reinforce the learning that has already occurred, and to assist youth to maintain more healthy behaviors.

The Rap'n Contest was open to any interested youth, and participants were Black, White, Latino and Asian. In this sense, the focus was a general one. However, there is particular importance in the use of a form of expression developed and prominent in Black culture. By making rap'n an object of positive attention, we endorsed and validated a characteristic of Black culture. Non-Black youth, composing and performing their own raps, had an opportunity to express admiration for this element of Black culture, and Black youth were further encouraged to feel pride in their culture. Connecting these lessons about AIDS prevention to a positive, esteem-building cultural activity was a strategy that strengthened the overall educational message, particularly for Black youth.

Our general education messages about AIDS are typically offered in the vernacular of the dominant culture. The Rap'n Contest demonstrated how a Black cultural phenomenon could also be used effectively as a vehicle for a general education message. We hope other minority communities will similarly be involved in AIDS prevention education for the general population based on culture-specific approaches.

Community-based Prevention

For AIDS prevention messages to effectively impact Black youth, general education programs must be reinforced by culture-specific programs based in and provided by Black community agencies. In one such agency in the San Francisco area, a variety of approaches has been developed, targeting youth, parents and other adults. This agency had been active in the black community for several years before the AIDS epidemic, so they began their AIDS prevention work having already obtained respect and credibility.

Young people have been actively involved in setting up and evaluating prevention activities. A teen theater group has written and performed scripts on drug abuse, sexuality and AIDS prevention. Youth consultants have helped develop a series of radio messages about AIDS prevention, which are being broadcast over a popular radio station with a predominantly Black audience. A comic book series featuring Black and Latino protagonists who advocate AIDS prevention is being distributed to young adults. The texts and storylines of these comics are reviewed and critiqued by teenagers before the materials go to press.

Enlisting the participation of Black youth in such programs requires meaningful incentives. In particular, we find the provision of cash prizes for contests or wages for youth who consult with us in program development has been very helpful. This communicates to these young people that what they are doing is important work that is valued by the community. Once a teen is involved in the program, other rewards—praise, gratitude, status in the community and a sense of being purposeful—are also quite useful. But without the initial monetary incentive our recruitment efforts would be less successful.

This lively involvement of young people in the prevention programs helps guarantee the efficacy of approaches used. The teens are quite vocal in their criticisms if they think an idea is not very good. It also helps build the self-esteem of those youth who participate in program planning. They appreciate being included as expert consultants and enjoy the respect commanded by this role. Finally, the messages carry particular strength for other Black youth as they are known to come from within the community and so are especially trustworthy.

Other Possibilities: Activities in the Black Church
Though the Black church generally has been hesitant to take an active role in AIDS prevention so far, a few congregations have begun some impressive work in this area. The church is remarkably well-suited to carry forth such programs, both because of its historical role as a resource for community education and activism, and because of its present ability to involve large numbers of youth and their families. Many different approaches are possible through the church. For example, the church could host community forums addressing a variety of issues of high concern to the Black community. Health and AIDS would certainly be among these. Using a "train the trainer" model, Black professionals could volunteer their time to educate selected delegates about particular issues. These delegates could then facilitate discussions with parents and youth. If such a model were used in discussing AIDS-related issues, we could see parent-to-parent and youth-to-youth education take place. Parents could be encouraged and taught how to bring up the topic with their children. Full family involvement, supported by the church, could set forth an ethic about AIDS and AIDS prevention that would resonate powerfully throughout the rest of the community. We would like to see the church take advantage of its unique role, speaking clearly to the needs and responsibilities of the Black community.

Funding
While it is tiresome to always come back to the old refrain, "If funds were available...," the fact is that we desperately need to see evaluation projects which will assess the efficacy of

these and other programs for AIDS prevention among youth. We would like to engage young people in a program and then follow a cohort over time to measure short- and long-term changes in knowledge, attitudes and behavior. Such projects are particularly essential for Black youth, since it appears thus far that the mainstream messages about AIDS are not effectively reaching this group and we know for some the risks are extraordinarily high.

Conclusion

Clearly, there are special concerns for Black youth regarding AIDS. We encourage greater participation from the Black community in planning and carrying forth AIDS prevention programs for youth. We endorse the establishment and evaluation of youth programs that will focus specifically on the Black community. We advocate that greater funding be made available to develop Black and multicultural AIDS education programs throughout the country, in rural as well as urban areas. And we support collaboration in these efforts among various community, governmental and professional organizations.

Our own efforts to educate and change AIDS-risk behavior are based on several principles applicable to *all* young people:

- Didactic education, while necessary, is not sufficient to change behavior.
- Educational strategies must be multifaceted if they are to appeal to youth.
- Programs must involve youth as teachers, and employ their own methods for transmitting information.
- Learning must take place in culturally sensitive and linguistically appropriate ways, both at the family and community level.

- Programs will succeed only if there is viable collaboration between local governmental entities and community agencies.

In our initial conversations about writing this chapter, we felt overwhelmed by the task of addressing the issues of Black youth and AIDS. As we talked further, we realized we were behaving and reacting the way other institutions and systems do—as if our youth cannot be reached.

One of the conclusions we came to as we continued our discussions is that, as parents of teenage children, we do believe they can be reached. There are successful ways to deliver difficult messages, and those ways need to be stated so that others also believe it is possible. We searched our own minds, exploring our relationships with our children and their friends. What is successful? What makes them achieve? Our answer was high self-esteem, the single crucial key to going forth into the world, the single gift so often missing with Black youth. There is nothing that builds self-esteem more than being loved by family and community.

We know the greatest risks to our youth are behaviors involving drug use and sex. If the quality that encourages Black youth to learn, to respond to a nurturing environment, to believe in themselves and their future, is missing, we cannot reasonably expect that they will hear our warnings about AIDS.

But if we love our children well, if our community embraces all of us, if our church accepts us, if we can build and strengthen our own and our youth's self-esteem, and if we learn to listen to what children have to tell us about their vulnerabilities and sensitivities, our work will be effective and our efforts to stop this epidemic will be successful.

359

References

Centers for Disease Control. 1986. Acquired immunodeficiency syndrome (AIDS) among Blacks and Hispanics - United States. *Morbidity and Mortality Weekly Report* 35:655-666.

DiClemente, R.J., Boyer, C.B. and Morales, E.S. 1988. Minorities and AIDS: Knowledge, attitudes and misconceptions among Black and Latino adolescents. *American Journal of Public Health* 78:55-57.

Institute of Medicine, National Academy of Sciences. 1986. *Confronting AIDS: Directions for public health, health care, and research.* Washington, DC, Author.

Johnston, L.D., O'Mally, P.M. and Bachman, J.G. 1985. *Use of licit and illicit drugs by America's high school students 1975-1984.* U.S. Department of Health and Human Services. DHHS Publications No. (ADM) 85-1394.

Louis Harris and Associates, Inc. 1986. American teens speak: Sex, myths, TV and birth control. New York: Planned Parenthood Federation of America, Inc.

National Longitudinal Survey of Youth. 1983. Center for Human Resources Research. Columbus, OH: Ohio State University.

O'Reilly, K.R. and Aral, S.C. 1985. Adolescence and sexual behavior: Trends and implications for STD. *Journal of Adolescent Health Care* 6:262-272.

Special Populations

at Risk

Special Populations at Risk

Young people are all individuals, each with his or her own particular history and concerns. In designing AIDS prevention programs, we usually want to be flexible enough to respond to individual needs but general enough to effectively reach large numbers of youth. The need is great and our resources are often limited.

There is no doubt that sound, general approaches, broad-based and widely implemented, are an important tool of prevention education. There are, however, groups of young people whose risks may be greater or more specialized and whose needs are different enough from the "general" population to require special attention or approaches.

There are two important points to remember about the young people discussed in this section. The first is that in any "general" assembly of young people, members of some of these groups may well be present. If we keep this in mind, we are less likely to make insensitive comments that discount the experiences of runaways, denigrate gay youth, ostracize youth with hemophilia, or overlook the potential for risk activities among those with developmental or physical disabilities. It is possible for *any* youth to engage in risk activities. Likewise, in a typical classroom or community setting, even with a group perceived as "low risk," some youth may have a history of risk exposures about which they are very concerned. When we are perceived as sensitive educators, these young people are more likely to heed our advice about prevention and seek out further support.

The second point is that there are, at present, few specific AIDS education programs or resources for most of these groups. Those that do exist, some of which are described here, are pioneers. We hope to see future materials developed and more funding provided for programs for these young people soon.

26

Runaways, Homeless and Incarcerated Youth

Renee S. Woodworth, MSW

G rowing up has never been easy. Successfully making the passage from child to adult in the 1980s is no exception. For many adolescents, coping with life and living is difficult at best. The transition is especially troublesome for youth with few skills, limited options and little or no support for positive choices.

Young people living with or in an intolerable situation may develop dangerous coping mechanisms in order to find their way through the transition. These coping skills vary in risk but are all potentially harmful. Included in this group are running away, living on the streets, and acting out criminal behavior. None of these behaviors is a safe method for dealing with anger, confusion, abuse at home, or the search for love. But the fact remains that our country and communities have not provided families or young people in crisis many safe alternatives.

Young people are making these choices out of desperation,

believing flight is their only option. Most runaways, homeless youth, street kids, and juvenile offenders would rather be "home": happy, loved, safe, and healthy. They do not, however, see "home" as that place. Families in crisis often have neither the support to provide that kind of environment nor the skills to seek out safe alternative living arrangements.

Young people living on the fringes of society are more vulnerable to high-risk HIV transmission behaviors. Paying for acceptance and love with their bodies and muting reality with drugs puts these youth into a distorted world in which dangerous sexual relationships and drugs are seen as solutions rather than problems.

These behaviors are not exclusive to runaways, street kids and homeless youth, but are certainly more prevalent among them. The issue of daily survival—where to sleep, how to find food—are all time consuming. Living this way is not new for these children. What is new is that these behaviors are now potential modes of transmission for the AIDS virus.

These young people are disconnected from most support systems that can provide accurate AIDS information, education and prevention skills. AIDS is a disease that has challenged us all to examine our behaviors, not just our youth in crisis. Runaway, homeless and incarcerated youth, however, are making dangerous life choices with misinformation. They have little or no knowledge of the risks they are taking.

Who Are These Young People?

Runaways, like persons with AIDS, are often characterized as an "us vs. them" syndrome in people's minds. Runaways and homeless youth historically have been seen as "them." These young people, coming from all ethnic and socioeconomic backgrounds, share some common behaviors and life experiences, and the isolation and rejection they have experienced at home are a significant part of the reason they find themselves on the streets of America. We cannot allow this labeling and separation to continue to set these youth apart. These are our children and our responsibility. Discrimination against them now will only further complicate the barriers to reaching them.

Definitions

Runaways
are children and youth who are away from home at least overnight without parental or caretaker permission.

Homeless
are youth who have no parental, substitute foster or institutional home. Often, these youth have left, or been urged to leave, with the full knowledge or approval of legal guardians and have no alternative home.

Street kids
are long-term runaway or homeless youth who have become adept at fending for themselves "on the street," usually by illegal activities.

Systems kids
are youth who have been taken into the custody of the state due to confirmed child abuse and neglect or other serious family problems. Often these children have been in a series of foster homes, have had few opportu-

nities to develop lasting ties with any adult, are school dropouts, and have few independent living skills.

Incarcerated youth are young people who have been placed in a secure setting (institution/placement) due to criminal behavior or an unstable mental/emotional condition.

These are working definitions (from Bucy, J. 1985. *To Whom Do They Belong?* Washington, DC: The National Network of Runaway and Youth Services, Inc.). A young person may fall within more than one grouping or may move from one group to another. Vulnerability to AIDS high-risk behaviors is a common factor with all the groupings and probably increases with the young person's disconnectedness from their family or other support systems.

Finding These Young People Is Not a Problem

It is not difficult to locate runaway and homeless youth. Not only do we know where they are, there is also a network of programs through which they can be reached. For over twenty years, local, community-based runaway centers have been working with this population of young people and their families. Runaway programs are not the crash pads of the sixties. Rather, they are sophisticated programs working to reunite families whenever possible, and when not possible, to locate other appropriate living arrangements for the youth.

Incarcerated youth are also easy to find, of course. By definition, these youth are placed in a secure setting and are, therefore, a captive audience. One has only to go to the local juvenile hall or youth authority to find incarcerated youths in abundant numbers.

These agencies and institutions now need to develop programs to educate staff and clients in AIDS education and prevention. More than that, we need to provide long-term assistance to all families and youth in crisis, in or out of these specific settings, and include AIDS education in those services.

Linkages are essential between runaway-youth-service providers and others working on the issues of AIDS. Public health officials, educators, mental health providers and policy makers all need to work together to reach these young people. The bandage will not work any more. We cannot simply give these youth a condom and bottle of bleach and pretend the problem has gone away. Neither can the problem be solved by having young people "just say no." Ongoing, repeated contacts, skills-based teaching approaches, and powerful commitment to the task are essential elements of AIDS prevention for this population.

Barriers to AIDS Education/Prevention

People often speak of the significant barriers to providing effective AIDS education to runaway, homeless and incarcerated youth. While we agree that this is a challenging population to work with, we feel that providers are unnecessarily discouraged by statements proclaiming the "hopelessness" or "futility" or "exceptional difficulty" of reaching these youth. Too often these arguments are used as excuses to avoid embarking on a difficult task. We are defeated by our own attitudes. In fact, these youth can be reached; they can be affected; and these "insurmountable barriers" can be overcome.

We explore below some of the common barriers cited in describing AIDS education programs for high risk youth.

While locating these young people is not a problem, reaching them is difficult and may be costly.

It is true that our usual modes of education will not work. For the most part, these young people do not attend school and are not connected to traditional support systems. Community-based programs working with this population have the best chance of providing accurate AIDS information. Programs that work at getting young people off the streets and reuniting families provide a necessary link. We need to go to where the young people are, build those relationships, and talk about AIDS. We need to provide AIDS training for the providers working directly with these youth. We must also set up programs where troubled youth feel comfortable seeking assistance.

These young people have trust issues with adults and "helping systems," and will not believe our information about AIDS.

Young people in this circumstance have a history of being lectured to and given unwanted information. They will not listen to rhetoric or accept information without a base of support and trust. Many come from backgrounds in which the "system" (child welfare, juvenile justice, schools) made promises that were broken or never carried out. Hope has been offered them, only to be withdrawn or denied. This has occurred not only in their contacts with systems, but also in their relationships with family, peers and other adults. There is an underlying mistrust of anyone perceived to be representing the interests of their families, the establishment, school or judicial systems, or other governmental entities.

We must not continue to make the same mistakes with these young people. To build a useful relationship with them, we must be honest in all we say, forthright in our manner, and trustworthy in our commitments. We must offer them something of value—a new set of skills with which to survive. AIDS information provided in this context—explicitly, earnestly, genuinely—can have an impact.

Adolescents feel they are not vulnerable.

Whatever the trauma, many adolescents continue to believe that somehow they will not be affected by it. They believe, "It won't happen to me." This is as true of runaways, homeless and incarcerated youth as it is of any other group of adolescents. Because of this, AIDS information needs to be personalized. Adolescents must believe *themselves* to be at risk of contracting the virus, and learn to care what happens to them. Educational efforts must focus on high-risk behaviors, rather than on simply labeling or stigmatizing high-risk populations. Emphasizing behaviors instead of singling out populations assists young people to identify and be responsible for their own personal behavior and that of others they care about. A young person living on the streets who gets a place to stay at night by sleeping with the owner of an apartment may deny being a juvenile prostitute but may be able to acknowledge engaging in unsafe sexual practices. Similarly, an IV drug user may deny being a junkie but can identify that his shooting behavior is high-risk.

Lack of future motivation is a significant barrier to AIDS education and prevention being accepted by these young people.

Looking to the future is difficult for any teenager. It is even more difficult for young people who feel they have little to live for. For them, a more immediate concern is simply making it through the night. Asking them seriously to consider changing a behavior that may make them deathly ill in five years but which today makes them feel loved and accepted or buys tonight's dinner is asking for a great deal.

Part of what we are teaching in our outreach programs to these youth, however, is that they do have a future. Programs that have been in place for some time may be able to bring successful "graduates" back to talk with current clients. Many programs hire former street youth as outreach workers. This demonstrates powerfully that another destiny is possible. Learning to believe in the future is a skill like any other, and since these youth have not been allowed the privilege of developing that skill in their home environment, we must do all we can, step by step, to help them do so now. AIDS becomes a part of that message: "We want you to protect yourself from AIDS because we believe you have a future to look forward to that is worth protecting."

These are not only barriers to providing AIDS education and prevention but also the dilemmas we face when asking for behavioral change in an adolescent. Behavioral change is, after all, what we want to accomplish. We hope that through AIDS education and an increase in prevention knowledge, a change in behavior can be fostered.

Overcoming these barriers may appear an overwhelming task, but it is not. One-time programs are not the answer. The process will take time and long-term commitment from the service professionals working with young people.

Approaches to Providing AIDS Education and Prevention

There are many possible approaches to providing AIDS education and prevention information to this population. No single method will be adequate. We must reach out on many levels, through many different routes, over and over again. We review some successful approaches here.

Educate the professionals working with runaway, homeless and incarcerated youth about AIDS and about behaviors that will put themselves and their clients at risk of infection. The education for both staff and young people must dispel myths while sharing preventive methods. The entire staff must be comfortable with AIDS discussions. Everyone should be educated on this issue to avoid the problem that arises when one provider is designated as "the AIDS person." When this is the case, youth may be stigmatized if they are seen talking to him or her. Questions will not be asked and education will not be effective.

Provide information and materials in the vernacular of the young people. Materials should be directed to those service providers with most access to the youth. Consider innovative strategies for delivery of the material, taking into account reading abilities, trust concerns, attention spans, access to precautionary materials (i.e. condoms, clean needles), and time constraints. The use of activities such as role plays, computer formats, puzzles, videos, and peer-to-peer groups have proved to be effective in the transfer of knowledge and understanding.

Reinforce the AIDS message at every possible level of interaction, not just in group-discussion settings. Group settings are not always possible. Information must be shared and repeated whenever appropriate: on street corners, while having coffee or a sandwich with the youth. Aim at and look for small steps in behavior change. We see progress when a young man hooking on the streets tapes a condom to his underwear in an effort to protect himself and others. These small steps must be supported and encouraged, even if the behaviors still pose a risk.

Focus on high risk behaviors, not high risk populations. All discussions and materials should address the issue of AIDS from the perspective of behaviors, rather than singling out a population of infected people who are to be avoided. Such a perspective will empower youth to know they can make choices and do something positive to protect themselves and others.

Be prepared to deal with the issues of death and dying. Some of these children are dying of HIV or other illnesses. The young people will be dealing with dying friends and with the very real fear that they may themselves have HIV infection. Staff will also need assistance in resolving their feelings of anger and helplessness as they watch some clients die. Anger and fear are two separate but related issues that staff and the young people must learn to identify and deal with. Anger may be a large part of how this fear is expressed by both staff and young people.

Help these young people and their families believe they can have a healthy, productive future. We need to be able to offer them real, concrete, alternatives to drugs, life on the streets, incarceration and abuse at home. AIDS is a disease that has further complicated the plight of these families and their children. The solutions to their problems must go far beyond the answers that AIDS education seeks to provide. We need to provide an impetus for change, a belief that they have other options, and the reality that the services are there.

Empower youth to know they can protect themselves and others they care about. A key to this issue may be the degree to which we can empower this group of young people. They feel quite powerless. They feel decisions are made for them, usually without much consideration for their own wishes. Running away can often be a young person's statement about wanting to take control of his or her life. AIDS education can help give a young person a sense of real control over their willingness to take risks with possible contraction of HIV.

Mandatory Testing and the Runaway, Homeless, Incarcerated or Street Youth

Some individuals and institutions have recommended mandatory HIV antibody testing for this high-risk population as a prevention tactic. Such approaches raise important legal and ethical concerns (see Chapter 20). They would also damage our prevention efforts without improving the situation.

An adult working for a mandatory testing program would soon be known to the street population. That individual and any agency with which he or she was identified would be avoided by the youth. Other programs would be suspect as well. A crisis of trust would arise, and we would be more hindered than ever in our efforts to help young people get off the streets. Their fears of testing would force them deeper into the abandoned buildings of our large cities and further from the reaches of programs that could help them.

We must remember that there is, at present, no successful therapy for an asymptomatic, seropositive person. The young person informed of a positive test result must somehow understand and integrate that information, even though he or she may have little ego strength and few coping skills with which to do this. The prognosis for such an individual is bleak, and he or she knows it. We have seen street youth given this information attempt suicide, threaten homicide, and increase high-risk behaviors. These are not unusual reactions. We do not have the resources available to offer such youth the careful, intensive long-term counseling they need to handle the information.

We will work much more productively with these young people by our efforts to change their high-risk behaviors. We do not help them or anyone else by giving them what they will perceive as a death sentence should they test antibody positive. We further obstruct our efforts when a young person gains a false sense of security from a negative antibody test.

We recommend strongly against general antibody testing in this population at this time.

Recommendations

We endorse, then, a number of recommendations for AIDS prevention education with high-risk youth.

Running away, living on the streets, and pushing the law and rules to the point of incarceration are all last resort behaviors. Young people behaving this way often see no other option. Our task is to provide alternatives. Included in the alternatives is empowerment through AIDS education and long-term transitional services.

AIDS education must include prevention techniques, some of which do not ask for a complete change in lifestyle but a modification that minimizes the risk for transmission. Working toward abstinence is an ideal that can only be achieved in small steps.

Collaboration is necessary between all agencies working with these young people. Key to this effort is the network of runaway centers around the country and the training of their staffs about AIDS. All agencies need to be giving the same message to youth, one that is nonjudgmental and includes listening to what they are saying.

Expect the process to take time. We are building relationships as well as hoping to change behavior. This is difficult and time consuming. We are asking more from these youth than any adult or agency has ever given them.

Systems must change so that our youth do not feel their only option is to run away from life. Families and communities need support in providing services to assist children and youth in crisis. Long-term programs offering care, support, education, and counseling are needed for youth wishing to leave the street or prevent them from ever entering that life.

Conclusions

Even if AIDS were not an issue, these young people are worth the effort. For far too long, we have said it was okay to discard a portion of our youth. Recently more attention is being paid to what can be done on their behalf. What can be frustrating is that the upsurge of care and concern for their well-being is partially cloaked in the fear that the runaways, homeless and incarcerated youth may infect the "good" folk of this country. What should sober us is the realization that regular kids, not bad kids, run away.

Youth in crisis are deserving of our care and attention with or without the complications of AIDS. This means we must make long-term commitments to assisting families and youth in crisis. We must also accept partial responsibility for any young person feeling the only way to survive is by selling his or her body and soul. We must acknowledge that while we are demanding that these young people care about themselves and others, the message from our society is often that we do not care about them. With AIDS now a real threat, we must, more than ever before, show homeless and runaway youth that we do care for them, body as well as soul.

AIDS Prevention and Education with Gay and Lesbian Adolescents

A. Damien Martin, EdD

E ducation, particularly education directed toward special groups, is more than a matter of disseminating information. It is a process in which the characteristics of the population to be educated, the context in which the program will take place, the information to be disseminated, the goals of the program, and the characteristics of those who do the training, must interact. The form and content of the AIDS education program proposed here depends to a large extent on the specification of these general factors and their interaction (Martin and Hetrick, 1987). The experience of educators and social service personnel in developing programs directed toward Blacks, Hispanics, and other minority groups has demonstrated the necessity of integrating the group's experience into program planning and execution (Bell et al., 1983). This chapter addresses how these and other concerns are considered in providing AIDS education for gay and lesbian adolescents.

Like most teenagers, gay and lesbian adolescents believe they are immortal. The implications of disease, even life threatening diseases like AIDS, are difficult or impossible for them to imagine. Attempts to break through this wall of immaturity and inexperience with a didactic approach alone may result in either denial or phobic behavior. An educational program, therefore, must disseminate the needed information in a manner that will permit the knowledge to be processed without negative effects but with the desired impact. I suggest that while a specialized curriculum for the group is important, it can be effective only within the context of a larger effort that takes into consideration the social and emotional realities of the gay and lesbian population.

There are significant inadequacies in most national and local proposals for AIDS education with children and adolescents. They virtually never mention gay and lesbian youth. Considering the statistics on sexual activity among teenagers, the emphasis on "fidelity in marriage" and "wait until you are married" in certain national campaigns is insufficient and inappropriate. It is also dangerous for the homosexually oriented young person, especially the adolescent male. It gives the mistaken message that marriage and marriage alone is the only and the best protection against AIDS. Two possible responses to these messages are very disturbing: the gay adolescent who has no desire or possibility for heterosexual activity may simply give up and indulge in unnecessarily dangerous behavior; the adolescent may be encouraged to marry when this is socially and psychologically inappropriate.

Even with teachers and program personnel who are sympathetic or knowledgeable, programs in schools and agencies usually assume the heterosexuality of the population, thus ignoring at least 10 percent of the young people addressed by these programs. The danger arises not only from ignoring the

380

specific needs of the young person who is gay, but in the possibility of giving incorrect and damaging information.

At the Hetrick-Martin Institute, Inc. we are able to develop and direct our AIDS prevention efforts specifically toward gay or lesbian adolescents since this is the population we serve. Nevertheless, our clients represent only a very small percentage of gay and lesbian youth. Most others in this population are in schools or programs in which they are a hidden group. If, in the development of AIDS education programs for adolescents in general, we do not recognize that gay and lesbian adolescents are part of that population, we will continue to neglect their needs.

The following discussion will be divided into two parts: the first will address special problems and characteristics of gay and lesbian youth. The second will describe a proposed program for dealing with this population.

Problems and Issues for Gay and Lesbian Youth

Problems faced by homosexually oriented adolescents do not stem from sexual orientation per se, but from society's stigmatization of the homosexual (Martin, 1982a, 1982b; Hetrick and Martin, 1984, 1987; Hunter and Schaecher, 1987; Martin and Hetrick, 1988.) This is not to say, of course, that, like their heterosexual counterparts, gay and lesbian adolescents do not face other issues as well. Problems specifically related to stigmatization, however, often become manifest as self-destructive or dangerous behaviors, that may be directly related to high risk for AIDS (Martin, 1982a; Martin and Hetrick, 1987). For example, we have worked with young gay men who, responding to episodes of harassment or ostracism, have gone where they feel wanted—neighborhoods where they can cruise or hustle, and where they may engage in unsafe sex.

In a review of the presenting problems of gay and lesbian youth requesting services at the Hetrick Martin Institute, Inc. (formerly The Institute for the Protection of Lesbian and Gay Youth, Inc.) three were the most frequent: isolation, family problems and violence. These problems, and the programs we have developed to address them, are addressed in detail elsewhere (Martin 1982a; Hetrick and Martin, 1987; Martin and Hetrick, 1988). The most important for this discussion, however, is the cognitive, social and emotional isolation suffered by the majority of gay and lesbian youth.

Gay and lesbian adolescents differ from their heterosexual counterparts in other minority groups in two important ways. First, the homosexually oriented enter adolescence with no preparation for the social identity that homosexuality carries with it (Martin, 1982a; Hetrick and Martin, 1984; Dank, 1971.) No matter how deleterious the environment in which Jews, Hispanics, Blacks, and other minority group adolescents are raised, they have had preparation for their status through shared learning with the family. They gain a sense of the important "we" versus "they" that is essential to the social and personal recognition of group membership (Allport, 1958.) Gay or lesbian adolescents have no such recognition with relation to social identity as a homosexual. Nor can they can expect much help in reaching it from the most important social unit from which children and adolescent draw support, the family. To give but one example, a young Black or Jew who is beaten up by peers because he or she is Black or Jewish can go home and share that experience with the family. The family can deal with it in a number of ways, all based on its own and the group's experiences within a hostile society. The young boy who is beaten up for being a faggot, the young girl who is taunted for being a dyke, often cannot share this with the family. Indeed, the family may mirror the reaction of the general society and enforce the stigmatization of the homosexual.

Secondly, unlike Black, Hispanic, and other minority group adolescents, gay and lesbian youth run the risk of expulsion from their families, their churches, their peer groups and any other group to which they have been socialized if their sexual orientation is discovered. Therefore, when other adolescents are learning the bases for developing adult social networks, many homosexually oriented adolescents are learning to hide their sexual identity. In the process, gay male adolescents in particular often develop those behaviors that later place them at high risk for AIDS. Sexual encounters, often in the most degrading and dangerous contexts, become their only way to make contact with a member of their group and to escape the desperate social and emotional isolation involved in, as Goffman (1963) so aptly put it, "the management of a spoiled identity." Aside from the direct exposure to sexually transmitted diseases, drugs, and violence that such behavior entails, these adolescents are socialized to use sexual behavior as a means to make social contact. Nor is it only gay males who place themselves at high risk. We have seen teenage lesbians who become pregnant in an attempt to hide their orientation. They feel, usually correctly, that families will accept an unwanted pregnancy sooner than a lesbian daughter. Lesbian teenagers, like heterosexual teenagers, may also experiment with their sexual identity, having sexual experiences with men on occasion. Since young gay men may be more accepting of this sort of behavior than other men, they become likely sexual partners for young lesbians involved in such explorations. Thus, while lesbians are generally considered to be at lowest risk for AIDS, the teenage lesbian who acts out heterosexually may be at risk for HIV infection.

The basic problems, then, are to reach a hidden population

whose most serious problem is cognitive, social and emotional isolation; to develop an appropriate learning environment that reflects the needs of these young people; and to develop programs that will give them accurate information and appropriate strategies for avoiding high-risk behavior. In addition, the strategies must be such that the AIDS education program does not exacerbate the already existing stigmatization of this population, with the resulting possibility of denial, phobic behavior, or increased self-hatred.

There are three interrelated and mutually necessary ways to approach these issues. First, develop a program for youth-serving professionals who must deal with these problems. Second, create an appropriate learning environment coupled with an adequate curriculum. Third, create special programs for gay and lesbian youth. The last cited approach may not be possible immediately in most areas of the country, but the first two can and should be initiated immediately. Indeed, there is some indication that the denial of appropriate educational programs to gay and lesbian youth as a group may be illegal (Dennis and Harlow, 1986).

Teacher Training

Societal stigmatization does not affect only the targeted minority group; the resulting socialization has an equal, though different, effect on the dominant group. It is not surprising, therefore, that medical, educational, and social service professionals who provide services to stigmatized populations may have negative attitudes that will have a deleterious effect on the delivery of services. Negative attitudes are usually reinforced when there is little or no information available to counteract them (Allport, 1958; Goffman, 1963; Hetrick and Martin, 1984). Therefore, the first step in the development of AIDS education and prevention programs for particular populations is the training and education of those who will deliver such programs in the nature and experience of the groups to be served. This is especially true in the development of AIDS education programs for gay and lesbian youth.

In a needs survey of youth-serving professionals, over 80 percent reported they had had little or no education or training in homosexuality or issues related to delivery of services to the homosexually oriented (Robinson and Martin, 1983). A follow up nationwide survey conducted over a five-year period (1983-1988) confirmed this finding (Martin and Northrop, 1988). In informal interviews, teachers and guidance counselors in the New York City public school system reported to The Hetrick-Martin Institute, Inc. that difficulty in dealing with the issue of homosexuality was the major problem they had in their AIDS education programs. This problem operated on two levels. First, they felt they were unprepared to address issues surrounding homosexuality. Secondly, most students believed AIDS to be a homosexual disease and the homophobia of the students prevented their accepting the dangers they might face.

A first priority, therefore, must be the education and training of those who will be conducting AIDS education and prevention programs in the issues and problems related to gay and lesbian youth. Programs should be implemented for those already working in the field; such programs should also be introduced in professional and paraprofessional training programs. In the needs survey cited above (Robinson and Martin, 1984), 61 percent of the professionals responding stated they were afraid they would endanger their jobs if they addressed the needs of gay and lesbian youth. Professional and community support for those who will be entrusted with these special programs must be initiated.

The development and delivery of such educational and

training programs has been a priority of the Hetrick-Martin Institute, Inc. We provide training and education to agencies and schools all over the country. We believe firmly that since the majority of gay and lesbian youth are in mainstream educational and social service systems, it is the system that must be affected.

Learning Environment and Curriculum

As mentioned above, the cognitive isolation of gay and lesbian youth is overwhelming. They have little or no access to correct, factual information about homosexuality. Yet such information is essential to combat the cognitive dissonance that results from their realization of their homosexual orientation (Festinger, 1957; Martin, 1982a). It is also essential to any AIDS prevention program directed toward gay and lesbian adolescents. Gay and lesbian youth have had little or no exposure to anything but the grossest slanders about the homosexuality oriented. They often have an extremely poor self-image, especially relating to their sexual identity. Any AIDS education program that is not sensitively designed runs the danger of reinforcing that damaged self-esteem. Any AIDS education program directed toward gay adolescents must be offered in a setting and context that provides and reinforces a positive self-image. Two long term strategies can make major inroads in this dissonance. First, ensure that school and community libraries have adequate and appropriate gay-related reading material. This includes novels, histories and literature as well as technical treatises. Second, try to develop role models for these young people. Having openly gay and lesbian adults as teachers is important. But also include as role models those heterosexual teachers who are openly and clearly not homophobic and who willingly address issues of homosexuality without condemnation or embarrassment. The creation of an environment in which sexuality can be discussed, and in which homosexuality is not automatically a matter of snickers or hostility, is essential. This is also important for the heterosexually oriented youngsters. They have the right to accurate information about the 10 percent of the population having a gay orientation, and this information can further help to dispel the myth that AIDS is only a gay disease and that they, as heterosexuals, are not at risk.

Third, curricula should place AIDS within a total health context. It must be treated as a disease like other diseases. The history of disease, and the ways in which some groups were targeted and blamed for plagues and health problems should be highlighted. Again, while this serves a purpose in taking some of the stigma away from homosexuals, thus decreasing the likelihood of denial, phobic behavior, and exacerbation of self-hatred, it also will serve to point out to the nonhomosexually oriented students that it is risk behavior not risk groups that are important.

Attempts to introduce family planning and sexuality education curricula in the public schools demonstrate that cultural, religious and social attitudes toward sex, especially sex among adolescents, are perhaps the most severe stumbling blocks toward the development of an ideal learning environment on this issue. Yet it is too important to allow such difficulties to become an excuse for ignoring the needs of this special population. Again, it is critical that support systems be created to help and protect those teachers, social workers, youth-serving professionals, and administrators who try to implement an adequate program.

Community Group Programs

The emphasis so far has been on the development of programs in school systems and, to a certain extent, in social service agencies. Community groups, including those that have
social service delivery as a focus, have perhaps greater freedom
to develop programs that will serve gay and lesbian youth.
Community center programs should have the following goals:
(1) to provide the homosexually oriented adolescent, especially
the male, the opportunity to interact with peers in other than
sexual situations; (2) to prevent the development of those sexual and social behaviors that have been identified as predispos-
ing and enabling factors for AIDS risk activities, and to do so in
part, by fostering the acquisition of social skills that allow positive relationships to develop that are not necessarily based on
sexual contact; (3) to provide general health information related to sexual activity, and especially health information related to AIDS; (4) to provide such information within a context
that will be appropriate for this population.

Suggestions for an AIDS Education Program

The core of an AIDS education and prevention program for
any population must, of course, be accurate and up-to-date information about the disease, its transmission and its prevention.
This is not so easy as it sounds since ongoing research today
modifies much of what we thought yesterday. Therefore, the
first informational component should be the establishment of a
means whereby information is constantly examined and modified when necessary.

A major point in this chapter has been the context within
which this information is presented. The context itself can and

should carry basic information essential to the group needs. A number of strategies can be used to provide this informational context.

One strategy used at The Institute is a film club in which commercial films are shown and discussions following the films address issues relating to the group and to AIDS. A film like *Boys in the Band*, though stereotypical and negative in many ways, can provide a number of topics that, while not apparently directly related to AIDS, are relevant. For example, the film contains two characters who are lovers. One man wants a monogamous relationship, the other wants an "open" relationship in which he can have sex with other partners when he wants. Discussions have focused on the concept of relationships, an issue of great concern to the gay and lesbian adolescent. Nevertheless, in the context of the discussion, we have been able to raise health issues through questions like: "What is he exposing his lover to by sleeping around like that?" "How can the lover protect himself?" It is important to stress that while there was talk of safer sex techniques and the use of condoms, some of the discussion involved the nature of the relationship and the possibility of ending it. Similarly, a discussion of the film *Lady Sings the Blues* focused on racism, internalized self-hatred and the self-destructive behaviors that result. We were still able to bring in a discussion of drugs and their relationship to AIDS.

One point should be stressed here. The discussion leaders must be prepared to go beyond the usual connections like the relationship of IV drug use and needle sharing. In one of our discussions, we made the point that drugs could impair judgment and perceptions to the point that someone might do something dangerous without realizing it. A request by one young man that we be more specific triggered a discussion of the concept of "thresholds of pain" and how even so-called "rec-

389

reational drugs" like poppers or marijuana might raise that threshold to the point where a person might be being hurt without realizing it.

We also hold "condom comfort" classes in which young people get the chance to handle condoms, practice putting them on bananas, have "races" to see who can put one on the banana correctly in the shortest time, blow them up, and so on. There usually is much giggling and joking, behaviors we encourage because the point is to familiarize them with the condom, desensitize them to viewing it solely as a joke, and, in a sense, to make it seem very commonplace. We also make condoms freely available with cookie jars filled with condoms scattered throughout the agency.

The condom comfort classes usually lead into discussion of the issues as viewed by the young people. How do you negotiate the use of a condom? How do you deal with a partner who refuses to use one? What if you have already agreed to have sex? We found that role playing as well as intensive discussion by the young people themselves is an ideal strategy for addressing these issues.

A favorable learning context can also be created by imaginative use of the environment. Posters, articles, pictures and other visual materials can be posted in the setting. We have poster and slogan contests in which prizes are offered for the best posters and slogans created by the young people.

While many of the posters we use are AIDS specific, they need not be. One of the more effective posters we have seen, published at one time by SIECUS showed a rainbow made up of the words "HUMAN SEXUALITY HETEROSEXUALITY HOMOSEXUALITY BISEXUALITY HUMAN SEXUAL-ITY." The message was that sexuality was not a taboo subject, that young people could discuss it among themselves and with others.

390

The development of materials appropriate to the population is also an essential component of any program. We have started one project that seems to be meeting with some success. We have planned a series of ten comic books with an ongoing set of gay and lesbian teenage characters. The first three books address the three problems identified as paramount by our clients: isolation, family and violence. The last seven will address health issues, especially AIDS, but again within the context of the needs of this population. For example, one comic book will relate the story of a teenage lesbian who gets pregnant as a means to hide. The emphasis will still be on the need to hide, one of the most debilitating problems faced by this population, but the appropriate AIDS information will be incorporated. The character will enroll in a teenage pregnancy outreach program in which there will be young women who must face the issue of a sero-positive diagnosis.

Individualized instruction must also play a part. Such instruction usually is best conducted in long term counseling during which specific short and long term goals can be set and achieved. For example, one of our workers counseled a 17-year-old young man who had had nothing but anonymous sexual encounters since he was 14. These encounters took place in abandoned piers on the riverfront. She set as a limited short term goal his having sex in a bed. While working on this, she constantly raised issues of safer sex, the danger of certain sexual acts, the use of condoms, and other related concerns. This was not the major focus of the counseling and was usually raised in an offhand manner as information while the concerns of the young man were being addressed. Eventually he did meet someone and insist that the sex take place in a setting other than the piers. He was so excited by the experience that his own goal for counseling changed, and he asked for advice on how he could meet people in places other than the piers. He began to incorporate the information his counselor had given him in the sessions and, three years later, apparently has completely changed his sexual behavior. It must be stressed again that such an individualized program is possible only when the professional concerned feels the freedom and protection to conduct the sessions as he or she sees fit.

Two final notes. All information about AIDS should be given in a general context of health information. To single out AIDS while ignoring pregnancy, personal hygiene, syphilis, gonorrhea and Hepatitis B not only neglects important health issues related to sexual behavior, it emphasizes AIDS to the point that many youth will begin to tune out the message from overexposure. AIDS education is a health education issue and must be addressed as such.

The second point is that all our programs include our young female clients. The tendency is to think of AIDS as a male issue, especially in a gay population, but that is not strictly true. While lesbians may be a "low risk group," the emphasis must always be on high and low risk behaviors, not groups. Lesbian teenagers in particular may indulge in high risk behaviors.

As should be apparent, most of the suggestions made here can be adapted for other populations of teenagers.

The proposed program outline follows:

- Develop a program that is sensitive to the needs of the specific group of teenagers. In this case, the overriding need is for programs that allows for the development of a healthy and mature gay or lesbian social identity.
- Train professional personnel who interact with gay and lesbian youth in the following areas: (1) problems and issues in service delivery to gay and lesbian youth; (2) specific social and emotional problems of this population, especially those related to stigmatization; (3) health-related information, particularly AIDS-related

information; (4) strategies for incorporating the latter information into all activities with gay and lesbian youth.

- Develop support systems for professional dealing with gay and lesbian youth that will protect them from political, economical and other social reprisals.
- Establish an appropriate context for the dissemination of information through a recognition of the nature of the group.

Conclusion

Schools and community organizations often find it expedient to believe "we don't have lesbian or gay youth here." Administrators further confirm this opinion by stating that, when asked directly, that no student or client identified him or herself as being homosexual. What is clear from our research and our experience is that these young people most certainly *do* exist and they are present in school and community settings. But they will not easily self-identify as gay unless they know they will be supported and accepted. For the sake of these youths' mental and social well being we must establish an atmosphere of support and acceptance in our society. As we consider the particular risks of AIDS for this group, it only reinforces the critical need to advocate for and protect lesbian and gay adolescents.

References

Allport, G. 1958. *The nature of prejudice*. Garden City, NY: Doubleday & Co., Inc.

Bell, C.C., Bland, I.J., Houston, E. and Jones, B.E. 1983. Curriculum development and implementation:Enhancement of knowledge and skills for the treatment of the Black population. In *Mental health and people of color: Curriculum development and change*. Chunn, J.C., Dunston, P.J., and Ross-Sheriff, F. (Eds.) Washington, DC: Howard University Press.

Dank, B.M. 1971. Coming out in the gay world. *Psychiatry* 34:180-197.

Dennis, D.I. and Harlow, R.E. 1986. Gay youth and the right to education. *Yale Law and Policy Review* IV, 2:446-478.

Festinger, L. 1957. *A theory of cognitive dissonance*. Evanston Il: Row, Peterson.

Goffman, E. 1963. *Stigma: Notes on the management of spoiled identity*. Englewood Cliffs, NJ: Prentice Hall.

Hetrick, E.S. and Martin, A.D. 1984. Ego dystonic homosexuality: a developmental view. In *Innovations in psychotherapy with homosexuals*. E.S. Hetrick and T.S. Stein (Eds.) Washington, DC: American Psychiatric Press.

Hetrick, E.S. and Martin, A.D. 1987. The development of the gay and lesbian adolescent. *Journal of Homosexuality* 14, 1-2:25-44.

Hunter, J. and Schaecher, R. 1987. Stresses on gay and lesbian adolescents in schools. *Social Work in Education* 9:180-190.

Martin, A.D. 1982a. Learning to hide: The socialization of the gay adolescent. In Feinstein, S.C., Looney, J.G., Schwartzberg, A. and Sorosky, A. *Adolescent Psychiatry: Developmental and Clinical Studies 10*, 52-65.

Martin, A.D. 1982b. The minority question. *etcetera:Journal of General Semantics* 39:22-42.

Martin, A.D. and Hetrick, E.S. 1987. Designing an AIDS risk reduction program for gay teenagers: Problems and proposed solutions. In *Biobehavioral control of AIDS*. Ostrow, D. (Ed.) 137-152. New York, NY: Irvington Publishers.

Martin, A.D. and Hetrick, E.S. 1988. The stigmatization of the gay and lesbian adolescent *Journal of Homosexuality* 15.

Martin, A.D. and Northrop, A. 1988. Needs survey of problems and issues in service delivery to gay and lesbian youth - 1984-1987 (In Press).

Robinson, G. and Martin, A.D. 1984. *Needs survey of problems and issues in service delivery to gay and lesbian youth.* New York, NY: IPLGY.

Troiden, R. 1979. Becoming homosexual: A model of gay identity acquisition. *Psychiatry* 42:362-373.

28

AIDS Education
for the Hemophilic Youth

Donna DiMarzo, ACSW, MPH

P roviding sensitive, informative AIDS education to hemophilic youth presents a unique challenge for teachers, administrators, community groups and parents. Although the risk
of AIDS in adolescents is of great concern worldwide, currently no other group of young people has experienced the
impact of human immunodeficiency virus (HIV) infection and
the AIDS threat as personally as adolescents with hemophilia.

Since the early 1970s, advances in hemophilia care have
enabled people with hemophilia to lead nearly normal, full and
productive lives (National Hemophilia Foundation, 1987).
With the advent of new treatment products and comprehensive
Hemophilia Treatment Centers, life expectancy increased dramatically until 1981, when it became evident that the AIDS
virus could be transmitted through infusion of blood and blood
products (McGrady, Jason and Evatt, 1987).

It is believed that as early as 1978, and to a greater degree in

1981-82, the majority of the hemophilic population in the United States were exposed to the AIDS virus through the use of factor concentrates (Hilgartner, 1987; McGrady, Jason and Evatt, 1987). Concentrates of clotting factor are produced from large plasma donor pools, which are obtained from as many as 10,000-15,000 individuals (Williams and Glader, 1987). Due to this process, many viruses have been found in pooled factor product, including the AIDS virus.

In October of 1984, heat-treated factor concentrates became available to the hemophilia community and were officially recommended as products of choice for most hemophilia patients requiring treatment. This recommendation, coupled with antibody screening of donated blood and plasma begun in March of 1985, have significantly reduced and possibly eliminated the risk of exposure to the AIDS virus for people with hemophilia (McGrady, Jason and Evatt, 1987).

As of March 28, 1988, 571 cases of AIDS in adults and adolescents with hemophilia, and 50 cases of AIDS in children with hemophilia have been reported by the Centers for Disease Control (1988). Although this absolute number of persons with hemophilia who have acquired AIDS is small relative to other high risk groups, the incidence of AIDS among the hemophilic population is higher than for any other group (Agle, Gluck and Pierce, 1987).

Seroprevalence rates for antibody to HIV among the estimated 20,000 hemophiliacs in the United States have been reported to be 70 percent, and are believed to be as high as 90 percent for individuals with severe hemophilia (Andrews et al., 1987). It is important to note that researchers have found the course of the AIDS epidemic in the hemophilic population to differ from that of others who have been exposed to the AIDS virus. Most persons with hemophilia who have been exposed remain well and are asymptomatic. Some researchers speculate that this difference may reflect the route of transmission of the AIDS virus in persons with hemophilia—intravenous infusion of commercially prepared factor concentrates, which results in a less even pattern of exposure to the AIDS virus than for sexual transmission (McGrady, Jason and Evatt, 1987).

Until 1985, the threat of AIDS in the hemophilia community was primarily confined to the person with hemophilia. It is now evident that mass educational efforts must focus on preventing transmission to sexual partners of hemophilic men and youth. Heterosexual and perinatal transmission of the AIDS virus in the hemophilia community have become a sobering reality.

A recent survey by the Centers for Disease Control of all United States Hemophilia Treatment Centers gathered information on 2,276 spouses/sexual partners of HIV seropositive hemophilic men. Seven hundred and seventy-two (34 percent) of these partners were known to have had HIV antibody tests. Of that group, 77 (10 percent) were reported seropositive. Among all sexual partners, 280 (12 percent) were reported to have been pregnant during the period January 1985 through March 1987. One hundred and seventy (61 percent) of these women have been tested for HIV antibody. Twenty-two (13 percent) of those tested were seropositive for HIV prior to pregnancy, during pregnancy or at delivery and 20 children were born to them. Fully adequate seroprevalence data is not available for the infants, but at the time of this report, four had tested seronegative and nine were seropositive (Centers for Disease Control, 1987).

The implications of these statistics and those for heterosexual and IV-drug-use-related transmission of HIV infection pose a special challenge for educators to disseminate accurate, up-to-date, informative and sensitive AIDS education to children and youth. Perhaps equally important, educators must dispel inaccurate information about AIDS, HIV infection, homosexuality and hemophilia.

Adolescents with hemophilia, like many of their peers, may have misinformation about AIDS and transmission of HIV. Like other adolescents and preadolescents, they also may be experimenting both sexually and with drugs. For the hemophilic youth, specific, detailed information about *how* the AIDS virus can be transmitted and about *which* body fluids have been found to contain the AIDS virus is especially critical. In our pediatric hemophilia clinic (University of California, San Francisco Medical Center), for example, we have found that some hemophilic youth maintain that as long as there is no exchange of blood during intercourse, their sexual partner will not be at risk for transmission of the AIDS virus.

In talking with hemophilic youth, it is also apparent that their own misinformation and that of their peers can have an enormous psychological impact and can create a heightened sense of concern about their health and the possibility of transmitting the virus to others. For example, beliefs by hemophilic youth that HIV infection can be transmitted casually (i.e., through sharing of food, utensils or toilet seats) may isolate them from family and peers. Similar beliefs on the part of peers may result in withdrawal from, and stigmatization of the youth with hemophilia.

In classroom and other settings, AIDS education often includes discussion of high-risk groups and statistics of the number of persons who have AIDS or who have died from AIDS. For an adolescent with hemophilia, identification of high-risk groups including persons with hemophilia and transfusion recipients may further isolate them from their peers. Cases like that of the Ray children in Florida (whose family home was destroyed by arson after it became known that the three hemophilic sons were HIV infected), demonstrate that discrimination is a very real threat to the hemophilia community (*American Medical News*, 1987). Our experience in working with hemophilic youth suggests that, even for those adolescents who are coping adaptively with the AIDS epidemic, hearing about or reading statistics may engender feelings of fear, despair, despondency and hopelessness.

The implications of a hemophilic youth either being singled out or perceiving that he is identified as being at high risk for AIDS are far-reaching. Many parents of children with hemophilia are no longer willing to share with peers or school personnel their child's medical condition for fear of discrimination and ostracism. Hemophilic youth may also hide their hemophilia from friends and teachers. This presents a serious medical dilemma for youth who may require treatment during school hours, and for school staff who are responsible for their well-being while in attendance.

What we have found to be particularly useful in educating hemophilic youth about AIDS and transmission of HIV is to focus away from their identification with "a high-risk group" (hemophilic adolescents seem to be particularly concerned about being identified with homosexuals because of the association between AIDS and homosexuality), and instead, focus on high-risk behaviors and the need for *all* adolescents to be well-informed about AIDS transmission and prevention. By normalizing the need for all individuals to incorporate safer sex practices into their lives, hemophilic youth will not feel identified as being different from their peers.

In approaching AIDS education with a group that includes an adolescent known to have hemophilia, sensitivity to the possibility that this individual may be experiencing a myriad of emotions related to being seropositive, including fears and concerns about stigmatization, discrimination, illness, loss of body image and death and dying, is vital.

The future for many hemophilic youth is uncertain, but sensitive, accurate and informative AIDS education can provide these adolescents what they need to know to prevent transmission to others, and to cope more effectively with AIDS-related concerns and issues.

References

Agle, D., Gluck, H. and Pierce, G. 1987. The risk of AIDS: Psychologic impact on the hemophilic population. *General Hospital Psychiatry* 9:11-17.

American Medical News. 1987, Sept. 25. MD regrets HIV test for boys.

Andrews, C. A., Sullivan, J.L., Brettler, D. B., Brewster, F.E., Forsberg, A.D., Scenney, S., Levine, P.H. 1987. Isolation of human immunodeficiency virus from hemophiliacs: Correlation with clinical symptoms and immunologic abnormalities. *Pediatrics* 3:5.

Centers for Disease Control. 1987, September. HIV infection and pregnancies in sexual partners of HIV-seropositive hemophilic men-United States. *Morbidity and Mortality Weekly Report* 36:35.

Centers for Disease Control. 1988, January 25. *AIDS Weekly Surveillance Report - United States.*

Hilgartner, M. 1987. AIDS and hemophilia. *New England Journal of Medicine* 317:1153-54.

McGrady, G.A., Jason, J.M., Evatt, B.L. 1987. The course of the epidemic of acquired immunodeficiency syndrome in the United States hemophilia population, 1987. *American Journal of Epidemiology* 126:1.

National Hemophilia Foundation. 1987. AIDS and HIV infection fact sheet. *NHF Publication.*

Williams, J. and Glader, B. 1987, February 21. Statement before the House Select Committee on Children, Youth and Families. Berkeley, CA.

29

AIDS Education for Individuals with Developmental, Learning or Mental Disabilities

Lynne Stiggall

As a sex education consultant who has worked in the field of disabilities for the better part of two decades, I find the task of writing about AIDS education for persons with developmental/learning disabilities to be both a professional honor and a humbling responsibility. The need for sex education that my colleagues and I have been championing all these years (with varying degrees of success, in a climate of continued controversy) has found a new ally in AIDS. It is an ally no one invited and no one welcomes. Nevertheless, the fear of AIDS has created an environment in which sex education is "in." From schools and agencies, which formerly banished sex education as being too controversial, we are now hearing cries for help.

In looking at AIDS education and this special population, one is at first struck with a dilemma. All people are *people first*. The mere categorization of special groups serves to discriminate, separate and isolate. In the last 20 years, great strides have been taken to break down the old labeling, to assist persons with developmental and other learning disabilities to blend and integrate into generic service systems so that they will not be separate, but be truly equal. This is juxtaposed with the recognition that special needs for special groups do exist. Needs that are legitimately unique must be met in unique ways. In education we do our best to integrate and mainstream students while providing special tutors, speech and behavior specialists as necessary to help those who learn differently or more slowly than other students.

This difficulty is an old story: finding the delicate balance between equal, nondiscriminatory services and effective, appropriately specialized services. It is easy for the very persons about whom we speak to get lost in the debate. We must be careful not to leave this population of students out in the provision of critical education about AIDS.

Another consequence of this labeling dilemma has to do with data collection. Retrieving meaningful data that might help in assessing the extent of the AIDS problem in this population is practically impossible. No statistics that identify people with AIDS as persons who have also been classified developmentally, learning or mentally disabled are currently being kept (the only exception is when a person with AIDS is a resident of a state hospital, or is in some way known to the state bureaucracy).

Whether the data exists to prove a special need for this group or not, we agree with Surgeon General Koop in his advocacy for sex education. All people need to know about sexuality. People with developmental and other learning disabilities especially need this education. Many individuals in these groups have poor self-esteem and are at greater risk than their nondisabled counterparts to be sexually abused or exploited (Blomberg, 1986). Reading skills are typically limited, so obtaining information from magazines, books or brochures is difficult. Many lead very protected lives and demonstrate poor judgment in relationship development. Separating fact from fantasy in media, hard for all of us, is even more difficult for these individuals.

Sex education including information about AIDS and its prevention is vitally important. How should AIDS education be provided? What are the essentials? What are the effective methods and materials to use?

What Do Students with Learning or Developmental Disabilities Need to Know About AIDS?

Students and young people in this special population need the same information as everyone else. Millicent Kellogg, a public health nurse in San Jose, California and a pioneer in AIDS services, declares that we need to teach all of our young people four things:
- AIDS is dangerous.
- It can happen to you.
- A person can have AIDS and not know it.
- You can prevent AIDS.

To assist young people in understanding these four concepts, classes should include the following topics: reproductive anatomy; how one can and cannot contract the virus; information about relationships, values and decision making; skills in assertiveness; the possibility of choosing abstinence; how to prevent sexual abuse; where and how to obtain and use condoms; what the antibody test means and where to go for testing, counseling, treatment; what an individual's rights and responsibilities are; and the meaning of informed consent.

This education, to be effective, should not come as an isolated unit on AIDS. Rather, it should be a part of a comprehensive, positive family life/sex education program. Human sexuality is a part of life. Being taught only about a tragic virus that can be acquired as a result of a sexual act would reflect a slanted, negative impression of sexuality.

Persons with developmental/learning disabilities are especially influenced by authority opinions. AIDS education insensitively offered may create unnecessary fear and distress. Educators must strive for balance: present factual information, be explicit and honest. One should not teach in a manner that frightens, engenders paranoia, or promotes homophobia. Incorporating this critical education about AIDS in a positive family life education framework sets the stage for maintaining this balance.

The desired basic information is the same for all groups of people. It is the methods of teaching and the materials used that may be different when offering this education to students with developmental, learning or mental disabilities. Winifred Kempton was the first to outline specific techniques necessary for teaching sex education to persons with disabilities that hinder learning (Kempton, 1988). Her work and the work of those who have followed help us know that for such education to be effective it must meet several criteria.

- Teachers should "draw out" from the students what they already know, to assess understanding and areas of interest.
- Statements, messages and materials should be as concrete, as real, as explicit as possible.
- Teaching approaches must not rely on reading skills for imparting information. Audiovisual materials, models and pictures are essential and effective.
- Learning should take place over a longer period of time,

with short sessions offered over several different days.

- Teachers should allow for repetition and use simple language.
- Lessons should include the opportunity to practice saying no, talking about lower risk practices, etc., through role plays.
- Lessons should include ways to check learning and get feedback from students.
- Materials should be as practical and relevant as possible to the learner's life experiences.
- The education should be offered in a nonjudgmental manner.

While these may be sound teaching techniques for all students, they are absolutely essential for people who do most of their learning by means other than reading. Emphasis must be on practical and behavioral matters rather than on understanding the medical make-up of HIV.

Special Issues

In addition to the need for especially concrete education, there are additional concerns.

Sexual Abuse/Exploitation

Statistics tell us that this population is one of the more vulnerable to sexual abuse, and that most perpetrators are known to the victim. Many persons who are developmentally disabled reside in group homes or institutional settings and are likely candidates for abuse by persons in caretaking roles. It is possible that individuals in this population are being exposed to the AIDS virus through sexual activity in their own homes, perpetrated either by other residents or by the very people hired to be their "helpers." The conspiracy of silence that operates here keeps these activities secret. Because care providers may not suspect sexual activity is taking place, there may be no AIDS education offered.

Antibody Testing, Informed Consent and Other Issues

Group home or institutional settings raise other concerns. Typically, this population is not only vulnerable to sexual abuse, but also to undue authoritarian influence. If caretakers require residents to participate in mandatory testing for HIV the residents will probably comply without protest. There would certainly be a question, however, of the legality and ethics of such a policy. Informed consent is an extremely important and sensitive issue for the developmentally, learning or mentally disabled.

Antibody testing may lead to other difficulties. Who receives the test results and how are they recorded in an individual's file? Who else has access to this information? Will an antibody-positive individual's activities be monitored in a different manner than those of other clients or residents (to make sure, for example, that he or she is not posing a threat to other residents through unsafe sexual exchanges)? Is so, does this constitute discrimination? How would a positive test result be explained to a person with limited ability to understand its meaning, and who would provide that information? What information would be given to other clients in the program?

These are challenging questions, many without clear answers at present. We believe programs should think very carefully before recommending testing for any enrolled individuals, and that policies should be considered and set before any testing takes place.

410

Is the Principle of Normalization and
Least Restrictive Environment in Jeopardy?

One of the most worrisome concerns is that fear of AIDS will foster a return to attitudes supporting more restricted and overprotective living environments for persons with developmental and other learning disabilities. Freedom to engage in healthy, normalizing community activities may be at stake. Rather than educate about reduced-risk sexual activities, some schools, agencies and homes may be inclined to discriminate by severely restricting independent activities, increasing supervision and ignoring needs for privacy. Ultimately such a course will not be in the best interests of the people these agencies seek to serve.

Teach, Don't Terrorize

Will AIDS frighten this population so completely that healthy, loving relationships are impossible? We hope not. Again, information about how one can contract HIV must be balanced with the fact that it is not easy to catch. Education can reduce unnecessary panic and fear.

Special Issues in Educating Those People Who Provide Services

Uniquely, this group of learners generally has a larger group of caretakers, or helping persons, than other students. In addition to parents and family, others are usually involved and may include group home staff, special education teachers and aides, court-appointed guardians, social workers, special tutors, physical and recreation therapists, and even special bus drivers. Incorrect beliefs and myths about the sexuality of this special group—that they are supersexed and dangerous, or that they are asexual and we mustn't put ideas into their heads by offering sex education—continue to prevail in the general community and with many of their care providers. Convincing the doubters that all people are sexual, that sex education promotes responsible behaviors and reduces risks for exploitation and AIDS transmission, and that everyone can learn using various methods and at different rates, is a major and essential task.

The explicitness necessary to reach some students identified as learning or developmentally disabled may set forth an extra obstacle that interferes with the provision of this critical education. Most teachers will require special training in order to be comfortable and knowledgeable enough to teach about AIDS and HIV infection. Direct, explicit teaching in this subject area can be hard for many teachers. They must be able to use words like penis, vagina, intercourse, anal and oral sex, condoms, rubbers. They must be able to listen well and encourage classroom discussions that may reveal a wide range of values and attitudes among the students, and do so without being critical or judgmental.

Similarly, teachers must be able to conduct sensitive discussions with parents and care providers and respect their values and attitudes. Parents and care providers need assistance in understanding the AIDS virus. Correct information can dispel myths and combat overreactive fears. Parents need to learn everything they can about the virus, and be given ways to reinforce student learning at home. The home and the school must work together to effectively educate this group of learners.

School boards must be helped to see that all students need education in this area. Further, they need to recognize the critical importance of explicit materials for these learners. This may require more latitude in approval for special education teaching materials than for the nonspecial education population.

Coordination and collaboration between the mainstream

412

and special education teachers is necessary to decide whether AIDS education is best presented in the mainstream class or the special class. Methods and materials useful in educating the student with limited reading skills must be appropriate and relevant, and may not be as helpful to the nondisabled learner. Presently, most schools are mobilizing to teach AIDS education to the "regular" student and this may in fact be the setting in which the special education student first receives this instruction. We would strongly encourage further lessons and review for these students in their special classes.

Risks to These Students

No conclusive data exists to verify that there is either more or less vulnerability of this population to AIDS, but we think there are some important considerations to keep in mind that suggest the risk may be higher. First, as was stated earlier, this group is vulnerable to sexual abuse, thus probably increasing the risk factor of contracting AIDS. In addition, many individuals in this group are less aware of physical concerns than other students. They may have, but not recognize, symptoms of sexually transmitted diseases. If these symptoms go unreported and the STD is not diagnosed, the fact that this individual is engaging in risk behavior may go unnoticed, and valuable opportunities for prevention education may be lost.

Another consideration in assessing risk has to do with group or institutional living, and the historical problems faced in effectively controlling epidemic diseases in such settings. Proper care with body fluids protects against the spread of infections like hepatitis or HIV, but these precautions must be effectively monitored in the institution. There may also be several shared sexual partners in group living environments, which could increase risk. Finally, poor self-esteem is a characteristic that this group of people generally share. This may lead to drug use and/or multiple sexual partners, both high-risk activities.

Just as it is difficult for many people to imagine that individuals with developmental or learning disabilities are sexual, there is often an assumption that disabled people don't "do" drugs. This assumption can prevent recognition of potential risk behaviors. In fact, many individuals, while able to interact and socialize with people they meet on the street, have little impulse control or understanding of activities suggested to them. If they are invited to share drugs or offered money for sexual favors, they may eagerly comply as a way to feel accepted. Sadly, and with complete support for the dignity of risk, as disabled individuals are integrated into the community, they become exposed to and perhaps involved with the unhealthy habits of some nondisabled citizens.

Current Efforts and Resources

There are several states that demonstrate some recognition of the need for sex education for special education students. Schools and agencies in these locations are beginning to incorporate AIDS education into already-existing family life/sex education programs. We presently see these efforts in California, New York, New Jersey, Pennsylvania, Michigan, Washington and Oregon.

In California, the Committee on the Sexuality of Persons with Developmental Disabilities has been advocating for appropriate sex education and counseling services since 1975. The Committee's 1988 Annual Symposium concentrated heavily on AIDS and the potential impact it carries for this population. This group has written a philosophy statement (Committee, 1975) citing an individual's right to privacy and to assistance in developing their sexuality to a level consistent with their ability to accept responsibility. The Committee provides training and consultation to all agencies and schools interested in providing sex education or AIDS education to persons with developmental disabilities.

Resource materials to assist in teaching special learners are also becoming available. A few are listed here.

An Easy Guide to Loving Carefully (McKee, Kempton and Stiggall, 1987) is a simple, reproductive health care book, with chapters on AIDS and other STDs. It includes graphic illustrations of reproductive parts of the body, and of putting on condoms.

Circles: SAFER Ways (Walker-Hirsch and Champagne, 1988) is an audiovisual package that can easily integrate AIDS information into a health education/communicable disease unit for special learners. It consists of filmstrips, slides and audio tapes and is accompanied by a comprehensive teacher's guide. The guide is written behaviorally, and offers developmental lesson plans with each story.

Life Horizons I & II (Kempton and Stanfield, 1988) is a comprehensive audiovisual curriculum guide that will enhance a teacher's ability to provide information in a meaningful way. This package offers the most complete aid to family life education ever attempted.

AIDS: Teaching People with Disabilities How to Better Protect Themselves is from Young Adult Institute (1987). It consists of a videocassette training tape and manual designed to help individuals with disabilities learn about reduced risk sexual activities and AIDS. As the title implies, the target population is young adults. Its very graphic illustrations of sexual activity and condom use, while appropriate for some groups, may be difficult or inappropriate for others. There is good information about HIV and its transmission sexually. It does not deal with AIDS and IV drugs use. The tape uses simple language and repeats appropriately.

AIDS: Prevention and Management of Persons with Developmental Disabilities At-Risk Concerning Acquired Immunodeficiency Syndrome: A Handbook (Lynn-Hill, 1987) is a well-written booklet citing history, policy development, maintaining confidential policy, prevention, reduced-risk sexual education, condoms, and condom use.

For combating the general lack of understanding regarding this special population's need for sex education, the following may be helpful: *Sex Education and Counseling of Special Groups* (Johnson and Kempton, 1987) and the film "Learning to Talk About Sex When You'd Rather Not," (1984).

References

Blomberg, P. 1986. *Vulnerability issues of children with developmental disabilities: Sexual exploitation, the problems, solutions and assessments.* Paper presented at the California Consortium of Child Abuse Councils, Sacramento, CA.

Committee on the Sexuality of the Developmentally Disabled, Inc. 1975. *Statement of philosophy on sexual rights of the developmentally disabled.* Danville, CA: Author.

Johnson, W. and Kempton, W. 1982. *Sex education and counseling of special groups.* Springfield, IL: Charles C. Thomas.

Kempton, W. 1988. *Sex education for persons with disabilities that hinder learning.* Revised edition. Philadelphia:Planned Parenthood of Southeast Pennsylvania.

Kempton, W. and Stanfield, J. 1988. *Life horizons I & II.* Santa Monica, CA: James Stanfield & Co.

Learning to talk about sex when you'd rather not. 1984. Aptos, CA: Special Purpose Films.

Lynn-Hill, D. 1987. *Prevention and management of persons with developmental disabilities at-risk concerning acquired immuno deficiency syndrome: A handbook.* Newport Beach, CA: Author.

Lynn-Hill, Erickson and Durby. 1987. *Persons with developmental disabilities as chemically-impaired: Deployment and mobilization of services.* Paper presented at the 111th AAMD Annual Meeting.

McKee, L., Kempton, W., and Stiggall, L. 1987. *An easy guide to loving carefully.* Revised edition. Santa Cruz, CA:Network Publications.

Walker-Hirsch, L. and Champagne, M. 1988. *Circles: Safer ways.* Santa Monica, CA:James Stanfield Publishing Co.

Young Adult Institute of New York. 1987. *Teaching people with disabilities how to better protect themselves.* New York, NY: Author.

Teaching About AIDS: Youth with Sensory or Physical Disabilities

Katherine M. Simpson, MA, MFCC

D isabled youth, like their able-bodied counterparts, have sexual feelings, enjoy intimacy, want to be accepted in their peer group, and may experiment with sex or drugs. They are as influenced by peer pressure as other youth. However, adults often have a difficult time imagining that young people with disabilities could—or should—be sexually active.

Adult resistance to acknowledging this is one of the greatest risks facing these young people. If the assumption is that they are not likely to engage in risky behavior, no explicit and specialized information on AIDS prevention will be offered. The curriculum for able-bodied students will be employed, and the disabled youth's specific questions will go unanswered. While this approach may protect adults from some awkwardness and discomfort and schools or community groups from greater controversies, it is a dangerous disservice to disabled youth.

Special Concerns for the Disabled

The assumption that people with disabilities are not or should not be sexual is a source of many problems for disabled youth. From early childhood on, a boy or girl may get negative messages about his or her sexuality, or the messages may be significant by their absence—no mention is made of future marriage or parenting. The young person may be discouraged from dressing to attract and rarely sees disabled adults as sexy role models in television, movies or literature.

These concerns can be complicated by the nature of a youth's disability. Young people with visual impairment need help learning to dress attractively, along with assistance in finding alternatives to the visual flirting cues our society depends on. Hearing impaired youth may not feel comfortable in a stereotypical romantic atmosphere—with soft music, which cannot be heard, and low lights, which make it difficult to read sign. If adults are not willing to help young people find appropriate ways to express their attractiveness and interest in romantic relationships, it may be hard for the youth to develop a positive sense of self in this regard.

Finally, many disabled youth receive little or no sexuality education. Almost none of the students in segregated institutions, and few in special education classes, are taught human sexuality. Accessibility to information elsewhere is very limited for visually and hearing impaired youth, and sometimes for those with motor impairment as well. If students are isolated with other similarly disabled peers in schools for the visually and hearing impaired, the possibilities for sexual misinformation to circulate are great.

The lack of education, the negative messages about their own sexuality, and the social difficulties sometimes posed by their disabilities, can make these teenagers especially likely to engage in risk-taking behavior. While disabled youth must cope with all the usual sexual feelings of normal teenagers, they may be doing so without the reassurance that what they experience is normal; without the understanding that they have many choices about how to respond to such feelings, including the choice to be abstinent; and without the acknowledgment from adults that having these feelings and figuring out what to do with them may be a big point of interest at this time of their lives.

Like other youth, disabled youth may engage in high risk or rebellious behaviors because they are emotionally troubled. Some of this behavior can certainly be damaging for the young person psychologically. If it is carried out without knowledge of AIDS risks and prevention strategies, it can be deadly.

We should also note that it is not only the troubled disabled youth who may be sexually active. Disabled teens, like able-bodied teens, may also have sex because they have deep feelings of love and attraction for their partner. These young people have just as great a need for information about human sexuality and AIDS prevention.

Teaching Disabled Youth About AIDS Prevention

Needs

It will be most productive to teach young people basic information about sexuality before discussing AIDS and its prevention. There are many good sexuality education curricula available. (Bibliographies on sex education for the physically disabled and visual and hearing impaired are available from SIECUS, 80 Fifth Avenue, Suite 801, New York, NY 10010.) As with all teen-oriented materials, language should be simple and clear, and graphics should be stylish and pleasing.

Many students have disabilities that affect their capacity to communicate. Cerebral palsy often affects speech. The student with severe speech handicaps may be learning delayed because communication has been slower, or literacy was achieved later. These young people will need careful and repeated lessons on AIDS prevention.

Students with visual impairments need braille or large print materials. Slides or films may not be especially helpful. But, many word processors can print in large type, and some print can be enlarged using photocopiers without losing much quality (Hughes, 1981). Resourceful educators may be able to develop appropriate materials desk-top style to assist such students.

Youth with hearing impairments often have information deficits. Because of their isolation in separate classes or schools, they may lack accurate information about sexuality and AIDS. American Sign Language (ASL) is the primary language for many people with hearing impairments, and it is best to teach about life-threatening issues such as AIDS in the student's primary language. Unfortunately, most AIDS education is based on English, a second language to these youth. Students in many public schools are instructed in C-sign, or finger spelling (of English). Students who have been taught to lip read instead of sign may have poor language skills; the best lip readers can only read about 20 percent of what is spoken. ASL is a very graphic language and lends itself well to the concrete and explicit descriptions of HIV transmission and safer sex practices that young people need to learn. This powerful resource for hearing impaired youth needs to be used more (Daughten, Minkin and Rosen, 1978; Woodward, 1979).

Issues

Discussing myths about AIDS can be a good way to begin talking about the subject. This would include the myth that people with disabilities are not at risk for AIDS. (Some people may believe another myth—that people with disabilities are "sick" and therefore more at risk for AIDS.)

It is essential to use simple, clear and explicit language whenever possible, especially with students who have communication handicaps. Sex is not an easy subject to understand for any one—most if us keep learning about it our whole lives. A teacher can compensate for communication handicaps and students' lack of basic knowledge about sexuality by using materials in as many sensory modes as possible. This would include the use of tactile as well as visual materials, role plays, small and large group discussions, and any other innovative techniques that vary the mode of delivering a lesson while maintaining appropriate guidelines in a classroom or other setting.

A useful resource is lifelike, lifesize models of the genitals (available from Jim Jackson and Co., 33 Richdale Ave., Cambridge, MA 02140). They are ideal for teaching proper condom use, helpful to all students, and especially helpful for the visually impaired. Use of anatomically approximate dolls can also help if a group's basic knowledge is limited.

Use of such explicit educational materials may cause controversy. Educators know that teen sexual activity is quite high. While most of us would prefer that teens delay sexual activity, we certainly want those teens who are sexually active to protect themselves from unwanted pregnancies and sexually transmitted diseases including AIDS by proper use of condoms and contraceptive foams. For many disabled youth, such explanations will need to be more explicit or lengthy than might be true for the able-bodied. The youth with communication difficulties may need to hear information several times, so a lesson would need to continue at some length. The visually impaired youth will not understand condom use well without an opportunity to actually touch a condom and practice unrolling it over a genital model. Similar practice is needed to understand how to fill and discharge foam applicators properly. These are challenging issues that need to be addressed by advocates for young people.

Some students with physical disabilities may have difficulty using condoms or foam. Disabilities that can affect ability to use a condom include amputations, spinal cord injury, stroke, muscular sclerosis, polio, arthritis, cerebral palsy, short stature and sickle cell anemia. Everyone is different and it is hard to generalize about specific adaptions. Medical providers should be encouraged to offer careful education in the use of these materials to all youth, but particularly to the disabled. In the privacy of a clinic office, the disabled individual can practice applying foam, putting on a condom or, if necessary, working with a partner to use these methods properly. A family planning educator or clinician may be able to train individuals or couples in the comfortable, effective use of condoms and foam. If the help of an assistant is needed, that individual may need some guidance, and the client may benefit from counseling about how to communicate such needs to an assistant.

Some men and women with spinal cord or other injuries may not choose penis/vagina intercourse as their primary mode of sexual expression. It is important, therefore, to point out risk factors associated with oral sex. Such discussions will be of benefit to any sexually active teen or adult, disabled or not.

Finally, in these educational sessions ask for constant feedback from students or clients. Be sure they understand you and the materials you are using. If time is limited, and it usually is, teach the essentials; it is more important that young people learn about AIDS transmission and prevention than that they understand the functioning of the human immune system.

Approaches to Teaching

Much of AIDS prevention involves communication—
learning how to talk with potential partners about safer sex,
being assertive about what activities one will and will not practice, discussing satisfaction or concerns with actual partners.
People with disabilities have had a lot of practice communicating about their needs and concerns, asserting their rights and
desires. Some of the films and books written about sexuality of
the disabled give wonderful examples of communication skills
that can help people adhere to safer sex guidelines (Bullard and
Knight, 1981). These could be used in general classroom settings, not to focus on disability, but to discuss how all people
can communicate about sexuality.

Such approaches are taken far too infrequently. Most often,
the sexual concerns of the disabled are simply ignored. In other
instances, the disabled youth may feel he or she is put on the
"hot seat," with the suggestion that his or her issues are isolated
and separated from others. AIDS prevention curricula should
integrate the concerns of the disabled with those of the nondisabled.

There are other ways this can be accomplished as well. A
good example is the use of role plays. These exercises, in which
teens practice dealing with challenging situations, are some of
the best ways for young people to build assertiveness and communication skills. Group discussions about the situations can
help teens find their own ways to deal with peer pressures. Incorporating role plays that bring up disability issues can set the
stage for greater acceptance and understanding of disability for
all students. Two examples of possible role play situations are
offered below.

Situation: Tom was in a serious automobile accident some
months ago and is paralyzed as a result of his injuries. He is

now a quadriplegic. He is still recovering from the accident and experiencing quite a bit of pain. His doctor has stopped his prescription for pain killers. Tom complains to his friend Randy at school, and Randy says he can fix Tom up with some good dope that will take care of his pain. What do you think Tom should do?

Situation: Jerry and Janet are young adults who have been dating for four months. Jerry has cerebral palsy. They are becoming very close and are thinking of marrying. Though they have not been sexual so far, it is clear that each feels strongly about the other and would like to be sexual. Janet has not suggested it because she feels it would be better for Jerry to bring it up. Jerry, in turn, is very nervous about bringing it up. He would want to use a condom to protect both of them from unwanted pregnancy or sexually transmitted diseases, but the lack of motor control in his hands would make it very difficult for him to put on a condom. What do you think Janet should do? What do you think Jerry should do?

Dealing with specific situations like these can be tricky if you have disabled students in the class who would feel singled out by such an exercise. It is important that materials used be general enough that this does not happen.

Conclusion

Advocacy for better sexuality and AIDS education for young people with disabilities is important—in schools, in agencies concerned with AIDS, and in agencies serving those young people. The comments of a woman with cerebral palsy are encouraging:

Figuring things out and getting the giggles over

things that didn't work are some of the intimate things that we have together that help to hold the relationship together...My disability kind of makes things more interesting. We have to try harder and I think we get more out of it because we do. We both have to be very conscious of each other—we have to take time. That makes us less selfish and more considerate of each other, which helps the relationship in other areas besides sexuality (Task Force on Concerns for Physically Disabled Women, 1984).

Communication is the key to safer sex, greater intimacy and effective AIDS prevention.

References

Bullard, D.G. and Knight, S.E. 1981. *Sexuality and physical disability: Personal perspectives.* St. Louis, MO: C.V. Mosby Co.

Daughten, S.D., Minkin, M.B. and Rosen, L.E. 1978. *Signs for sexuality: A resource manual.* Seattle, WA: Planned Parenthood of Seattle/King County.

Hughes, Katrine. 1981. *Large print birth control information packets.* San Francisco, CA: Planned Parenthood of Alameda/San Francisco.

Task Force on Concerns of Physically Disabled Women. 1984. *Family planning and sexuality concerns of physically disabled women.* New York: Human Science Press.

Woodward, J. 1979. *Signs of sexual behavior: An introduction to some sex-related vocabulary in American Sign Language.* Silver Springs, NY: T.J. Publishers, Inc.

Appendixes

Appendix A

Introduction to Guidelines

The following guidelines for AIDS education and curriculum evaluation are produced by two organizations—the Centers for Disease Control, and the National Coalition of Advocates for Students (a national network of 23 child advocacy organizations). These materials are similar in many ways, but some differences also exist, and we felt it would be useful to give readers an opportunity to compare the documents. Most significantly, under current federal laws, the CDC must advocate that the major emphasis in AIDS prevention programs be placed on sexual abstinence until a mutually monogamous relationship within the context of marriage is established. The NCAS also urges that students who choose abstinence be supported in that choice. Overall, however, the NCAS guidelines are somewhat broader in nature. For example, they address the need for curricula that "affirm that people have natural sexual feelings," something the CDC guidelines do not make reference to.

We believe both sets of guidelines offer clear and constructive suggestions for AIDS education. Please see Appendix E for further ideas on emphasizing abstinence in AIDS education settings.

CDC Guidelines for Effective School Health Education to Prevent the Spread of AIDS

Introduction

Since the first cases of acquired immunodeficiency syndrome (AIDS) were reported in the United States in 1981, the human immunodeficiency virus (HIV) that causes AIDS and other HIV-related diseases has precipitated an epidemic unprecedented in modern history. Because the virus is transmitted almost exclusively by behavior that individuals can modify, educational programs to influence relevant behavior can be effective in preventing the spread of HIV (*1-5*).

The guidelines below have been developed to help school personnel and others plan, implement, and evaluate educational efforts to prevent unnecessary morbidity and mortality associated with AIDS and other HIV-related illnesses. The guidelines incorporate principles for AIDS education that were developed by the President's Domestic Policy Council and approved by the President in 1987 (see Appendix I).

The guidelines provide information that should be considered by persons who are responsible for planning and implementing appropriate and effective strategies to teach young people about how to avoid HIV infection. These guidelines should not be construed as rules, but rather as a source of guidance. Although they specifically were developed to help **school personnel**, personnel from other organizations should consider these guidelines in planning and carrying out effective education about AIDS for youth who do **not** attend school and who may be at high risk of becoming infected. As they deliberate about the need for and content of AIDS education, educators, parents, and other concerned members of the community should consider the prevalence of behavior that increases the risk of HIV infection among young people in their communities. Information about the nature of the AIDS epidemic, and the extent to which young people engage in behavior that increases the risk of HIV infection, is presented in Appendix II.

Information contained in this document was developed by CDC in consultation with individuals appointed to represent the following organizations:

American Academy of Pediatrics
American Association of School Administrators
American Public Health Association
American School Health Association
Association for the Advancement of Health Education
Association of State and Territorial Health Officers
Council of Chief State School Officers
National Congress of Parents and Teachers
National Council of Churches

433

National Education Association
National School Boards Association
Society of State Directors of Health, Physical Education,
   Recreation and Dance
U.S. Department of Education
U.S. Food and Drug Administration
U.S. Office of Disease Prevention and Health Promotion

Consultants included a director of health education for a state department of education, a director of curriculum and instruction for a local education department, a health education teacher, a director of school health programs for a local school district, a director of a state health department, a deputy director of a local health department, and an expert in child and adolescent development.

Planning and Implementing Effective School Health Education about AIDS

The Nation's public and private schools have the capacity and responsibility to help assure that young people understand the nature of the AIDS epidemic and the specific actions they can take to prevent HIV infection, especially during their adolescence and young adulthood. The specific scope and content of AIDS education in schools should be locally determined and should be consistent with parental and community values.

Because AIDS is a fatal disease and because educating young people about becoming infected through sexual contact can be controversial, school systems should obtain broad community participation to ensure that school health education policies and programs to prevent the spread of AIDS are locally determined and are consistent with community values.

The development of school district policies on AIDS education can be an important first step in developing an AIDS education program. In each community, representatives of the school board, parents, school administrators and faculty, school health services, local medical societies, the local health department, students, minority groups, religious organizations, and other relevant organizations can be involved in developing policies for school health education to prevent the spread of AIDS. The process of policy development can enable these representatives to resolve various perspectives and opinions, to establish a commitment for implementing and maintaining AIDS education programs, and to establish standards for AIDS education program activities and materials. Many communities already have school health councils that include representatives from the aforementioned groups. Such councils facilitate the development of a broad base of community expertise and input, and they enhance the coordination of various activities within the comprehensive school health program (*6*).

AIDS education programs should be developed to address the needs and the developmental levels of students and of school-age youth who do not attend school, and to address specific needs of minorities, persons for whom English is not the primary language, and persons with visual or hearing impairments or other learning disabilities. Plans for addressing students' questions or concerns about AIDS at the early elementary grades, as well as for providing effective school health education about AIDS at each grade from late elementary/middle school through junior high/senior high school, including educational materials to be used, should be reviewed by representatives of the school board, appropriate school administrators, teachers, and parents before being implemented.

Education about AIDS may be most appropriate and effective when carried out within a more comprehensive school health education program that establishes a foundation for understanding the relationships between personal behavior and health (*7-9*). For example, education about AIDS may be more effective when students at appropriate ages are more knowledgeable about sexually transmitted diseases, drug abuse, and community health. It may also have greater impact when they have opportunities to develop such qualities as decision-making and communication skills, resistance to persuasion, and a sense of self-efficacy and self-esteem. However, education about AIDS should be provided as rapidly as possible, even if it is taught initially as a separate subject.

State departments of education and health should work together to help local departments of education and health throughout the state collaboratively accomplish effective school health education about AIDS. Although all schools in a state should provide effective education about AIDS, priority should be given to areas with the highest reported incidence of AIDS cases.

Preparation of Education Personnel

A team of representatives including the local school board, parent-teachers associations, school administrators, school physicians, school nurses, teachers, educational support personnel, school counselors, and other relevant school personnel should receive general training about a) the nature of the AIDS epidemic and means of controlling its spread, b) the role of the school in providing education to prevent transmission of HIV, c) methods and materials to accomplish effective programs of school health education about AIDS, and d) school policies for students and staff who may be infected. In addition, a team of school personnel responsible for teaching about AIDS should receive more specific training about AIDS education. All school personnel, especially those who teach about AIDS, periodically should receive continuing education about AIDS to assure that they have the most current information about means of controlling the epidemic, including up-to-date information about the most effective health education interventions available. State and local departments of education and health, as well as colleges of education, should assure that such in-service training is made available to all schools in the state as soon as possible and that continuing in-service and pre-service training is subsequently provided. The local school board should assure that release time is provided to enable school personnel to receive such in-service training.

Programs Taught by Qualified Teachers

In the elementary grades, students generally have one regular classroom teacher. In these grades, education about AIDS should be provided by the regular classroom teacher because that person ideally should be trained and experienced in child development, age-appropriate teaching methods, child health, and elementary health education methods and materials. In addition, the elementary teacher usually is sensitive to normal variations in child development and aptitudes within a class. In the secondary grades, students generally have a different teacher for each subject. In these grades, the secondary school health education teacher preferably should provide education about AIDS, because a qualified health education teacher will have training and experience in adolescent development, age-appropriate teaching methods, adolescent health, and secondary school health education methods and materials (including methods and materials for teaching about such topics as human sexuality, communicable diseases, and drug abuse). In secondary schools that do not have a qualified health education teacher, faculty with similar training and good rapport with students should be trained specifically to provide effective AIDS education.

Purpose of Effective Education about AIDS

The principal purpose of education about AIDS is to prevent HIV infection. The content of AIDS education should be developed with the active involvement of parents and should address the broad range of behavior exhibited by young people. Educational programs should assure that young people acquire the knowledge and skills they will need to adopt and maintain types of behavior that virtually eliminate their risk of becoming infected.

School systems should make programs available that will enable and encourage young people who **have not** engaged in sexual intercourse and who **have not** used illicit drugs to continue to—

- Abstain from sexual intercourse until they are ready to establish a mutually monogamous relationship within the context of marriage;

- Refrain from using or injecting illicit drugs.

For young people who **have** engaged in sexual intercourse or who **have** injected illicit drugs, school programs should enable and encourage them to—

- Stop engaging in sexual intercourse until they are ready to establish a mutually monogamous relationship within the context of marriage;

- To stop using or injecting illicit drugs.

Despite all efforts, some young people may remain unwilling to adopt behavior that would virtually eliminate their risk of becoming infected. Therefore, school systems, in consultation with parents and health officials, should provide AIDS education programs that address preventive types of behavior that should be practiced by persons with an increased risk of acquiring HIV infection. These include:

- Avoiding sexual intercourse with anyone who is known to be infected, who is at risk of being infected, or whose HIV infection status is not known;

- Using a latex condom with spermicide if they engage in sexual intercourse;

- Seeking treatment if addicted to illicit drugs;

- Not sharing needles or other injection equipment;

- Seeking HIV counseling and testing if HIV infection is suspected.

State and local education and health agencies should work together to assess the prevalence of these types of risk behavior, and their determinants, over time.

436

Content

Although information about the biology of the AIDS virus, the signs and symptoms of AIDS, and the social and economic costs of the epidemic might be of interest, such information is not the essential knowledge that students must acquire in order to prevent becoming infected with HIV. Similarly, a single film, lecture, or school assembly about AIDS will not be sufficient to assure that students develop the complex understanding and skills they will need to avoid becoming infected.

Schools should assure that students receive at least the essential information about AIDS, as summarized in sequence in the following pages, for each of three grade-level ranges. The exact grades at which students receive this essential information should be determined locally, in accord with community and parental values, and thus may vary from community to community. Because essential information for students at higher grades requires an understanding of information essential for students at lower grades, secondary school personnel will need to assure that students understand basic concepts before teaching more advanced information. Schools simultaneously should assure that students have opportunitites to learn about emotional and social factors that influence types of behavior associated with HIV transmission.

Early Elementary School

Education about AIDS for students in early elementary grades principally should be designed to allay excessive fears of the epidemic and of becoming infected.

AIDS is a disease that is causing some adults to get very sick, but it does not commonly affect children.

AIDS is very hard to get. You cannot get it just by being near or touching someone who has it.

Scientists all over the world are working hard to find a way to stop people from getting AIDS and to cure those who have it.

Late Elementary/Middle School

Education about AIDS for students in late elementary/middle school grades should be designed with consideration for the following information.

Viruses are living organisms too small to be seen by the unaided eye.

Viruses can be transmitted from an infected person to an uninfected person through various means.

Some viruses cause disease among people.

Persons who are infected with some viruses that cause disease may not have any signs or symptoms of disease.

AIDS (an abbreviation for acquired immunodeficiency syndrome) is caused by a virus that weakens the ability of infected individuals to fight off disease.

People who have AIDS often develop a rare type of severe pneumonia, a cancer called Kaposi's sarcoma, and certain other diseases that healthy people normally do not get.

About 1 to 1.5 million of the total population of approximately 240 million Americans currently are infected with the AIDS virus and consequently are capable of infecting others.

People who are infected with the AIDS virus live in every state in the United States and in most other countries of the world. Infected people live in cities as well as in suburbs, small towns, and rural areas. Although most infected people are adults, teenagers can also become infected. Females as well as males are infected. People of every race are infected, including whites, blacks, Hispanics, Native Americans, and Asian/Pacific Islanders.

The AIDS virus can be transmitted by sexual contact with an infected person; by using needles and other injection equipment that an infected person has used; and from an infected mother to her infant before or during birth.

A small number of doctors, nurses, and other medical personnel have been infected when they were directly exposed to infected blood.

It sometimes takes several years after becoming infected with the AIDS virus before symptoms of the disease appear. Thus, people who are infected with the virus can infect other people—even though the people who transmit the infection do not feel or look sick.

Most infected people who develop symptoms of AIDS only live about 2 years after their symptoms are diagnosed.

The AIDS virus cannot be caught by touching someone who is infected, by being in the same room with an infected person, or by donating blood.

Junior High/Senior High School

Education about AIDS for students in junior high/senior high school grades should be developed and presented taking into consideration the following information.

The virus that causes AIDS, and other health problems, is called human immuno-deficiency virus, or HIV.

The risk of becoming infected with HIV can be virtually eliminated by not engaging in sexual activities and by not using illegal intravenous drugs.

Sexual transmission of HIV is not a threat to those uninfected individuals who engage in mutually monogamous sexual relations.

HIV may be transmitted in any of the following ways: a) by sexual contact with an infected person (penis/vagina, penis/rectum, mouth/vagina, mouth/penis, mouth/rectum); b) by using needles or other injection equipment that an infected person has used; c) from an infected mother to her infant before or during birth.

A small number of doctors, nurses, and other medical personnel have been infected when they were directly exposed to infected blood.

The following are at increased risk of having the virus that causes AIDS and consequently of being infectious: a) persons with clinical or laboratory evidence of infection; b) males who have had sexual intercourse with other males; c) persons who have injected illegal drugs; d) persons who have had numerous sexual partners, including male or female prostitutes; e) persons who received blood clotting products before 1985; f) sex partners of infected persons or persons at increased risk; and g) infants born to infected mothers.

The risk of becoming infected is increased by having a sexual partner who is at increased risk of having contracted the AIDS virus (as identified previously), practicing sexual behavior that results in the exchange of body fluids (i.e., semen, vaginal secretions, blood), and using unsterile needles or paraphernalia to inject drugs.

Although no transmission from deep, open-mouth (i.e., "French") kissing has been documented, such kissing theoretically could transmit HIV from an infected to an uninfected person through direct exposure of mucous membranes to infected blood or saliva.

In the past, medical use of blood, such as transfusing blood and treating hemophiliacs with blood clotting products, has caused some people to become infected with HIV. However, since 1985 all donated blood has been tested to determine whether it is infected with HIV; moreover, all blood clotting products have been made from screened plasma and have been heated to destroy any HIV that might remain in the concentrate. Thus, the risk of becoming infected with HIV from blood transfusions and from blood clotting products is virtually eliminated. Cases of HIV infection caused by these medical uses of blood will continue to be diagnosed, however, among people who were infected by these means before 1985.

Persons who continue to engage in sexual intercourse with persons who are at increased risk or whose infection status is unknown should use a latex condom (not natural membrane) to reduce the likelihood of becoming infected. The latex condom must be applied properly and used from start to finish for every sexual act. Although a latex condom does not provide 100% protection—because it is possible for the condom to leak, break, or slip off—it provides the best protection for people who do not maintain a mutually monogamous relationship with an uninfected partner. Additional protection may be obtained by using spermicides that seem active against HIV and other sexually transmitted organisms in conjunction with condoms.

Behavior that prevents exposure to HIV also may prevent unintended pregnancies and exposure to the organisms that cause Chlamydia infection, gonorrhea, herpes, human papillomavirus, and syphilis.

*Persons who believe they may be infected with the AIDS virus should take precautions not to infect others and to seek counseling and antibody testing to determine whether they are infected. If persons **are not** infected, counseling and testing can relieve unnecessary anxiety and reinforce the need to adopt or continue practices that reduce the risk of infection. If persons **are** infected, they should: a) take precautions to protect sexual partners from becoming infected; b) advise previous and current sexual or drug-use partners to receive counseling and testing; c) take precautions against becoming pregnant; and d) seek medical care* *and counseling about other medical problems that may result from a weakened immunologic system.*

More detailed information about AIDS, including information about how to obtain counseling and testing for HIV, can be obtained by telephoning the AIDS National Hotline (toll free) at 800-342-2437; the Sexually Transmitted Diseases National Hotline (toll free) at 800-227-8922; or the appropriate state or local health department (the telephone number of which can be obtained by calling the local information operator).

Curriculum Time and Resources

Schools should allocate sufficient personnel time and resources to assure that policies and programs are developed and implemented with appropriate community involvement, curricula are well-planned and sequential, teachers are well-trained, and up-to-date teaching methods and materials about AIDS are available. In addition, it is crucial that sufficient classroom time be provided at **each** grade level to assure that students acquire essential knowledge appropriate for that grade level, and have time to ask questions and discuss issues raised by the information presented.

Program Assessment

The criteria recommended in the foregoing "Guidelines for Effective School Health Education To Prevent the Spread of AIDS" are summarized in the following nine assessment criteria. Local school boards and administrators can assess the extent to which their programs are consistent with these guidelines by determining the extent to which their programs meet each point shown below. Personnel in state departments of education and health also can use these criteria to monitor the extent to which schools in the state are providing effective health education about AIDS.

1. To what extent are parents, teachers, students, and appropriate community representatives involved in developing, implementing, and assessing AIDS education policies and programs?
2. To what extent is the program included as an important part of a more comprehensive school health education program?
3. To what extent is the program taught by regular classroom teachers in elementary grades and by qualified health education teachers or other similarly trained personnel in secondary grades?
4. To what extent is the program designed to help students acquire essential knowledge to prevent HIV infection at each appropriate grade?
5. To what extent does the program describe the benefits of abstinence for young people and mutually monogamous relationships within the context of marriage for adults?
6. To what extent is the program designed to help teenage students avoid specific types of behavior that increase the risk of becoming infected with HIV?
7. To what extent is adequate training about AIDS provided for school administrators, teachers, nurses, and counselors—especially those who teach about AIDS?

8. To what extent are sufficient program development time, classroom time, and educational materials provided for education about AIDS?
9. To what extent are the processes and outcomes of AIDS education being monitored and periodically assessed?

References
1. US Public Health Service. Coolfont report: a PHS plan for prevention and control of AIDS and the AIDS virus. Public Health Rep 1986;101:341.
2. Institute of Medicine. National Academy of Sciences. Confronting AIDS: directions for public health, health care, and research. Washington, DC: National Academy Press, 1986.
3. US Department of Health and Human Services, Public Health Service. Surgeon General's report on acquired immune deficiency syndrome. Washington, DC: US Department of Health and Human Services, 1986.
4. US Public Health Service. AIDS: information/education plan to prevent and control AIDS in the United States, March 1987. Washington, DC: US Department of Health and Human Services, 1987.
5. US Department of Education. AIDS and the education of our children, a guide for parents and teachers, Washington, DC: US Department of Education, 1987.
6. Kolbe LJ, Iverson DC. Integrating school and community efforts to promote health: strategies, policies, and methods. Int J Health Educ 1983;2:40-47.
7. Noak M. Recommendations for school health education. Denver: Education Commission of the States, 1982.
8. Comprehensive school health education as defined by the national professional school health education organizations. J Sch Health 1984;54:312-315.
9. Allensworth D, Kolbe L (eds). The comprehensive school health program: exploring an expanded concept. J Sch Health 1987;57:402-76.

Appendix I

The President's Domestic Policy Council's
Principles for AIDS Education

The following principles were proposed by the Domestic Policy Council and approved by the President in 1987:

Despite intensive research efforts, prevention is the only effective AIDS control strategy at present. Thus, there should be an aggressive Federal effort in AIDS education.

The scope and content of the school portion of this AIDS education effort should be locally determined and should be consistent with parental values.

The Federal role should focus on developing and conveying accurate health information on AIDS to the educators and others, not mandating a specific school curriculum on this subject, and trusting the American people to use this information in a manner appropriate to their community's needs.

Any health information developed by the Federal Government that will be used for education should encourage responsible sexual behavior—based on fidelity, commitment, and maturity, placing sexuality within the context of marriage.

Any health information provided by the Federal Government that might be used in schools should teach that children should not engage in sex and should be used with the consent and involvement of parents.

Appendix II

The Extent of AIDS and Indicators of Adolescent Risk

Since the first cases of acquired immunodeficiency syndrome (AIDS) were reported in the United States in 1981, the human immunodeficiency virus (HIV) that causes AIDS and other HIV-related diseases has precipitated an epidemic unprecedented in modern history. Although in 1985, fewer than 60% of AIDS cases in the United States were reported among persons residing outside New York City and San Francisco, by 1991 more than 80% of the cases will be reported from other localities (1).

It has been estimated that from 1 to 1.5 million persons in the United States are infected with HIV (1), and, because there is no cure, infected persons are potentially capable of infecting others indefinitely. It has been predicted that 20%-30% of individuals currently infected will develop AIDS by the end of 1991 (1). Fifty percent of those diagnosed as having AIDS have not survived for more than about 1.5 years beyond diagnosis, and only about 12% have survived for more than 3 years (2).

By the end of 1987, about 50,000 persons in the United States had been diagnosed as having AIDS, and about 28,000 had died from the disease (2). Blacks and Hispanics, who make up about 12% and 6% of the U.S. population, respectively, disproportionately have contracted 25% and 14% of all reported AIDS cases (*3*). It has been estimated that during 1991, 74,000 cases of AIDS will be diagnosed, and 54,000 persons will die from the disease. By the end of that year, the total number of deaths caused by AIDS will be about 179,000 (*1*). In addition, health care and supportive services for the 145,000 persons projected to be living with AIDS in that year will cost our Nation an estimated $8-$10 billion in 1991 alone (*1*). The World Health Organization projects that by 1991, 50-100 million persons may be infected worldwide (*4*). The magnitude and seriousness of this epidemic requires a systematic and concerted response from almost every institution in our society.

A vaccine to prevent transmission of the virus is not expected to be developed before the next decade, and its use would not affect the number of persons already infected by that time. A safe and effective antiviral agent to treat those infected is not expected to be available for general use within the next several years. The Centers for Disease Control (*5*), the National Academy of Sciences (*6*), the Surgeon General of the United States (*7*), and the U.S. Department of Education (*8*) have noted that in the absence of a vaccine or therapy, educating individuals about actions they can take to protect themselves from becoming infected is the most effective means available for controlling the epidemic. Because the virus is transmitted almost exclusively as a result of behavior individuals can modify (e.g., by having sexual contact with an infected person or by sharing intravenous drug paraphernalia with an infected person), educational programs designed to influence relevant types of behavior can be effective in controlling the epidemic.

A significant number of teenagers engage in behavior that increases their risk of becoming infected with HIV. The percentage of metropolitan teenage girls who had ever had sexual intercourse increased from 30%-45% between 1971 and 1982. The average age at first intercourse for females remained at approximately 16.2 years between 1971 and 1979 (*9*). The average proportion of never-married teenagers who have ever had intercourse increases with age from 14 through 19 years. In 1982, the percentage of never-married girls who reported having engaged in sexual intercourse was as follows: approximately 6% among 14-year-olds (*10*), 18% among 15-year-olds, 29% among 16-year-olds, 40% among 17-year-olds, 54% among 18-year-olds, and 66% among 19-year-olds (*11*). Among never-married boys living in metropolitan areas, the percentage who reported having engaged in sexual intercourse was as follows: 24% among 14-year-olds, 35% among 15-year-olds, 45% among 16-year olds, 56% among 17-year-olds, 66% among 18-year olds, and 78% among 19-year olds (*9,12*). Rates of sexual experience (e.g., percentage having had intercourse) are higher for black teenagers than for white teenagers at every age and for both sexes (*11,12*).

Male homosexual intercourse is an important risk factor for HIV infection. In one survey conducted in 1973, 5% of 13- to 15-year-old boys and 17% of 16- to 19-year-old boys reported having had at least one homosexual experience. Of those who reported having had such an experience, most (56%) indicated that the first homosexual experience had occurred when they were 11 or 12 years old. Two percent reported that they currently engaged in homosexual activity (*13*).

Another indicator of high-risk behavior among teenagers is the number of cases of sexually transmitted diseases they contract. Approximately 2.5 million teenagers are affected with a sexually transmitted disease each year (*14*).

443

Some teenagers also are at risk of becoming infected with HIV through illicit intravenous drug use. Findings from a national survey conducted in 1986 of nearly 130 high schools indicated that although overall illicit drug use seems to be declining slowly among high school seniors, about 1% of seniors reported having used heroin and 13% reported having used cocaine within the previous year (*15*). The number of seniors who injected each of these drugs is not known.

Only 1% of all the persons diagnosed as having AIDS have been under age 20 (*2*); most persons in this group had been infected by transfusion or perinatal transmission. However, about 21% of all the persons diagnosed as having AIDS have been 20-29 years of age. Given the long incubation period between HIV infection and symptoms that lead to AIDS diagnosis (3 to 5 years or more), some fraction of those in the 20- to 29-year-age group diagnosed as having AIDS were probably infected while they were still teenagers.

Among military recruits screened in the period October 1985-December 1986, the HIV seroprevalence rate for persons 17-20 years of age (0.6/1,000) was about half the rate for recruits in all age groups (1.5/1,000) (*16*). These data have lead some to conclude that teenagers and young adults have an appreciable risk of infection and that the risk may be relatively constant and cumulative (*17*).

Reducing the risk of HIV infection among teenagers is important not only for their well-being but also for the children they might produce. The birth rate for U.S. teenagers is among the highest in the developed world (*18*); in 1984, this group accounted for more than 1 million pregnancies. During that year the rate of pregnancy among sexually active teenage girls 15-19 years of age was 233/1,000 girls (*19*).

Although teenagers are at risk of becoming infected with and transmitting the AIDS virus as they become sexually active, studies have shown that they do not believe they are likely to become infected (*20,21*). Indeed, a random sample of 860 teenagers (ages 16-19) in Massachusetts revealed that, although 70% reported they were sexually active (having sexual intercourse or other sexual contact), only 15% of this group reported changing their sexual behavior because of concern about contracting AIDS. Only 20% of those who changed their behavior selected effective methods such as abstinence or use of condoms (*20*). Most teenagers indicated that they want more information about AIDS (*20,21*).

Most adult Americans recognize the early age at which youth need to be advised about how to protect themselves from becoming infected with HIV and recognize that the schools can play an important role in providing such education. When asked in a November 1986 nationwide poll whether children should be taught about AIDS in school, 83% of Americans agreed, 10% disagreed, and 7% were not sure (*22*). According to information gathered by the United States Conference of Mayors in December of 1986, 40 of the Nation's 73 largest school districts were providing education about AIDS, and 24 more were planning such education (*23*). Of the districts that offered AIDS education, 63% provided it in 7th grade, 60% provided it in 9th grade, and 90% provided it in 10th grade. Ninety-eight percent provided medical facts about AIDS, 78% mentioned abstinence as a means of avoiding infection, and 70% addressed the issues of avoiding high-risk sexual activities, selecting sexual partners, and using condoms. Data collected by the National Association of State Boards of Education in the summer of 1987 indicated that a) 15 states had mandated comprehensive school health education; eight had mandated AIDS education; b) 12 had legislation pending on AIDS education, and six had state board of education actions pending; c) 17 had developed curricula for AIDS education, and seven more were developing such materials; and d) 40 had developed policies on admitting students with AIDS to school (*24*).

The Nation's system of public and private schools has a strategic role to play in assuring that young people understand the nature of the epidemic they face and the specific actions they can take to protect themselves from becoming infected — especially during their adolescence and young adulthood. In 1984, 98% of 14 and 15 year-olds, 92% of 16 and 17 year-olds, and 50% of 18 and 19 year-olds were in school (*25*). In that same year, about 615,000 14- to 17-year-olds and 1.1 million 18- to 19-year-olds were not enrolled in school and had not completed high school (*26*).

References
1. US Public Health Service. Coolfont report: a PHS plan for prevention and control of AIDS and the AIDS virus. Public Health Rep 1986;101:341.
2. CDC. Acquired immunodeficiency syndrome (AIDS) weekly surveillance report — United States. Cases reported to CDC. December 28, 1987.
3. CDC. Acquired immunodeficiency syndrome (AIDS) among blacks and Hispanics — United States. MMWR 1986;35:655-8, 663-6.
4. World Health Organization. Special program on AIDS: strategies and structure projected needs. Geneva: World Health Organization, 1987.
5. CDC. Results of a Gallup Poll on acquired immunodeficiency syndrome — New York City, United States. MMWR 1985;34:513-4.
6. Institute of Medicine. National Academy of Sciences. Confronting AIDS: directions for public health, health care, and research. Washington, DC: National Academy Press, 1986.
7. US Department of Health and Human Services, Public Health Service. Surgeon General's report on acquired immune deficiency syndrome. Washington, DC: US Department of Health and Human Services, 1986.
8. US Department of Education. AIDS and the education of our children, a guide for parents and teachers. Washington, DC: US Department of Education, 1987.
9. Zelnick M, Kantner JF. Sexual activity, contraceptive use, and pregnancy among metropolitan-area teenagers: 1971-1979. Fam Plann Perspect 1980;12:230-7.
10. Hofferth SL, Kahn J, Baldwin W. Premarital sexual activity among United States teenage women over the past three decades. Fam Plann Perspect 1987;19:46-53.
11. Pratt WF, Mosher WD, Bachrach CA, et al. Understanding US fertility: findings from the National Survey of Family Growth, cycle III. Popul Bull 1984:39:1-42.
12. Teenage pregnancy: the problem that hasn't gone away. Tables and References. New York: The Alan Guttmacher Institute. June 1981.
13. Sorensen RC. Adolescent sexuality in contemporary America. New York, World Publishing, 1973.
14. Division of Sexually Transmitted Diseases, Annual Report, FY 1986. Center for Prevention Services, Centers for Disease Control, US Public Health Service, 1987.
15. Johnston LD, Bachman JG, O'Malley PM. Drug use among American high school students, college, and other young adults: national trends through 1986. Rockville, Md: National Institute on Drug Abuse, 1987.
16. CDC. Trends in human immunodeficiency virus infection among civilian applicants for military service — United States, October 1985-December 1986. MMWR 1987;36:273-6.
17. Burke DS, Brundage JF, Herbold JR, et al. Human immunodeficiency virus infections among civilian applicants for United States military service, October 1985 to March 1986. N Engl J Med 1987;317:131-6.
18. Jones EF, Forrest JD, Goldman N, et al. Teenage pregnancy in developed countries: determinants and policy implications. Fam Plann Perspect 1985;17:53-63.
19. National Research Council. Risking the future: adolescent sexuality, pregnancy, and child-bearing (vol. 1). Washington, DC: National Academy Press, 1987.
20. Strunin L, Hingson R. Acquired immunodeficiency syndrome and adolescents: knowledge, beliefs, attitudes, and behaviors. Pediatrics 1987;79:825-8.

21. DiClemente RJ, Zorn J, Temoshok L. Adolescents and AIDS: a survey of knowledge, attitudes, and beliefs about AIDS in San Francisco. Am J Public Health 1986;76:1443-5.
22. Yankelovich Clancy Shulman. Memorandum to all data users from Hal Quinley about Time/Yankelovich Clancy Shulman Poll findings on sex education, November 17, 1986. New York City: Yankelovich Clancy Shulman, 1986.
23. United States Conference of Mayors. Local school districts active in AIDS education. AIDS Information Exchange 1987;4:1-10.
24. Cashman J. Personal communication on September 8, 1987, about the National Association of State Boards of Education survey of state AIDS-related policies and legislation. Washington, DC: National Association of State Boards of Education.
25. US Department of Commerce, Bureau of the Census. Statistical abstract of the United States, 105th ed. Washington, DC: US Department of Commerce, 1985.
26. US Department of Commerce, Bureau of the Census. School enrollment — social and economic characteristics of students: October 1984. Current Population Reports. Washington, DC: US Department of Commerce, 1985 (Series P-20, No. 404).

Centers for Disease Control. Guidelines for Effective School Health Education To Prevent the Spread of AIDS. *MMWR* 1988;37 (suppl. no. S-2):[inclusive page numbers].

National Coalition of Advocates for Students: Guidelines for Selecting Teaching Materials

Devon Davidson

T he National Coalition of Advocates for Students (NCAS) is a network of 23 experienced child advocacy organizations working on issues of access and equity in the public schools. NCAS acts to protect the educational rights of the most vulnerable students—the poor, minority or disabled. Its goal is fair and excellent public education for all children.

In late 1986 and early 1987, NCAS reviewed AIDS education materials developed by a number of state and local education agencies. Because this review uncovered serious problems with quality, NCAS convened a group of experienced sex educators and child development specialists to develop criteria which parents, advocates and school personnel could use to evaluate educational materials on AIDS. To help assure cultural appropriateness of the criteria, NCAS created Black and Latino review panels, and incorporated the comments of these panel members into the criteria. The following document, revised in 1988, is the result of this work. Copies are available in Spanish from NCAS.

Criteria for Evaluating an AIDS Curriculum

Adolescents and young adults are now a primary risk group for contracting Acquired Immune Deficiency Syndrome (AIDS). At least 50% of all teenagers are sexually active; most will have more than one sexual partner, and some will be experimenting with drugs. Regardless of whether adults approve of this behavior, young people's lives may be at risk. Public schools must assume a key role in giving youth the information they need to avoid contracting this deadly disease.

Teaching about AIDS should take place within the context of a comprehensive health education or family life/sex education course. Such a course should present the positive aspects of sexuality as well as its dangers. An AIDS curriculum must be appropriate to the chronological and developmental age of the student, and should be taught in small groups of 20 or fewer students.

Below is a checklist for parents, child advocates, school board members, teachers and administrators to evaluate existing AIDS curricula and to advocate for the establishment of high quality curricula. An effective AIDS curriculum should elicit "yes" answers to the following questions:

Curriculum Content

_____For students in grades 6 and up, does the curriculum give simple, clear, and direct information about AIDS transmission and prevention?

_____Does the curriculum help students acquire the necessary self-esteem and assertiveness to choose to abstain from sexual intercourse?

_____Does the curriculum inform all students about effective ways to prevent infection when they become sexually active, including information about condoms and their correct use?

_____Does the curriculum focus on teaching students how to make healthy sexual decisions and not just on the medical aspects of AIDS?

_____By emphasizing high-risk behaviors rather than high-risk groups, does the curriculum strongly convey the message that anyone can get AIDS regardless of race, sex, age, or sexual orientation?

_____Does the curriculum affirm that people have natural sexual feelings?

_____Are several class periods provided to give each student multiple opportunities to rehearse making decisions based on the information they have learned about AIDS?

_____Does the curriculum allay young children's fears of AIDS?

_____Does the curriculum give young children a foundation for more detailed discussion of sexuality and health at the 6th grade level and later?

Development and Implementation

_____Does the program provide for adequate staff training to teach the curriculum?

_____ Are staff helped to examine their own attitudes about sexuality and AIDS?

_____Are staff given accurate and detailed information about AIDS?

_____Are staff trained in the concrete skills needed to effectively teach an AIDS curriculum?

_____Is the same information given to limited English proficient students in their own language?

_____Is the information provided appropriately to students with hearing and visual impairments and to students with severely disabling conditions?

_____Is the curriculum updated regularly to incorporate new information as it becomes available?

_____Has sufficient community and parental support been generated to give teachers the backing they need to teach sensitive material in a direct manner?

_____Does the curriculum facilitate an ongoing dialogue with parents on these issues?

Matching Approaches to AIDS Education with Childhood Development

Students in a particular grade may vary widely in their emotional development. Teachers are urged to individualize their teaching where appropriate, keeping in mind that the following statements are apt to characterize the vast majority of their students.

Developmental Characteristics of Students
Grades K through 3 Students Are Likely to Be:
- egocentric;
- developing some independence from parents and gradually orienting toward peers;
- able to relate to their own bodies/be curious about body parts;
- highly competitive and capable of unkindness to each other;
- able to understand information if it relates to their own experiences.

Grades 4 and 5 Students Are Likely to Be:
- aware of sexual feelings and desires either in themselves or in others, and confused about them;
- increasingly sensitive to peer pressure;
- capable of concern for others;
- exploring sex roles;
- in different stages of pre-puberty and early puberty and usually very interested in learning about sexuality and human relationships;
- quite comfortable discussing human sexuality;
- confused between fact and fancy (between hypothesis and reality);

- able to internalize rules and know what is right or wrong according to those rules.

Grades 6 through 9
Students Are Likely to Be:

- engaged in search for identity (including sexual identity); asking "Who am I?" and "Am I normal?"; very centered on self;
- influenced by peer attitudes;
- concerned about and experimenting with relationships between boys and girls;
- confused about the homosexual feelings many of them will have experienced;
- worried about the changes in their bodies;
- able to understand that behavior has consequences, but may not believe the consequences could happen to them;
- fearful of asking questions about sex which might make them appear uninformed.

Grade 10 through 12
Students Are Likely to Be:

- still struggling for a sense of personal identity, especially those who are confused about their sexual identities;
- thinking that they "know it all";
- seeking greater independence from parents;
- open to information provided by trusted adults;
- near end of this period, beginning to think about establishing more permanent relationships;
- experiencing an illusion of immortality;
- sexually active.

Appropriate Approaches to AIDS Education
Grades K through 3

The primary goal is to allay children's fears of AIDS and to establish a foundation for more detailed discussion of sexuality and health at the 6th grade level.

- Information about AIDS should be included in the larger curriculum on body appreciation, wellness, sickness, friendships, assertiveness, family roles and different types of families.
- Children should be encouraged to feel positively about their bodies and to know their body parts and the difference between girls and boys. Teachers should answer questions about how babies are developed and born.
- AIDS should be defined simply as a very serious disease that some adults and teenagers get. Students should be told that young children rarely get it and that they do not need to worry about playing with children whose parents have AIDS or with those few children who do have the disease.
- Children should be cautioned never to play with hypodermic syringes found on playgrounds or elsewhere and to avoid contact with other people's blood.
- Questions should be answered directly and simply; responses should be limited to questions asked.
- Children should be taught assertiveness about refusing unwanted touch by others, including family members.

Grades 4 and 5

It is appropriate to use the same approach as for grades K-3 with an increased emphasis on:
- affirming that bodies have natural sexual feelings;
- helping children examine and affirm their own and their families' values;

In addition, teachers of 4th and 5th graders should:
- Continue providing basic information about human sexuality—helping children understand puberty and the changes in their bodies,
- Be prepared to answer questions about AIDS and AIDS prevention.

Grades 6-12

The primary goal is to teach students to protect themselves and others from infection with the AIDS virus.
- Students should learn the information outlined below in "What Adolescents Should Know About AIDS."
- AIDS issues should be made as real as possible without overly frightening students. Movies about or classroom visits from people with AIDS have helped students in some schools overcome their denial of the disease and give AIDS a human face.
- The focus should be on healthy behaviors rather than on the medical aspects of the disease.
- Students should examine and affirm their own values.
- Students should rehearse making responsible decisions about sex, including responses to risky situations.
- Students should know they have a right to abstain from sexual intercourse or to postpone becoming sexually active. They should be helped to develop the skills to assert those rights.
- It must not be assumed that all students will choose abstinence.
- Information about AIDS should be presented in the context of other sexually transmitted diseases (STDs).
- It is important to be honest and to provide information in a straightforward manner. Be explicit. Use simple, clear words. Explain in detail. Use examples.

454

- Sexual vocabulary should be connected with slang, if necessary, to be certain students understand the lesson.
- It is important to be non-threatening and to work to alleviate anxiety.
- Students should be given the opportunity to ask questions anonymously.
- Discussion of dating relationships can provide opportunities to teach decision-making skills. Students should be helped to think through how to make responsible decisions about sex before questions arise in a dating context.
- Teaching about AIDS is often enhanced by:
  - movies and other visual aids;
  - role plays and other participatory exercises;
  - same-sex groupings (to encourage more candid discussion) *followed* by sharing in a mixed-sex group (to increase comfort level in discussing sexual subjects with members of the opposite sex);
  - involvement of students in planning and teaching—let young people speak the message to each other whenever possible.
- AIDS education should also include discussion of critical social issues raised by the epidemic, such as protecting the public health without endangering individual liberties.
- Teachers should have resources to help students find answers to detailed medical questions.
- Students should be taught skills that will enable them to continue to evaluate the AIDS crisis.

What Adolescents Should Know About AIDS

The information adolescents need is simple and straightforward. Home and school instruction should emphasize prevention through teaching safe behaviors. While adolescents need only minimal knowledge of the medical aspects of the disease, some may seek a more in-depth understanding of the virus and its manifestations. Teachers and parents should be prepared to answer their questions. **This is what should be appropriately communicated to all adolescents:**

Definition of AIDS

A disease triggered by infection with the human immunodeficiency virus (HIV) which weakens the immune system, causing the infected person to catch certain diseases that healthy people can fight off, but that can be fatal to a person with AIDS. Unlike most infections, HIV infection does not go away. The virus remains in the person's body for the rest of his or her life.

Transmission of HIV

HIV is extremely difficult to catch. It is *not* transmitted by casual contact such as hugging, sneezing, or sharing bathrooms.

There is no danger of getting AIDS by donating blood. A few years ago, some people became infected with HIV through receiving blood transfusions. Now, however, all blood donations are screened and tested so that the blood supply is quite safe.

HIV is transmitted in three main ways:

1. Through infected semen and vaginal secretions (by vaginal or anal sexual intercourse or, possibly, by oral sex);

2. Through infected blood (by sharing intravenous IV drug needles or using unsterile hypodermic needles for steroids or any other purpose);

3. From an infected mother to her child either before or during childbirth and, possibly, through breast milk.

Anyone who engages in risky behaviors can become infected—regardless of gender, sexual orientation, age or race.

Three Manifestations of Infection

1. Many people who are infected with the virus have no symptoms of disease. Since they look and feel healthy, these people may not know they are infected. They can, however, transmit HIV to others through unprotected sexual intercourse, sharing unsterile needles or childbirth. Many, if not all, of these carriers will eventually become symptomatic. Most of them, however, will not become sick for three to seven years or more after infection.

2. People who are infected with HIV may develop a set of specific symptoms related to AIDS. They are said to have AIDS Related Complex (ARC). They may be only mildly ill or very sick.

3. Manifestations of AIDS can include opportunistic infections and cancers as well as neurological and psychological problems.

Testing

It is now possible to test blood, in most cases, to determine if a person is a carrier of HIV. At this time, the Centers for Disease Control and the U.S. Surgeon General do not recommend testing of the general population. However, men and women who are considering parenting and who practice risky behaviors are advised to be tested. Anyone thinking of being tested should contact an alternative test site which tests anonymously and offers pre- and post-test counseling.

Adolescents Can Prevent AIDS By:

- abstaining from or postponing becoming sexually active;
- only having sexual relations within the context of a mutually faithful relationship with an uninfected partner;
- always using latex condoms (even in combination with other birth control) from beginning to end of all types of intercourse, preferably also using a spermicidal jelly containing nonoxynol 9;
- not using intravenous drugs. Those who do should NEVER share needles or syringes. They should be encouraged to enter a drug treatment program. Those who continue to share needles should be told how to sterilize their equipment. Tattoo needles and needles used for injecting body-building hormones or for piercing ears should also never be shared.

Local Telephone Number

Students should be given a local telephone number to call for additional information. Sources of AIDS information in other languages should also be provided. Some local AIDS hotlines have Spanish-speaking staff available during certain hours. Find out what these hours are and provide all this information to Spanish-speaking students. Health clinics and other community organizations serving the Latino, Chinese and other language minority communities may also be able to provide AIDS counseling in those languages.

National AIDS Hotline

1-800-342-7514
AIDS Information in English & Spanish
24 Hours

Staff Training

Staff training is a *must*. It should be provided at two levels:

Basic Information

All staff (teachers, administrators, custodians and clerical persons) should receive basic information about AIDS. They should understand its transmission and prevention and know where to turn in the school and in the community for more information and help.

Someone in each school should be designated as an AIDS resource person. Each school district should have a similar AIDS resource staff person at the central office level. AIDS education at this level can be conducted as a one or two session in-service workshop. Public health departments and local AIDS service agencies can usually provide knowledgeable workshop leaders.

Comprehensive Training

Those teachers and supervisory administrators who will be teaching AIDS education must receive comprehensive training. When feasible, participants should be offered graduate level credit.

Training should:
- help staff examine their own attitudes about sexuality and AIDS;
- provide accurate and detailed information about AIDS;
- provide concrete skills to effectively teach an AIDS curriculum.

Effective training may also involve significant participation of parents and students.

Teachers who are uncomfortable with the subject matter should not be required to teach an AIDS unit. Their confusion and discomfort will inevitably be conveyed to their students.

Teachers who do agree to teach AIDS units should be offered opportunities to team teach or to draw on outside resource people for support and assistance.

Family planning agencies can help identify sexuality educators to lead this training.

Parental and Community Involvement

It is important to include parents and community leaders in the development and implementation of AIDS curricula. By doing so, you will:
- educate key members about AIDS and the risks it poses to adolescents;
- involve parents in an important way in their children's education;
- develop a curriculum that considers the ethnic and cultural roots of sexual attitudes;
- build respect and a broad validation for the curriculum;
- build a solid base of supportive community members who can speak to opposition that may arise;
- give teachers the support they need to teach sensitive material in a direct manner.

Two effective means of facilitating parent/community participation are:

An AIDS Education Advisory Committee

Form an advisory committee to work with key school personnel to design a program, provide information to the community, and present the program to the local school board. The committee might include parents, religious leaders, student leaders, elected officials, and staff of community agencies. Be sure the committee reflects the true racial and ethnic diversity of the community. While it is important that all members concur on the importance of elective AIDS education, committee members should reflect a broad range of community perspectives.

While the primary mandate of the Advisory Committee is the timely implementation of an AIDS curriculum, it should also begin to lay the groundwork for a comprehensive health and sexuality education program. It is through such a comprehensive program that students can acquire the self-esteem and decision-making skills necessary to make healthy choices about AIDS and other important life issues.

Parental Component of the AIDS Curriculum

At the same time students are taught about AIDS, parents should also be educated about the disease, its transmission and prevention. A well-planned and publicized parent information night is one method. A second effective strategy is a parent/student communication component built into the curriculum itself. Students are then empowered to be educators themselves, perhaps assisted by a study guide to use in teaching their parents. The benefits of this approach include:

- reinforcement of classroom learning;
- education of parents about AIDS;
- facilitation of a dialogue between students and parents about sexuality issues.

———————— Appendix B ————————

CDC Guidelines for Education and Foster Care of Children Infected with Human T-Lymphotropic Virus Type III/ Lymphadenopathy-Associated Virus

—————————————

The information and recommendations contained in this document were developed and compiled by CDC in consultation with individuals appointed by their organizations to represent the Conference of State and Territorial Epidemiologists, the Association of State and Territorial Health Officers, the National Association of County Health Officers, the Division of Maternal and Child Health (Health Resources and Services Administration), the National Association for Elementary School Principals, the National Association of State School Nurse Consultants, the National Congress of Parents and Teachers, and the Children's Aid Society. The consultants also included the mother of a child with acquired immunodeficiency syndrome (AIDS), a legal advisor to a state education department, and several pediatricians who are experts in the field of pediatric AIDS. This document is made available to assist state and local health and education departments in developing guidelines for their particular situations and locations.

These recommendations apply to all children known to be infected with human T-lymphotropic virus type III/lymphadenopathy-associated virus (HTLV-III/LAV). This includes children with AIDS as defined for reporting purposes (Table 1); children who are diagnosed by their physicians as having an illness due to infection with HTLV-III/LAV but who do not meet the case definition; and children who are asymptomatic but have virologic or serologic evidence of infection with HTLV-III/LAV. These recommendations do not apply to siblings of infected children unless they are also infected.

BACKGROUND

The Scope of the Problem. As of August 20, 1985, 183 of the 12,599 reported cases of AIDS in the United States were among children under 18 years of age. This number is expected to double in the next year. Children with AIDS have been reported from 23 states, the District of Columbia, and Puerto Rico, with 75% residing in New York, California, Florida, and New Jersey.

The 183 AIDS patients reported to CDC represent only the most severe form of HTLV-III/LAV infection, i.e., those children who develop opportunistic infections or malignancies (Table 1). As in adults with HTLV-III/LAV infection, many infected children may have milder illness or may be asymptomatic.

Legal Issues. Among the legal issues to be considered in forming guidelines for the education and foster care of HTLV-III/LAV-infected children are the civil rights aspects of public

Appendix B

TABLE 1. Provisional case definition for acquired immunodeficiency syndrome (AIDS) surveillance of children

For the limited purposes of epidemiologic surveillance, CDC defines a case of pediatric acquired immunodeficiency syndrome (AIDS) as a child who has had:
1. A reliably diagnosed disease at least moderately indicative of underlying cellular immunodeficiency, and
2. No known cause of underlying cellular immunodeficiency or any other reduced resistance reported to be associated with that disease.

The diseases accepted as sufficiently indicative of underlying cellular immunodeficiency are the same as those used in defining AIDS in adults. In the absence of these opportunistic diseases, a histologically confirmed diagnosis of chronic lymphoid interstitial pneumonitis will be considered indicative of AIDS unless test(s) for HTLV-III/LAV are negative. Congenital infections, e.g., toxoplasmosis or herpes simplex virus infection in the first month after birth or cytomegalovirus infection in the first 6 months after birth must be exluded.

Specific conditions that must be excluded in a child are:
1. Primary immunodeficiency diseases — severe combined immunodeficiency, DiGeorge syndrome, Wiskott-Aldrich syndrome, ataxia-telangiectasia, graft versus host disease, neutropenia, neutrophil function abnormality, agammaglobulinemia, or hypogammaglobulinemia with raised IgM.
2. Secondary immunodeficiency associated with immunosuppressive therapy, lymphoreticular malignancy, or starvation.

---

school attendance, the protections for handicapped children under 20 U.S.C. 1401 et seq. and 29 U.S.C. 794, the confidentiality of a student's school record under state laws and under 20 U.S.C. 1232g, and employee right-to-know statutes for public employees in some states.

Confidentiality Issues. The diagnosis of AIDS or associated illnesses evokes much fear from others in contact with the patient and may evoke suspicion of life styles that may not be acceptable to some persons. Parents of HTLV-III/LAV-infected children should be aware of the potential for social isolation should the child's condition become known to others in the care or educational setting. School, day-care, and social service personnel and others involved in educating and caring for these children should be sensitive to the need for confidentiality and the right to privacy in these cases.

ASSESSMENT OF RISKS

Risk Factors for Acquiring HTLV-III/LAV Infection and Transmission. In adults and adolescents, HLTV-III/LAV is transmitted primarily through sexual contact (homosexual or heterosexual) and through parenteral exposure to infected blood or blood products. HTLV-III/LAV has been isolated from blood, semen, saliva, and tears but transmission has not been documented from saliva and tears. Adults at increased risk for acquiring HTLV-III/LAV include homosexual/bisexual men, intravenous drug abusers, persons transfused with contaminated blood or blood products, and sexual contacts of persons with HTLV-III/LAV infection or in groups at increased risk for infection.

The majority of infected children acquire the virus from their infected mothers in the perinatal period (1-4). In utero or intrapartum transmission are likely, and one child reported from Australia apparently acquired the virus postnatally, possibly from ingestion of breast milk (5). Children may also become infected through transfusion of blood or blood products that contain the virus. Seventy percent of the pediatric cases reported to CDC occurred among children whose parent had AIDS or was a member of a group at increased risk of acquiring HTLV-III/LAV infection; 20% of the cases occurred among children who had received blood or blood products; and for 10%, investigations are incomplete.

464

Appendix B

Risk of Transmission in the School, Day-Care or Foster-Care Setting. None of the identified cases of HTLV-III/LAV infection in the United States are known to have been transmitted in the school, day-care, or foster-care setting or through other casual person-to-person contact. Other than the sexual partners of HTLV-III/LAV-infected patients and infants born to infected mothers, none of the family members of the over 12,000 AIDS patients reported to CDC have been reported to have AIDS. Six studies of family members of patients with HTLV-III/LAV infection have failed to demonstrate HTLV-III/LAV transmission to adults who were not sexual contacts of the infected patients or to older children who were not likely at risk from perinatal transmission (*6-11*).

Based on current evidence, casual person-to-person contact as would occur among schoolchildren appears to pose no risk. However, studies of the risk of transmission through contact between younger children and neurologically handicapped children who lack control of their body secretions are very limited. Based on experience with other communicable diseases, a theoretical potential for transmission would be greatest among these children. It should be emphasized that any theoretical transmission would most likely involve exposure of open skin lesions or mucous membranes to blood and possibly other body fluids of an infected person.

Risks to the Child with HTLV-III/LAV Infection. HTLV-III/LAV infection may result in immunodeficiency. Such children may have a greater risk of encountering infectious agents in a school or day-care setting than at home. Foster homes with multiple children may also increase the risk. In addition, younger children and neurologically handicapped children who may display behaviors such as mouthing of toys would be expected to be at greater risk for acquiring infections. Immunodepressed children are also at greater risk of suffering severe complications from such infections as chickenpox, cytomegalovirus, tuberculosis, herpes simplex, and measles. Assessment of the risk to the immunodepressed child is best made by the child's physician who is aware of the child's immune status. The risk of acquiring some infections, such as chickenpox, may be reduced by prompt use of specific immune globulin following a known exposure.

RECOMMENDATIONS

1. Decisions regarding the type of educational and care setting for HTLV-III/LAV-infected children should be based on the behavior, neurologic development, and physical condition of the child and the expected type of interaction with others in that setting. These decisions are best made using the team approach including the child's physician, public health personnel, the child's parent or guardian, and personnel associated with the proposed care or educational setting. In each case, risks and benefits to both the infected child and to others in the setting should be weighed.

2. For most infected school-aged children, the benefits of an unrestricted setting would outweigh the risks of their acquiring potentially harmful infections in the setting and the apparent nonexistent risk of transmission of HTLV-III/LAV. These children should be allowed to attend school and after-school day-care and to be placed in a foster home in an unrestricted setting.

3. For the infected preschool-aged child and for some neurologically handicapped children who lack control of their body secretions or who display behavior, such as biting, and those children who have uncoverable, oozing lesions, a more restricted environment is advisable until more is known about transmission in these settings. Children infected with HTLV-III/LAV should be cared for and educated in settings that minimize exposure of other children to blood or body fluids.

465

4. Care involving exposure to the infected child's body fluids and excrement, such as feeding and diaper changing, should be performed by persons who are aware of the child's HTLV-III/LAV infection and the modes of possible transmission. In any setting involving an HTLV-III/LAV-infected person, good handwashing after exposure to blood and body fluids and before caring for another child should be observed, and gloves should be worn if open lesions are present on the caretaker's hands. Any open lesions on the infected person should also be covered.

5. Because other infections in addition to HTLV-III/LAV can be present in blood or body fluids, all schools and day-care facilities, regardless of whether children with HTLV-III/LAV infection are attending, should adopt routine procedures for handling blood or body fluids. Soiled surfaces should be promptly cleaned with disinfectants, such as household bleach (diluted 1 part bleach to 10 parts water). Disposable towels or tissues should be used whenever possible, and mops should be rinsed in the disinfectant. Those who are cleaning should avoid exposure of open skin lesions or mucous membranes to the blood or body fluids.

6. The hygienic practices of children with HTLV-III/LAV infection may improve as the child matures. Alternatively, the hygienic practices may deteriorate if the child's condition worsens. Evaluation to assess the need for a restricted environment should be performed regularly.

7. Physicians caring for children born to mothers with AIDS or at increased risk of acquiring HTLV-III/LAV infection should consider testing the children for evidence of HTLV-III/LAV infection for medical reasons. For example, vaccination of infected children with live virus vaccines, such as the measles-mumps-rubella vaccine (MMR), may be hazardous. These children also need to be followed closely for problems with growth and development and given prompt and aggressive therapy for infections and exposure to potentially lethal infections, such as varicella. In the event that an antiviral agent or other therapy for HTLV-III/LAV infection becomes available, these children should be considered for such therapy. Knowledge that a child is infected will allow parents and other caretakers to take precautions when exposed to the blood and body fluids of the child.

8. Adoption and foster-care agencies should consider adding HTLV-III/LAV screening to their routine medical evaluations of children at increased risk of infection before placement in the foster or adoptive home, since these parents must make decisions regarding the medical care of the child and must consider the possible social and psychological effects on their families.

9. Mandatory screening as a condition for school entry is not warranted based on available data.

10. Persons involved in the care and education of HTLV-III/LAV-infected children should respect the child's right to privacy, including maintaining confidential records. The number of personnel who are aware of the child's condition should be kept at a minimum needed to assure proper care of the child and to detect situations where the potential for transmission may increase (e.g., bleeding injury).

11. All educational and public health departments, regardless of whether HTLV-III/LAV-infected children are involved, are strongly encouraged to inform parents, children, and educators regarding HTLV-III/LAV and its transmission. Such education would greatly assist efforts to provide the best care and education for infected children while minimizing the risk of transmission to others.

Appendix B

References
1. Scott GB, Buck BE, Leterman JG, Bloom FL, Parks WP. Acquired immunodeficiency syndrome in infants. N Engl J Med 1984;310:76-81.
2. Thomas PA, Jaffe HW, Spira TJ, Reiss R, Guerrero IC, Auerbach D. Unexplained immunodeficiency in children. A surveillance report. JAMA 1984;252:639-44.
3. Rubinstein A, Sicklick M, Gupta A, et al. Acquired immunodeficiency with reversed T4/T8 ratios in infants born to promiscuous and drug-addicted mothers. JAMA 1983;249:2350-6.
4. Oleske J, Minnefor A, Cooper R Jr, et al. Immune deficiency syndrome in children. JAMA 1983; 249:2345-9.
5. Ziegler JB, Cooper DA, Johnson RO, Gold J. Postnatal transmission of AIDS-associated retrovirus from mother to infant. Lancet 1985;i:896-8.
6. CDC. Unpublished data.
7. Kaplan JE, Oleske JM, Getchell JP, et al. Evidence against transmission of HTLV-III/LAV in families of children with AIDS. Pediatric Infectious Disease (in press).
8. Lewin EB, Zack R, Ayodele A. Communicability of AIDS in a foster care setting. International Conference on Acquired Immunodeficiency Syndrome (AIDS), Atlanta, Georgia, April 1985.
9. Thomas PA, Lubin K, Enlow RW, Getchell J. Comparison of HTLV-III serology, T-cell levels, and general health status of children whose mothers have AIDS with children of healthy inner city mothers in New York. International Conference on Acquired Immunodeficiency Syndrome (AIDS), Atlanta, Georgia, April 1985.
10. Fischl MA, Dickinson G, Scott G, Klimas N, Fletcher M, Parks W. Evaluation of household contacts of adult patients with the acquired immunodeficiency syndrome. International Conference on Acquired Immunodeficiency Syndrome (AIDS), Atlanta, Georgia, April 1985.
11. Friedland GH, Saltzman BR, Rogers MF, et al. Lack of household transmission of HTLV-III infection. EIS Conference, Atlanta, Georgia, April 1985.

Centers for Disease Control. Education and Foster Care of Children Infected with Human T-Lymphotropic Virus Type III/Lymphadenopathy-Associated Virus. MMWR 1985;34:517-521.

467

Appendix C

AMERICAN ACADEMY
OF PEDIATRICS RECOMMENDATIONS
Committee on School Health
Committee on Infectious Diseases

School Attendance of Children and Adolescents with Human T Lymphotropic Virus III/Lymphadenopathy-Associated Virus Infection

As of October 15, 1985, there have been 204 cases of acquired immunodeficiency syndrome (AIDS) (or 1% of the total number of cases) reported in American children. Serologic testing has detected additional high-risk children (e.g., hemophiliacs) who are human T lymphotropic virus type III/lymphadenopathy-associated virus (HTLV-III/LAV) antibody positive and are apparently well. Some of these children are of school age; thus, a policy on school attendance of children with HTLV-III infection is required.

The present AAP recommendations are based on (1) a review of available data related to potential transmission of HTLV-III by school-aged children and (2) the Centers for Disease Control (CDC) statement of August 30, 1985.[1]

469

BACKGROUND

These recommendations apply to all children known to be infected with HTLV-III/LAV including (1) children with AIDS as defined for reporting purposes; (2) children determined to have an illness due to infection with HTLV-III/LAV but who do not meet the case definition, which has been called AIDS-related complex (ARC; symptoms may include chronic lymphadenopathy, weight loss, fever, chronic diarrhea, anemia, thrombocytopenia, and mild signs of opportunistic infections); (3) children who are asymptomatic but have virologic or serologic evidence of HTLV-III/LAV infection.

It is important that the serologic screening test for HTLV-III be confirmed by specific tests to eliminate false-positive results. True seropositive individuals have a high probability of being infected with HTLV-III and, therefore, are potentially capable of transmitting the virus to others.

The adult and adolescent cases, which constitute about 99% of all cases, are transmitted primarily through sexual contact (homosexual and heterosexual) and by intravenous injection of infected blood or blood products. Adults at increased risk for acquiring HTLV-III/LAV include homosexual/bisexual men, intravenous drug abusers, persons given transfusions of contaminated blood or blood products, and those who have sexual contact with persons with HTLV-III/LAV infection or with persons in groups that are at increased risk for infection (i.e., hemophiliacs).

In contrast, approximately 75% of the AIDS/ARC cases in children are due to maternal and perinatal transmission, and 19% of these cases are due to use of contaminated blood and blood products. In approximately 7% of cases, the source of HTLV-III is as yet unexplained. Although HTLV-III has been isolated from breast milk, saliva, tears, and urine, its presence

470

does not necessarily imply that these fluids are involved in the transmission of infection.

None of the reported cases of HTLV-III/LAV infection in the United States is known to have been transmitted in the school, in the day-care or foster-care setting, or through other casual person-to-person contact. Of the more than 13,500 cases of AIDS reported to the CDC to date, none has been attributed to household contacts. Serologic testing for HTLV-III infection has been performed on 251 household contacts of 94 patients with AIDS or ARC. Eighteen of the 251 contacts (8%) were infected. All 18 were determined to be at increased risk: 13 positive contacts were children born to infected mothers and five were positive adult contacts with a high-risk factor. Consequently, the possibility of transmission is likely to be extremely low under situations of casual contact and normal school behavior. Recommendations for management of the school-aged child with HTLV-III infection are based on these considerations. Information regarding the epidemiology, clinical manifestations, and management of infected children is evolving. The AAP will update and modify this statement as new information becomes available.

RECOMMENDATIONS

1. Most school-aged children and adolescents infected with HTLV-III should be allowed to attend school in an unrestricted manner with the approval of their personal physician. HTLV-III infection, in these recommendations, includes cases of AIDS, ARC, or seropositivity, in as much as the potential for transmission of the virus is present in any of these three clinical conditions. Based on present data, the benefits of unrestricted school attendance to these students outweigh the remote possibility

471

that such students will transmit the infection in the school environment.

2. Some infected students may pose a greater risk than others. Students who lack control of their body secretions, who display behavior such as biting, or who have open skin sores that cannot be covered require a more restricted school environment until more is known about the transmission of the virus under these conditions. Special education should be provided in these instances as required by PL 94-142.

3. School districts should designate individuals, including the student's physician, who have the qualifications to evaluate whether an infected student poses a risk to others. Evaluations to assess the need for alternatives to continuing in school should be performed regularly. Hygienic practices of an infected student may improve with maturation or deteriorate if the condition worsens. If it is determined that a risk exists, the student must be removed from the classroom, and an appropriate alternative education program must be established until a subsequent review determines that the risk has abated. A plan for periodic review should be established at the time a decision has been made to exclude a child from attending classes.

4. The number of personnel aware of the child's condition should be kept to the minimum needed to assure proper care of the child and to detect situations in which the potential for transmission may increase. It is essential that persons involved in the care and education of an infected student respect the student's right to privacy. Confidential records should be maintained.

5. All schools should adopt routine procedures for handling blood or body fluids, including sanitary napkins, regardless of whether students with HTLV-III infection are known to be in attendance. School health care workers, teachers, administrators, and other employees should be educated about procedures

that may be or may have been established by local codes. For example, soiled surfaces should be promptly cleaned with disinfectants, such as household bleach, diluted 1:10, one part bleach to ten (10) parts water. Persons involved in such cleaning should avoid exposure of open skin lesions or mucous membranes to blood or body fluids.

6. The physician of the student with HTLV-III infection should regularly assess the risk of school attendance. Students with HTLV-III may develop immunodeficiency, which places them at increased risk of experiencing severe complications from infections such as chickenpox, tuberculosis, measles, cytomegalovirus, and herpes simplex.

7. Routine screening of children for HTLV-III is not recommended.

COMMITTEE ON SCHOOL HEALTH,
1985-1986
Joseph R. Zanga, MD, Chair
Michael A. Donlan, MD
Jerry Newton, MD
Maxine M. Sehring, MD
Marin W. Sklaire, MD
Martin C. Ushkow, MD

Liaison Representatives
Marjorie Hughes, MD
Janice Hutchinson, MD
M. Ray Kelly, PhD
Betty McGinnis, MA, CPNP, NAPNA/P
Charles Zimont, MD

COMMITTEE ON INFECTIOUS DISEASES,
1985-1986
Philip A. Brunell, MD, Chair
Robert S. Daum, MD

G. Scott Giebink, MD
Caroline Breese Hall, MD
Martha L. Lepow, MD
George H. McCracken, Jr, MD
Andre S. Nahmias, MD
Carol F. Phillips, MD
Stanley A. Plotken, MD
Harry T. Wright, Jr, MD

Liaison Representatives
Alan R. Hinman, MD
William S. Jordan, Jr, MD
Paul Parkman, MD
David Scheifele, MD

Section Liaison
John A. Anderson, MD

REFERENCE

1. Centers for Disease Control: Education and foster care of children infected with human T-lymphotropic virus type III/lymphadenopathy-associated virus. MMWR 1985; 34:517-521

Reprinted with permission from *Pediatrics*, 77:3 (March 1986), published by the American Academy of Pediatrics, Elk Grove Village, IL.

The National PTA is on record

Resolution

ACQUIRED IMMUNODEFICIENCY SYNDROME

(Adopted by the 1986 National PTA convention delegates)

Whereas, One Object of the PTA is "to promote the welfare of children and youth in home, school, community, and place of worship;" and

Whereas, 183 of the reported cases of Acquired Immunodeficiency Syndrome (AIDS) were among children under the age of 18, as of August 1985; and

Whereas, None of the identified cases of AIDS infection in the United States is known to have been transmitted in the school, day care or foster care setting; and

Whereas, The Centers for Disease Control, in consultation with several health associations as well as the National Association of Elementary School Principals and the Board of Directors of the National Congress of Parents and Teachers, released the following statement in August, 1985, "These children should be allowed to attend school and after- school day care and can be placed in foster homes in an unrestricted setting;" therefore be it

Resolved, That the National Congress of Parents and Teachers believes that in the case of diagnosed Acquired Immunodeficiency Syndrome the child's physician, public health officials, the parents or guardians of that child and the appropriate school personnel should be responsible for determining the most suitable placement for that public school child; and be it further

Resolved, That the National Congress of Parents and Teachers discourage social displays that would seek to segregate, persecute or ban children with AIDS from school.

Resolution

AIDS—INFORMATION AND DISSEMINATION

(Adopted by the 1986 National PTA convention delegates)

Whereas, One Object of the PTA is "to promote the welfare of children and youth in the home, school, community and place of worship;" and

Whereas, The AIDS epidemic has rapidly become one of the most complex public health problems in our nation's history, affecting both adults and children of all ages; and

Whereas, Without education about how AIDS is transmitted, the disease will spread at an alarming rate; therefore be it

Resolved, That the National PTA make available to its constituent bodies information on Acquired Immunodeficiency Syndrome from medically related organizations such as the Centers for Disease Control, the American Academy of Pediatrics, the U.S. Public Health Service and the U.S. Department of Health and Human Services; and be it further

Resolved, That the National PTA encourage its states, districts or regions, councils and units, in cooperation with said medical groups and representatives of state departments of health and education, to conduct workshops and disseminate information on the disease's nature, transmission and legal, social and emotional consequences, so that parents, students, educators and the general public may be more knowledgeable as they encourage and/or consider state and local district policies addressing this issue; and be it further

Resolved, That the National PTA urge its constituent bodies to encourage health officials to support continued testing of supplies of blood in all blood banks prior to use, so that recipients of blood are not infected with AIDS.

National PTA
Position Statement

COMPREHENSIVE SCHOOL HEALTH EDUCATION

(Revised and reaffirmed 1987)

The National PTA has consistently supported the inclusion of various health topics in the school curriculum. These have included, but not been limited to, such broad health topics as dental, mental, environmental health, physical fitness, family life education, health supervision, nutrition and accident prevention as well as such specific health subjects as alcohol and drug abuse, smoking, sex and STD (Sexually Transmitted Diseases) including venereal disease and AIDS.

Limitation of time, overcrowded school curriculum and finances do not permit separate courses for each of the health topics. A unified, planned program of health instruction with scope, sequence, progression, and continuity is necessary for a coordinated total approach to health education.

The National PTA supports the concept of comprehensive school health education programs and believes these programs should have high priority at national, state, and local levels.

We, therefore, urge educators to develop and incorporate such programs in the schools and urge governmental agencies at all levels to provide the necessary funds to make this possible.

The Issue of Abstinence

Marcia Quackenbush and Pamela Sargent

We have heard a lot more talk about sexual abstinence since AIDS was first identified. Many people believe that teaching about abstinence is the best course for preventing the sexual transmission of AIDS among teenagers. There has been controversy about the issue, however, which we would like to address.

We couldn't agree more on the benefits of abstinence for teenagers. If more teens were abstinent, we would see fewer sexually transmitted diseases with their associated health problems (for example, pelvic inflammatory disease—PID—causes thousands of young women a year to become infertile). The rate of teenage pregnancy would also drop, and fewer young people would have to face the double burden of trying to complete their education while parenting a newborn or young child. And finally, we could expect the rate of AIDS infection to stay low in this age group. These are wonderful benefits, so promoting abstinence certainly has its place in teen education.

The problem arises when people suggest that abstinence is the *only* acceptable teaching for AIDS prevention. Adolescents are making their own decisions about sexual behavior, whether we want them to or not. American adolescents today are deciding in significant numbers *not* to be sexually abstinent. If we present abstinence as the only method of AIDS prevention, we are offering nothing to the twelve million teenagers in this country who *are* sexually active. We are essentially saying to them, "Be abstinent or die."

If we want to promote abstinence among teenagers, we must devote time, energy and effort to the task. Teens are surrounded by overt and covert messages from peers, in young adult fiction, in movies, television and advertising, and in popular music that endorse and encourage sexual activity. There are few resources in popular culture that suggest abstinence is a positive or desirable choice. To help teens balance the picture, we can teach them skills related to values clarification, decision making and assertiveness. To help them resist these compelling persuasions to be sexually active, we must promote teen self-esteem. These lessons are well beyond the scope of AIDS education alone. Careful planning of curricula in family life education and modern living skills, spanning the full course of a student's school career, can establish the foundation needed to develop such capabilities.

In providing teens a thorough and careful education about AIDS, we want to emphasize that abstinence is the only 100% effective method of preventing the sexual transmission of the AIDS virus. By also including a description of safer sex activities, we acknowledge that sexual activity does or might take place, now or in the future. We are not promoting teen sexual activity in these programs, however, and we can state this clearly to our students. What we are endorsing is care and thoughtfulness about decisions that affect oneself and one's friends or sexual partners. What we are supporting is health and longevity. What we hope to prevent is unnecessary suffering and death.

Teens (and adults) *deserve* full information about AIDS prevention. If we offer them less, we lose credibility as educators and as role models. If, in our AIDS education efforts, we neglect to acknowledge teenagers as people who may be sexually active, we lose a valuable opportunity to stem the spread of this devastating illness. If we fail to encourage those who are, or may someday be, sexually active to consider their choices carefully and reevaluate past decisions, we condemn them to a risk they might not otherwise choose to take.

We cannot afford to make these errors. The lives of our youth, of the adults they will become, and the children they will bear are much too precious. In our education efforts, we can present abstinence as the best of several possible choices for teens, but we must be honest and forthright about the full spectrum of prevention options for a population already quite active sexually.

AIDS Questionnaire

Editors' Note:

Surveys of knowledge, attitudes and behaviors concerning AIDS and risk reduction can be useful in many ways. A survey of teenagers that reveals poor knowledge about AIDS transmission, for example, can be a persuasive rationale for implementing AIDS education. A survey of teens' risk reduction practices can help evaluate how effective current education efforts are. Surveys of teacher attitudes may suggest areas of focus for staff trainings.

The questionnaire that follows can be used in these or other contexts, in full or in part, as written or with modification. The questionnaire is divided into five parts:

Part 1 (questions 1-25) addresses knowledge about AIDS transmission and prevention.

Part 2 (questions 26-36) explores attitudes toward AIDS education, persons with AIDS and public response to the epidemic.

Part 3 (questions 37-44) examines personal risk behaviors.

Part 4 (questions 45-52) explores beliefs about background risks for peer groups and sexual histories of those answering the questionnaire.

Part 5 (questions 53-56) provides demographic data.

Anonymity is essential in this kind of survey because it asks about opinions and personal sex and drug use history. Students should never be asked to sign their names to questionnaires of this sort.

AIDS Questionnaire

AIDS is a very serious health problem in our nation. Health officials are trying to find the best ways to teach people about AIDS. This survey has been developed so you can tell us what you know and how you feel about AIDS. The information you give will be used to develop better AIDS education programs for young people.

DO NOT write your name on this survey. The answers you give will be kept *private*. No one will know what you write. Answer the questions based on what you really know, feel, or do.

Thank you for your help.

PART 1 DIRECTIONS: Read each question carefully, then circle YES, NO, or UNSURE in response to the questions below.

Can a person get AIDS from ...
1. shaking hands with someone who has AIDS?

                                                 YES   NO   UNSURE
2. giving blood?   YES   NO   UNSURE

3. going to school with a student who has AIDS?

                                                   YES   NO   UNSURE

4. kissing on the mouth?   YES   NO   UNSURE

5. being bitten by mosquitoes or other insects?

                                                   YES   NO   UNSURE

6. sharing needles or syringes used to inject drugs?

                                                 YES   NO   UNSURE

7. using public toilets?　　　　　　YES　　NO　　UNSURE

8. having sexual intercourse?　　　　YES　　NO　　UNSURE

9. having a blood test?　　　　　　　YES　　NO　　UNSURE

Can people reduce their chances of becoming infected with the AIDS virus by ...

10. not having sexual intercourse (being abstinent)?
　　　　　　　　　　　　　　　　　YES　　NO　　UNSURE

11. using condoms (rubbers) during sexual intercourse?
　　　　　　　　　　　　　　　　　YES　　NO　　UNSURE

12. urinating after sexual intercourse?
　　　　　　　　　　　　　　　　　YES　　NO　　UNSURE

13. having sexual intercourse with only one person who is not infected with the AIDS virus?　　　YES　　NO　　UNSURE

14. not having sexual intercourse with a person who injects or has injected illegal drugs?　　　YES　　NO　　UNSURE

15. taking birth control pills?　　　　YES　　NO　　UNSURE

16. Can you protect yourself from becoming infected with the AIDS virus?　　　　　　　　　　YES　　NO　　UNSURE

17. Can you tell if a person is infected with the AIDS virus by looking at the person?　　　　　YES　　NO　　UNSURE

18. Can any person infected with the AIDS virus infect someone else during sexual intercourse?   YES   NO   UNSURE

19. Can a pregnant woman who has the AIDS virus infect her unborn baby with the virus?   YES   NO   UNSURE

20. Is there a cure for AIDS?   YES   NO   UNSURE

21. Are gay men the only people who can get AIDS?
                                YES   NO   UNSURE

22. With regard to AIDS, are blood transfusions now generally safe?   YES   NO   UNSURE

23. Do you think you can get AIDS?
                                YES   NO   UNSURE

24. Do you know where to get correct information about AIDS?   YES   NO   UNSURE

25. Do you know where to get tested for the AIDS virus?
                                YES   NO   UNSURE

PART 2 DIRECTIONS: Please circle the answer that best describes how you feel about each statement below. Use the following scale:

AGREE = I agree with this statement
DISAGREE = I disagree with this statement

26. Students my age should be taught about AIDS.
                                AGREE   DISAGREE

27. People should not be afraid of catching AIDS from casual contact, like hugging or shaking hands.

AGREE   DISAGREE

28. I think that people with AIDS get what they deserve.

AGREE   DISAGREE

29. The thought of being around someone with AIDS does not bother me.   AGREE   DISAGREE

30. No one deserves to have a disease like AIDS.

AGREE   DISAGREE

31. I would not be afraid to take care of a family member with AIDS.   AGREE   DISAGREE

32. The best way to get rid of AIDS is to get rid of homosexuality.   AGREE   DISAGREE

33. I would not avoid a friend if he/she had AIDS.

AGREE   DISAGREE

34. A list of people who have AIDS should be available to everyone.   AGREE   DISAGREE

35. Students with AIDS have a right to go to my school.

AGREE   DISAGREE

36. It would not bother me to attend class with someone who has AIDS.   AGREE   DISAGREE

PART 3 DIRECTIONS: **Read each question carefully. Circle the answer that is most appropriate.**

37. Have you injected cocaine, heroin, or other illegal drugs into your body?   YES   NO   NO RESPONSE

38. Have you shared needles or syringes used to inject drugs?
                         YES   NO   NO RESPONSE

39. Because of AIDS, have you stopped injecting illegal drugs?
                         YES   NO   NO RESPONSE

40. Because of AIDS, have you stopped sharing needles and syringes used to inject drugs?   YES   NO   NO RESPONSE

41. Because of AIDS, have you ever talked with your boyfriend or girlfriend about AIDS before having sexual intercourse?   YES   NO   NO RESPONSE

42. Because of AIDS, have you stopped having sexual intercourse?   YES   NO   NO RESPONSE

43. Because of AIDS, have you started using condoms during sexual intercourse?   YES   NO   NO RESPONSE

44. Because of AIDS, have you decreased the number of people you have sexual intercourse with?
                         YES   NO   NO RESPONSE

PART 4 DIRECTIONS: Read each statement carefully, then circle the answer that you think is best.

How many persons your age do you think are ...

45. having sexual intercourse?
a. ALMOST ALL   b. MOST   c. HALF   d. FEW
e. ALMOST NONE

46. using condoms (rubbers) during sexual intercourse?
a. ALMOST ALL   b. MOST   c. HALF   d. FEW
e. ALMOST NONE

47. injecting illegal drugs?
a. ALMOST ALL   b. MOST   c. HALF   d.FEW
e. ALMOST NONE

48. sharing needles or syringes used to inject drugs?
a. ALMOST ALL   b. MOST   c. HALF   d. FEW
e. ALMOST NONE

49. How many people have you had sexual intercourse with *in your life*?
a. 0   b. 1   c. 2   d. 3 OR MORE
e. NO RESPONSE

50. How many people have you had sexual intercourse with *in the last year?*
a. 0   b. 1   c. 2   d. 3 OR MORE
e. NO RESPONSE

51. How old were you the first time you had sexual intercourse?
a. 12 or less   b. 13-14   c. 15-16   d. 17-18
e. DOES NOT APPLY

52. When you have sexual intercourse, how often is a condom used?
a. ALWAYS b. SOMETIMES c. RARELY d. NEVER
e. DOES NOT APPLY

PART 5 DIRECTIONS: Read each question carefully. Circle the correct answer.

53. What grade are you in?
a. 8th   b. 9th   c. 10th   d. 11th   e. 12th

54. What is your sex?
a. FEMALE   b. MALE

55. How old are you?
a. 12 OR UNDER   b. 13-14   c. 15-16   d. 17-18
e. 19 YEARS OLD OR MORE

56. What is your race?
a. WHITE   b. BLACK   c. HISPANIC   d. ASIAN
e. OTHER

THE END

Thank you for your help. Please return this survey and your answer sheet to your teacher.

AIDS Questionnaire (Answers)

1.	No	13.	Yes
2.	No	14.	Yes
3.	No	15.	No
4.	No	16.	Yes
5.	No	17.	No
6.	Yes	18.	Yes
7.	No	19.	Yes
8.	Yes	20.	No
9.	No	21.	No
10.	Yes	22.	Yes
11.	Yes	23.	N/A—Personal Opinion
12.	No	24, 25.	N/A—Personal knowledge

Glossary

AIDS

Acquired Immune Deficiency Syndrome. A viral disease that damages the body's immune system, making the infected person susceptible to a wide range of serious diseases. May also involve neurologic symptoms.

antibody

Proteins produced in the blood in response to toxins or other foreign organisms. Antibodies in some cases can neutralize toxins and help eliminate infections, though in the case of AIDS, antibodies are not effective in combating the disease.

ARC

AIDS-related complex. A diagnosis given to people infected with the AIDS virus who have symptoms of illness related to this infection, but do not meet the diagnostic criteria necessary to be given a diagnosis of AIDS.

ARV

The name given the AIDS virus by Jay Levy of the University of California, San Francisco. Stands for AIDS-associated retrovirus.

blood transfusion

To put blood into the veins of an individual. First, blood is withdrawn from a donor. It may be stored for some period of time. Then, to treat injury or illness, a recipient is given this donated blood.

carcinoma

A malignancy, or cancer, made up of a particular kind of cell and with a tendency to metastasize, or spread. The cells of a carcinoma are epithelial cells, which cover the internal and external surfaces of the body.

casual contact

Normal day-to-day contact between people at home, school, work or in the community, which does not involve sexual interactions or the sharing of needles.

casual transmission

Transmission of disease through casual contact. Colds and flus are often casually transmitted. The AIDS virus is not transmitted casually.

CDC

The Centers for Disease Control, a federal agency based in Atlanta that studies and monitors the incidence and prevalence of disease in the U.S., and also provides health and safety guidelines for the prevention of disease.

cellular immunodeficiency

A defect in the immune system characterized by poor functioning of the T-cells. This is the kind of immune deficiency seen in HIV infection. Other immune deficiencies may affect the B-cells (antibody immunodeficiency), the phagocytes (phagocytic dysfunction disorders), or the lymphoid cells (combined immunodeficiency).

condoms

Also called rubbers or prophylactics. A latex sheath used to cover the penis during intercourse to prevent pregnancy and the transmission of sexual diseases. Latex condoms are effective in preventing the transmission of the AIDS virus. "Natural skin" condoms are not as reliable for the prevention of disease.

disease

A particular destructive process in an organ or organism with a specific cause and characteristic symptoms; an illness.

EIA

Another way to abbreviate "enzyme linked immunosorbent assay," hence the same thing as "ELISA."

ELISA

A test used to detect HIV antibodies in blood samples. The most inexpensive and widely used test to date. Stands for enzyme-linked immunosorbent assay.

epidemiology

The study of the distribution and causes of diseases.

false negative

In an AIDS antibody test, a result that reads negative when there is actually antibody in the blood. A type of erroneous result.

false positive

In an AIDS antibody test, a result that reads positive when there is actually no antibody in the blood. A type of erroneous result.

hemophilia

A rare, inherited bleeding disorder of males in which normal blood clotting is not possible. Treated with Factor VIII, a product made of human blood which allows normal clotting to occur.

HIV

The accepted scientific name for the AIDS virus, in most common usage now. Stands for human immunodeficiency virus. Also called HIV-1, since the discovery of HIV-2.

HIV-2

Another human immunodeficiency virus, discovered in 1985. Similar enough to HIV-1 to be considered a genetic cousin, but different enough to be considered a separate and distinct entity. Transmitted in a similar fashion to HIV-1 (sharing blood, sexual intercourse) and causes similar symptoms.

HTLV-III

The name given the AIDS virus by Robert Gallo of the National Cancer Institute. Stands for human T-cell lymphotropic virus, type three.

IFA

A test used to detect HIV antibodies in blood samples. More difficult to perform and more expensive than the ELISA. Also believed to be more specific (can accurately identify samples without antibody) than the ELISA, so sometimes used to verify ELISA results. Stands for immunofluorescent assay.

immortal cell line

A special cell line developed for research purposes which is easily reproduced and survives well in laboratory conditions. In AIDS research, it was necessary to discover and develop a line of T-cells which could be used to study HIV in laboratory settings.

immune system

The body's system of defense against disease, consisting of specialized cells and proteins in the blood and other body fluids.

incubation

In a medical context, the length of time between an individual first being infected with a disease-causing organism and the development of symptoms or diagnosis. The incubation period for AIDS averages over five years.

intercourse

A type of sexual contact involving one of the following:

(1) insertion of a man's penis into a woman's vagina, called "vaginal intercourse"; (2) placement of the mouth on the genitals of another person, called "oral intercourse"; or (3) insertion of a man's penis into the anus of another person, called "anal intercourse."

intravenous

"Within veins"; injection by needles directly into the blood veins.

Kaposi's sarcoma

KS, a cancer or tumor of the blood and/or lymphatic vessel walls, sometimes seen in persons with AIDS. Usually appears as pink or purple blotches on the skin.

LAV

The name given the AIDS virus by Luc Montagnier of the Institute Pasteur, Paris. Stands for lymphadenopathy associated virus.

lubricant

In this context, a substance applied to condoms or sexual organs which makes contact between condom and skin slippery. Lubricants can be purchased in most places where condoms are sold. Use only water based lubricants with condoms, and read labels carefully— any fats or oils will break down the latex and may cause the condom to tear.

lymphadenopathy

The condition of lymph nodes being swollen. Often a sign of infection or illness. People infected with the AIDS virus often have chronic lymphadenopathy.

lymphoreticular malignancy

A malignant cancer of the lymph system. A malignancy based in the lymph system and its connecting structures, including lymphocytic leukemias, multiple myeloma, and non-Hodgkin's lymphoma. Leukemias are cancers of the blood, myelomas are cancers of the bone marrow, and non-Hodgkin's lymphomas are a heterogeneous group of lymph system malignancies.

malignant

Tending to become progressively worse and to result in death.

neurologic

Pertaining to the nervous system or brain. Persons infected with the AIDS virus often develop neurologic infection with symptoms such as forgetfulness, confusion, perceptual problems, lack of coordination or loss of muscle control.

nonoxynol 9

A spermicide which has also been shown to kill the AIDS virus in laboratory studies. Available in some sexual lubricants which can be used with condoms, non-oxynol 9 is *not* an effective AIDS prevention method used on its own. Concentrations of 5% or more are recommended.

opportunistic infection

An infection caused by organisms that are not able to affect people with healthy immune systems.

parenteral

By injection. This can be subcutaneous, intramuscular, intravenous or through other entries.

pathogen

Any disease-producing microorganism.

perinatal

Pertaining to or occurring in the period shortly before or shortly after birth.

PGL

"Persistent generalized lymphadenopathy," a syndrome characterized by swollen lymph glands, usually in at least two sites for three months or longer. A common syndrome in persons who are HIV infected. Lymph glands will also become swollen in reaction to many other infections.

Pneumocystis carinii pneumonia

PCP, the most common life-threatening opportunistic illness diagnosed in AIDS. Caused by a protozoan parasite, it creates difficulty in breathing and is the most common cause of death for people with AIDS.

PWA

Person with AIDS. Many people with AIDS prefer this term to others like "AIDS victim," or "AIDS patient." They would rather see themselves as active participants in their treatment and healing, not helpless victims who passively wait to die. They are whole and complete persons, and the term "patient" reduces them to little more than a case of disease.

risk
> The chance of injury, damage or loss; dangerous chance; hazard.

safer sex
> Sexual activity which protects one from infection with the AIDS virus. In safer sex, no body fluids are shared.

secondary malignancies
> A malignancy that develops due to the metastases, or spread, of a primary (initial) malignancy; or a cancer which appears after but independent of a primary malignancy.

secondary opportunistic infections
> A secondary infection that develops after the immune system has been weakened by an initial infection. The initial infection is often viral.

secretion
> A substance generated from blood or cells which may have cleansing, lubricating or other characteristics.

seropositive
> In the case of AIDS, the condition of having AIDS virus antibodies found in the blood.

spermicide
> Any substance used to help prevent pregnancy because of its ability to kill sperm. One spermicide, nonoxynol 9, has also been shown to kill the AIDS virus in laboratory studies.

STD

Sexually transmitted disease, any of a number of diseases which can be transmitted through various forms of sexual contact. AIDS is a disease which is transmitted through sexual intercourse.

surveillance

In public health terms, monitoring and collecting data on incidence of disease—essentially, counting the number of cases.

T-cell

A specialized white blood cell which helps orchestrate the immune system's response to infection. The T-cell is invaded and disabled by the HIV virus.

transmission

Passed along. In the context of disease, passed from one individual to another.

vaccine

A preparation introduced to the body to produce immunity to disease. Historically, most vaccines have been made of weakened, or killed disease organisms themselves. In the future, we may see vaccines which are genetically engineered non-lethal forms of such organisms.

virus

An organism formed of genes surrounded by a protein coating. Technically not living, since it cannot reproduce itself. Smaller than any living organism.

Western blot

A test used to detect HIV antibodies in blood samples. More difficult to perform, and more expensive, than the ELISA. Also believed to be more specific (can accurately identify samples without antibody) than the ELISA, so sometimes used to verify ELISA results.

Selected Resources on AIDS

General Information Books

Bennett, W.J. 1987. *AIDS and the education of our children.* Washington, DC: U.S. Department of Education.

Includes facts, prevention recommendations and sources of information about AIDS. Some of the recommendations are fairly conservative in nature.

Callen, M., ed. 1987. *Surviving and thriving with AIDS: Hints for the newly diagnosed.* New York: People With AIDS Coalition.

A collection of essays and articles by persons with AIDS, covering emotional reactions to diagnosis; standard treatments and alternative therapy approaches to healing; how to develop productive relationships with doctors; how to

utilize social services if necessary; sex, love and friendships; telling friends and family; spirituality; politics; and
more. A wide variety of experience and opinion is represented.

Haffner, D.W. 1987. *AIDS and adolescents: The time for prevention is now.* Washington, DC: Center for Population
Options (CPO).

A summary of ideas about how to prevent the AIDS epidemic from reaching young people. From the first national
meeting on adolescents and AIDS, sponsored by CPO.

Hooper, S. and Gregory, G. 1986. *AIDS and the public schools.*
Alexandria, VA: National School Boards Association.

Includes a review of medical facts, information about the
legal complications of AIDS in the school setting, and an
overview of possible school board policy responses to
AIDS.

Institute of Medicine, National Academy of Sciences. 1986.
*Confronting AIDS: Directions for public health, health
care, and research.* Washington, DC: National Academy
Press.

One of the best general references books on AIDS to date.
Includes excellent background and history, along with
explanations of medical and care aspects of HIV infection.
Public health and policy recommendations are also made.
Language is fairly technical and some specific chapters
are very technical.

Koop, C.E. 1986. *Surgeon general's report on Acquired Immune Deficiency Syndrome.* Washington, DC: U.S. De-

partment of Health and Human Services.

Surgeon General's message describes the virus and discusses signs and symptoms, transmission, risks, prevention and fears. Recommends sex education begin in early elementary school and include information about AIDS.

Lagone, J. 1988. *AIDS: The facts*. Boston: Little, Brown and Company.

A well-written and readable general information book, including some good chapters on scientific issues related to AIDS ("What is the AIDS virus?"; "How does the virus cause infection?"). The author makes a strong case that heterosexual transmission will not be a major factor in the American AIDS epidemic. Ultimately, we feel he incorrectly minimizes the risk of transmission through heterosexual intercourse—it is essential to remember that a significant number of such cases have occurred, and that these are unequivocally documented.

Martelli, L.J. with Peltz, F.D. and Messina, W. 1987. *When someone you know has AIDS*. New York: Crown Publishers, Inc.

A comprehensive guide for partners, families or close friends of persons with AIDS who will be in a caretaking or major supportive role in their illness. Emotional, medical and practical aspects of care are covered. Sound and down to earth in its information and recommendations.

Moffat, B.C., Spiegel, J., Parrish, S. and Helquist, M., eds. 1987. *AIDS: A self-care manual*. Santa Monica, CA: IBS Press.

A broadbased collection of articles by various experts along with personal accounts by individuals affected by the AIDS epidemic. The focus is on prevention as well as on those with symptoms or a diagnosis of AIDS/ARC. Many areas are covered, including medical overview, spiritual issues, practical steps and treatment.

Norwood, C. 1987. *Advice for life: A woman's guide to AIDS risks and prevention*. New York: Pantheon Books.

A good source of general information, as well as a persuasive explanation of the realities of AIDS risks for women. Well written and readable, and also opinionated. Factually sound, though we would disagree with the author's assertion that people probably do not need to take precautions in the practice of oral sex. We are also apprehensive about recommendations for mandatory HIV antibody screening for hospital admissions and clients of VD clinics.

Peabody, B. 1986. *The screaming room: A mother's journal of her son's struggle with AIDS—a true story of love, dedication and courage*. New York: Avon Books.

A personal and moving story of what it is like to care day-to-day for someone who is very ill with AIDS. Readable but difficult because of the intensity of the subject.

Pierce, C. and VanDeVeer, D. 1988. *AIDS: Ethics and public policy*. Belmont, CA: Wadsworth Publishing Company.

An interesting anthology of articles addressing various ethical issues raised by the HIV epidemic. Includes sections on "Grounds for Restricting Liberty," "Law and Public Policy," and "Sexual Autonomy and the

Constitution." Good background resource for teachers or others wanting to teach classes on ethics.

U.S. Public Health Service. *AIDS school health education subfile on the combined health information database (CHID)*.

This database, managed by the CDC, contains descriptions of programs, curricula, guidelines, policies, regulations and materials. Addresses are included for items that can be purchased. For further information, contact Centers for Disease Control, Center for Health Promotion and Education, Division of Health Education, Attn: AIDS School Health Education Subfile, Atlanta, GA 30333; or call (404) 639-3492, or (404) 639-3824.

Teaching Resources

Berne, L.A. 1988. *AIDS and other sexually transmitted diseases*. Sunnyvale, CA: Scott, Foresman & Company. (Student and teacher books for grades 5 through 12.)

Meeks, L. and Heit, P. 1988. *AIDS: What you should know*. Websterville, OH: Merrill Publishing Company. (Student and teacher books for grades 6 through 8.)

Meeks, L. and Heit, P. 1988. *Understanding and Prevention*. Websterville, OH: Merrill Publishing Company. (Student and teacher books for high school classrooms.)

Oatman, E. 1988. *AIDS and your world*. New York: Scholastic, Inc. (Student and teacher books for grades 7 through 12.)

Pies, C.A. and Stoller, E.J. 1987. *Teacher's curriculum guide on AIDS.* San Francisco: San Francisco Department of Public Health in cooperation with the San Francisco Unified School District. (For middle and high school teachers.)

Post, J. and McPherson, C. 1988. *Into adolescence: Learning about AIDS.* Santa Cruz, CA: Network Publications, a division of ETR Associates. (For teachers of grades 5 through 8.)

Quackenbush, M. and Sargent, P. 1988 (rev. ed.). *Teaching AIDS: A resource guide on Acquired Immune Deficiency Syndrome.* Santa Cruz, CA: Network Publications. (For high school teachers.)

Quackenbush, M. and Villarreal, S. 1988. *"Does AIDS Hurt?" Educating Young Chidren About AIDS.* Santa Cruz, CA: Network Publications (For preschool through age 10.)

Sroka, S. 1987. *Educator's guide to AIDS and other STDs.* Lakewood, OH: Stephen T. Sroka, PhD, Inc. (For middle and high school teachers.)

Webster, C. 1988. *AIDS: The preventable epidemic.* Portland, OR: AIDS Education Program, Oregon Health Division. (For teachers of grades 4 through 12.)

Yarber, W.L. 1987. *AIDS: What young adults should know.* Reston, VA: American Alliance for Health, Physical Education, Recreation and Dance. (Student and teacher books for high school classrooms.)

Contributors

Jack Martin Balcer, PhD, is Cochair of the National Association of People with AIDS; a cofounder of the Columbus, Ohio AIDS Taskforce and remains on the board of that organization as Advocate for People with AIDS (PWA). He is also PWA Advocate for and Past President of the Ohio AIDS Coalition; a member of the Professional Activities Board of the Joshua Foundation, a home in Columbus for PWAs; a member of the Episcopal Diocese of Southern Ohio AIDS Taskforce; and a member of the Ohio State University AIDS Education and Research Committee.

Kenneth G. Castro, MD, is Medical Epidemiologist for the AIDS Program, Center for Infectious Diseases, Centers for Disease Control (CDC). He is also Consultant and Temporary Advisor, Health Situation and Trends Assessment, Pan American Health Organization. Since joining the Epidemic Intelligence Service at the CDC in 1983, Dr. Castro has made over forty presentations on various aspects of the AIDS epidemic, including presentations at each of the three International AIDS Conferences. He is a member of the American College of Physicians, the American Public Health Association and the American Medical Association and received a commendation medal from the U.S. Public Health Service in 1987 for his work in the field of AIDS.

Kay Clark is Editor-at-Large at ETR Associates, Santa Cruz, CA. She has worked in the area of family life and reproductive health education since 1984 and participated in the development of a number of ETR publications, including pamphlets, books and other AIDS prevention education materials.

Devon Davidson is the AIDS Education Coordinator for the National Coalition of Advocates for Students (NCAS), Boston, MA. She managed the development of NCAS' "Criteria for Evaluating an AIDS Curriculum" and has provided consultation on AIDS education to public school systems. Ms. Davidson is currently directing a CDC-funded AIDS prevention project for NCAS that serves migrant, immigrant and rural teenagers. Before coming to NCAS Ms. Davidson developed, implemented and supervised a number of community-based urban advocacy programs.

Donna DiMarzo, ACSW, MPH, is Clinical Social Worker in the Comprehensive Hemophilia Treatment Center at The University of California, San Francisco Medical Center, which serves adults and children with hemophilia and related bleeding disorders. She is also The Northern California Coordinator of the AIDS Help and Prevention Plan (AHPP), a risk and stress reduction project for the hemophilia community. In addition to

Ms. DiMarzo's current involvement in AIDS program development, evaluation and research for AHPP, she provides counseling to persons with hemophilia and their families, and consultation and inservice education in her role as a Clinical Social Worker. Her special interests include AIDS in women and children, psychosocial intervention with acutely and chronically ill children and child sexual abuse.

Abigail English, JD, is an attorney at the National Center for Youth Law in San Francisco and directs the Center's Adolescent Health Care Project. The National Center for Youth Law, established in 1970, is a nonprofit organization providing legal assistance to attorneys and other advocates for poor children and youth. The Adolescent Health Care Project works to protect the rights of adolescents to obtain health care services on a confidential and independent basis where appropriate.

Joyce V. Fetro, PhD, is Acting Research Director and Research Associate at ETR Associates, Santa Cruz, CA. She has extensive experience in qualitative and quantitative research methodology and statistics, as well as experience in applied research and instrument development. She has developed instruments to measure knowledge, attitudes and behaviors in various health related areas, has conducted content analyses, and is experienced in the development of needs assessments. Dr. Fetro has served on expert review panels for instrument validations. In addition, she taught health education at the middle school level for 13 years. Her field of research is adolescent alienation.

Glen Fischer is Codirector of the Center for AIDS and Substance Abuse Training in Falls Church, VA, which develops and coordinates the AIDS training agenda of the National Institute on Drug Abuse (NIDA). As a consultant to NIDA, he helped develop an AIDS curriculum for IV drug users and an AIDS and substance abuse curriculum for the New York correctional system. In 1982, Fischer designed and delivered the first New York City AIDS training to treatment personnel at the New York State Division of Substance Abuse Services Bureau of Training. He has been an advocate for people and families with AIDS, delivered AIDS workshops to high school students, and presented on AIDS and substance abuse at numerous national conferences.

Gilberto R. Gerald is Director of Minority Affairs of the National AIDS Network (NAN), Washington, DC. As the executive director of the National Coalition of Black Lesbians and Gays between 1983 and 1986, Gerald established a national reputation as one of the most visible and outspoken advocates for a community whose existence is frequently denied. In that capacity, he has played an important role in bringing national attention to the disproportionate incidence of AIDS in racial and ethnic minority communities. Gerald has written a number of articles on AIDS and about Black lesbians and gays. He has spoken extensively, appeared on radio and television programs, and received numerous awards for community service.

Debra W. Haffner, MPH, is Director of Information and Education for the Center for Population Options, Washington, DC. She is the author *of AIDS and Adolescents: The Time For Prevention Is Now*, and directs a Centers for Disease Control funded project on AIDS prevention for adolescents. Ms. Haffner serves on the Washington, DC AIDS Education Advisory Committee, the Advisory Committee on AIDS of the National Family Planning Reproductive Health Association, and the AIDS Advisory Council of the Girls Clubs of America. Ms. Haffner has been a sexuality educator for thirteen years.

Michael J. Helquist is a Program Officer for AIDSCOM, a federally funded AIDS prevention project focused on developing countries worldwide, Washington, DC. As an independent consultant Mr. Helquist has worked with the World Health Organization's Global Program on AIDS, the Centers for Disease Control, the San Francisco AIDS Foundation, and AIDS Project Los Angeles. In addition, he is the editor of several publications including *FOCUS: A Guide to AIDS Research*, an internationally distributed newsletter; *AIDS: A Self-Care Manual;* and *Working with AIDS: A Guide for Mental Health Professionals*. Mr. Helquist has been active in AIDS prevention efforts since the early days of the epidemic. He was one of the first medical science writers to chronicle the personal impact of the disease, the incidence among women, the connection with IV drug use, and the urgency to develop experimental treatments.

Sally Jo Jones is Codirector of the Center for AIDS and Substance Abuse Training in Falls Church, VA, which develops and coordinates the AIDS training agenda of the National Institute on Drug Abuse (NIDA). She has designed and delivered training workshops on AIDS to substance abuse treatment professionals, AIDS service workers, health educators and correctional system personnel. In 1985 she coordinated curriculum development, coauthored course materials and trained substance abuse counselors and administrators at the first NIDA AIDS training. She is consultant to the Health Education Resources Organization (HERO) of Baltimore and has presented on AIDS prevention strategies at numerous national conferences.

David L. Kirp, JD, is Professor of Public Policy and Lecturer

515

in Law at the University of California, Berkeley, and was the founder of the National Center on Law and Education at Harvard University. His books include *Gender Justice, Just Schools: The Idea of Racial Equality in American Education*, and *Doing Good by Doing Little*. Dr. Kirp's essays have appeared in *The New Republic*, *The Public Interest*, and *Harvard Educational Review*. Between 1983 and 1985, he was an associate editor at the *Sacramento Bee*. His weekly op/ed column for the *San Francisco Examiner* and the *Los Angeles Herald-Examiner* is syndicated by Copley News Service.

Sandra Orwitz Ludlow is Executive Director and Member of the Board of ETR Associates, Santa Cruz, CA. She has extensive experience in the field of family life and health education and is a member of the California State Legislative Task Force, the California State Department of Health Task Force and the Planned Parenthood Federation of America Task Force. She has been a consultant and advisor for the U.S. Department of Health and Human Services, the California State Department of Education, the Hawaii State Department of Health and the Mexican Department of Health-Office of Family Planning, and served as Chairperson of the California Family Planning Council.

Cathie Lyons, Convener of the AIDS Task Force of the National Council of Churches of Christ in the USA (NCC), is Assistant General Secretary of the United Methodist Church's Health and Welfare Ministries Department, New York, NY. She has initiated the department's work in the areas of AIDS ministries and women's health strategies and has planned national and international meetings on these topics. Ms. Lyons serves on a Roman Catholic/United Methodist bilateral dialogue team addressing end-of-life biomedical ethical issues and has written and lectured widely on these topics. She has authored two books, *Organ Transplants: The Moral Issues* and *Journey Toward Wholeness: Justice, Peace and Health in an Interdependent World*. Her writings on "A Woman's Health Is More than a Medical Issue" have been published in five languages and distributed worldwide.

Susan B. Manoff, MD, is Epidemic Intelligence Service Officer of the AIDS Program, Centers for Infectious Diseases, Centers for Disease Control (CDC). Before working with the AIDS Program, she was Medical Epidemiologist with the CDC's Division of Tuberculosis Control, assigned to the New York City Department of Health. Dr. Manoff has published two articles in CDC's *Morbidity and Mortality Weekly Report*: "Tuberculosis and Acquired Immunodeficiency Syndrome—New York City," (MMWR 1987;36:785-790,795) and "Human Immunodeficiency Virus Infection in the United States: A Review of Current Knowledge," (MMWR 1987;36 [suppl. no. S-6]:1-48). She is a member of the American Public Health Association.

A. Damien Martin, EdD, is the Executive Director and Cofounder of the Hetrick Martin Institute (Formerly The Institute for the Protection of Lesbian and Gay Youth, Inc.), New York, NY. He is also Associate Professor in the Department of Communication Arts and Sciences, School of Education, Health, Nursing and Arts Professions, New York, NY. He has published extensively on issues of concern for gay and lesbian adolescents, and has been active in advocacy for this population for more than 10 years.

Renetia Martin, MSW, LCSW, is Deputy Director of the AIDS Health Project, a mental health training and clinical services program of the University of California, San Francisco. Ms. Martin also conducts a private practice, providing organizational and management consulting and clinical supervision. She is a member and Treasurer of the San Francisco Black Coalition on AIDS, the San Francisco Department of Public Health's Third World Advisory Committee on AIDS, and the Health Department's General Advisory Committee on AIDS. She has a longstanding professional and personal interest in child and family health, and health concerns of Black and minority communities.

Ana Consuelo Matiella, MA, is Associate Director for the California AIDS Clearinghouse and Editor for Latino Educational Materials at ETR Associates, Santa Cruz, CA. Currently Ms. Matiella is writing Latino family life education curricula for middle school students focusing on cultural pride, the family and effective communication, and is developing AIDS educational materials for high risk minority populations. Before coming to ETR Associates, Ms. Matiella worked as an Hispanic marketing consultant, assisting nonprofit health and human service organizations in developing educational programs for Latinos. One of her particular interests and areas of expertise is fotonovela production.

Kathleen Middleton, MS, is Editor for Classroom Materials at ETR Associates, Santa Cruz, CA and is recognized as an expert in school health curricula. She is the former Director of the Office of School Health Programs for the National Center for Health Education. Ms. Middleton has been responsible for the authorship of ten major health-related curricula, including *Growing Healthy (K-7)* and the *California State Teacher's Guide for STDs*. In 1984, she coauthored with Dr. Marion B. Pollock a widely used college text, *Elementary School Health Instruction*

(2nd edition in press 1989). In her current position, she directs the development of curricula in elementary and secondary drug abuse prevention, family life education and AIDS and STD prevention. She currently serves on the National Management Committee for the CDC-funded project to integrate AIDS education into two existing curricula.

Mary Nelson, MLS, is Editorial Director of ETR Associates, Santa Cruz, CA. She has been responsible for the development and publication of many AIDS resources including "Teens and AIDS," "What Women Should Know About AIDS," "Talking with Your Teenager About AIDS," "Talking with Your Partner About Safer Sex," and "Condoms and STDs." In her capacity as Editor of *Family Life Educator* magazine, Ms. Nelson has been publishing AIDS information articles since 1983. She has worked in the field of family life and reproductive health since 1979.

Catherine Pickerel is Dean of Students at Presentation High School in San Francisco. She has taught in the Theology Department since 1976, and previously served as Campus Minister and Theology Department Chair. Ms. Pickerel has been involved in grief/loss education since 1977, and has given classes, workshops and talks around these issues. She was also a member of the San Francisco Archdiocesan Grief Care and Support Training Committee, training parish groups to respond to the needs of bereaved people.

Cheri Pies, MSW, MPH, has been working as a Health Education Specialist providing AIDS education in both Alameda and San Francisco counties since 1985. While working as a Health Educator with the San Francisco Department of Public Health, she collaborated with ETR Associates and the San Francisco

Unified School District to develop an AIDS education training program for teachers of grades 4-12. In addition, Ms. Pies is coauthor of the *Teacher's Curriculum Guide on AIDS*, which was written as part of a teacher training project funded by the Centers for Disease Control.

Jory Post, MA, is a teacher at Happy Valley Elementary School in Santa Cruz, CA. He has worked in education as a mentor teacher, project director and principal. Mr. Post has received a number of grants focusing on curriculum integration, two from the California Educational Initiatives Fund. He has also written feature stories and reviews for *Family Life Educator* magazine, and is the coauthor of *Communication for a Livable World*, a curriculum unit for grades 5-8 (1988) and *Into Adolescence: Learning about AIDS* (grades 5-8; 1988).

Marcia Quackenbush, MS, is the Coordinator of Youth and Women's Services for the AIDS Health Project, a program of the University of California, San Francisco, and the San Francisco Department of Public Health. She has been active in AIDS prevention education for youth since early 1984. In this capacity, she has worked directly with in-school and out-of-school youth (including street youth, juvenile prostitutes, incarcerated youth, runaways and young people using and dealing in intravenous drugs). She has trained teachers and other educators on AIDS prevention approaches with children and youth. She is the coauthor of *Teaching AIDS*, a resource guide for secondary teachers, and *"Does AIDS Hurt?" Educating Young Chidren About AIDS*. In her role as an advocate for AIDS education, she has appeared on national television, spoken on radio shows across the country, and testified before a Congressional Committee. She counsels persons with AIDS, ARC and HIV infection.

Jane Quinn, MA, is Director of Program Services for Girls Clubs of America, Inc., New York, NY. In this capacity she has developed and implemented national-level programs in pregnancy prevention, math and science, sports, health promotion, sexual abuse prevention and substance abuse prevention. Ms. Quinn's professional interest in youth-serving agencies dates from 1979, when she began consulting with 20 national youth organizations as part of a project she directed for the Center for Population Options. For the past six years, she has participated in the Program Directors Group of the National Collaboration for Youth, serving as Chairperson from 1984-86.

Andrew Rose, LCSW, is the AIDS Project Coordinator at Jewish Family and Children's Services in San Francisco. He has organized a broad educational effort reaching teens and adults in the Bay Area Jewish community, in addition to assisting people with AIDS and ARC and their families. Mr. Rose, who also serves on the Committee on AIDS of the Union of American Hebrew Congregations, has become a frequent speaker at national Jewish Conferences and among social service agencies. Prior to his current position he worked at AIDS Project Los Angeles, providing mental health services and coordinating interfaith efforts to respond to AIDS with knowledge and compassion.

George W. Rutherford, MD, is Medical Director of the AIDS Office of the San Francisco Department of Public Health and an Assistant Clinical Professor of Pediatrics and Epidemiology and International Health at the University of California, San Francisco. He has served on many local, state and national AIDS committees. Dr. Rutherford has published extensively on infectious disease epidemiology and the public health aspects of the AIDS epidemic.

Sandra K. Schwarcz, MD, MPH, is an Epidemic Intelligence Service Officer in the Division of Sexually Transmitted Diseases, Centers for Prevention Services, Centers for Disease Control. She was previously a preventive medicine resident in the AIDS Office and in the Bureau of Family Health of the San Francisco Department of Public Health and also served on the Pediatric and Perinatal AIDS Advisory Committee. Her areas of interest are sexually transmitted disease control, infectious disease epidemiology and maternal-child health.

Katherine M. Simpson, MA, MFCC, is Director of Education and Director of the Disability Program at Planned Parenthood Shasta-Diablo, Walnut Creek, CA. She has eight years experience as a counselor, educator, trainer, lecturer and consultant in the field of sexuality and disability, and was recently instrumental in starting a program to teach children in special education classes about sexuality and sexual abuse prevention.

Jack B. Stein, LCSW, is Executive Director of Health Education Resource Organization (HERO) in Baltimore, one of the first community-based AIDS service agencies in Maryland. He also coordinated the design, staff training, supervision and evaluation for all HERO programs. He is Project Director for a National Institute of Drug Abuse (NIDA) research project to evaluate the effectiveness of AIDS prevention through indigenous community educators, and he provides consultation to NIDA on a number of other AIDS projects. Mr. Stein's extensive training experience includes developing curricula and providing training for health care workers and state drug abuse administration treatment staff throughout the state of Maryland.

Lynne Stiggall, Sex Education Consultant, Stiggall & Associates, Los Gatos, CA, has worked with persons who are disabled in rehabilitation and family planning settings and schools for over 18 years. She has produced educational films on sexuality and mental retardation, and is coauthor of *An Easy Guide to Loving Carefully*, specially written and illustrated for adults with minimal reading skills. Ms. Stiggall has taught sexuality education to students with and without developmental and learning disabilities and has trained professionals nationwide on how to provide appropriate, relevant sex education to varied learner groups, including people with disabilities. Immediate past president of the California Committee on the Sexuality of the Developmentally Disabled, she currently edits the newsletter for this group, which advises the California State Department of Developmental Services in matters of sex education and counseling.

Florence Stroud, RN, MPH, is Deputy Director, Community Health Programs, San Francisco Department of Public Health.

Mary Lee Tatum, MEd, is a teacher at George Mason Junior-Senior High School in Falls Church, VA and also teaches at George Mason University and the University of Virginia. She is a consultant for program development for Alexandria City Public Schools and is involved in curriculum development and teacher training in a number of schools nationwide. Tatum received Planned Parenthood Association of Virginia's Vivian Roe Award for Outstanding Contribution in Sex Education in 1982 and the *Washington Post's* Agnes Meyer Award for Outstanding Teacher in 1984. She is a member of the American Association of Sex Educators, Counselors and Therapists (AASECT), the National Education Association (NEA) and serves on the Editorial Board of the *Sex Education Coalition News*.

Manya Ungar, National PTA President for 1987-89, has been involved with the PTA for nearly 30 years. Prior to being elected president, Ms. Ungar served as National PTA First Vice-President for 1985-87, and was Vice-President for Legislative Activity from 1981-84. She is the current Chair of the Task Force on Membership Inclusiveness, Emerging Issues and Headquarters Committees and former Chair of the Communications Committee. She has also served as a member of the Executive, Leadership, Legislative Program and Budget Committees, and on the Health and Welfare and Education Commissions on the National Board of Directors.

Sylvia F. Villarreal, MD, is Assistant Clinical Professor of Pediatrics and a staff member of the Children's Health Center at San Francisco General Hospital. She is Director of the Kempe High Risk Clinic and Early Childhood Services. Her community work includes membership on the San Francisco Department of Public Health AIDS Minority Task Force as well as the Department of Public Health's Refugee Task Force and the Community Forum for Children and Youth for the City of San Francisco. She is a member of the board of directors for the California Children's Lobby. Dr. Villarreal has published extensively on Hispanic health care issues and her field of research is nonorganic failure to thrive.

Paul A. Volberding, MD, is the Director of the AIDS Activities Division at San Francisco General Hospital. As a leader in the fight against AIDS, he has been named to many advisory committees and has served on the Organizing Committee for each of the three International AIDS Conferences. Dr. Volberding is Cochair of the AIDS Task Force of the University of California, San Francisco, a member of the San Francisco Mayor's AIDS Advisory Committee, and the California Medical Association AIDS Task Force. He is a member of the Executive Committee of the National Institutes of Health AIDS Clinic Trial Group, and is also on the AIDS Oversight Committee of the National Academy of Sciences/Institute of Medicine. He is Coeditor-in-Chief of the *Journal of the Acquired Immune Deficiency Syndrome.*

Ellen Wagman, MPH, is the Associate Director of ETR Associates, Santa Cruz, CA. In her former capacity as ETR Associates' Director of Training, she managed major family life education and substance abuse prevention education training and research programs and conducted prevention education training for educators throughout the United States. Ms. Wagman is an experienced family life educator of teens, college students, teachers and parents, and the author of several noted publications in the field including the *Family Life Education Teacher Training Manual.* She currently directs ETR Associates' planning efforts, including planning for new research, training and publications in family life education and AIDS prevention.

Claudia L. Webster has worked in the AIDS Education Program of the Oregon State Health Division since 1985. In 1986 she authored *AIDS: The Preventable Epidemic,* a state curriculum for grades 9-12. She has worked for many years in the fields of family planning and sexually transmitted disease education. As a certified sex educator with American Association of Sex Educators, Counselors and Therapists (AASECT), Ms. Webster has provided sexuality education in Oregon since 1971. During the 1960s, she and her family served as United Methodist missionaries in the Philippines, where she began a family planning clinic. Ms. Webster currently works in a volunteer capacity as the Family Life/Human Sexuality Coordinator for the Oregon-Idaho Conference of the United Methodist Church.

She also serves on the AIDS Task Force of Ecumenical Ministries of Oregon.

Judith C. Wilber, PhD, ABMM, directs the Virology Laboratory of the San Francisco Department of Public Health. She was instrumental in the planning of the San Francisco Alternate Test Site HIV antibody testing program, including developing ways of assuring anonymity, training counselors in the meaning of test results, and continuing evaluation of the accuracy of available tests. This program is recognized as a model, and her laboratory has so far been responsible for the voluntary testing of over 30,000 people. Dr. Wilber has served on several national committees dealing with the laboratory performance of HIV antibody tests and the interpretation of results.

Renee S. Woodworth, MSW, is Project Coordinator at the National Network of Runaway and Youth Services, Inc., Washington, DC. Ms. Woodworth has worked in the youth service field since 1978. During 1987, she was the Director of the Safe Choices Program, a cooperative agreement project operated by the National Network through the Centers for Disease Control. This grant focused on the development of AIDS policies at runaway centers. Ms. Woodworth has participated in and coordinated workshops nationwide since 1985 in areas such as AIDS, runaway services and policy development.